BIOSTATISTICS

BIOSTATISTICS
Experimental Design
and Statistical Inference

JAMES F. ZOLMAN

Department of Physiology and Biophysics
College of Medicine
University of Kentucky

New York   Oxford
OXFORD UNIVERSITY PRESS
1993

Oxford University Press

Oxford New York Toronto
Delhi Bombay Calcutta Madras Karachi
Kuala Lumpur Singapore Hong Kong Tokyo
Nairobi Dar es Salaam Cape Town
Melbourne Auckland Madrid

and associated companies in
Berlin Ibadan

Copyright © 1993 by Oxford University Press, Inc.

Published by Oxford University Press, Inc.,
200 Madison Avenue, New York, New York 10016

Oxford is a registered trademark of Oxford University Press

Library of Congress Cataloging-in-Publication Data
Zolman, James F.
Biostatistics : experimental design and statistical inference /
James F. Zolman.
p. cm.
Includes bibliographical references and index.
ISBN 0-19-507810-1
1. Biometry. 2. Experimental design. I. Title.
QH323.5.Z64 1993
574'.01'5195—dc20 92-22605

9 8 7 6 5 4 3 2 1

Printed in the United States of America
on acid-free paper

To Carolyn

PREFACE

As an experimental biologist you are concerned primarily with designing and interpreting your own experiments as well as critically evaluating articles and papers in your scientific area. Consequently, you must know whether an experiment is properly conceived, correctly controlled, adequately analyzed, and correctly interpreted. This book emphasizes experimental design and statistical literacy and focuses on a particular form of statistical inference, namely hypothesis testing using analysis of variance (ANOVA) techniques for between-subject, within-subject, and mixed factorial designs. The essentials of experimental design and statistical inference are first discussed briefly and then are reviewed by illustrating their applications and misapplications in 100 research design problems. Detailed critiques of these research design problems help identify the most common interpretative errors found in biological studies.

The logic of experimental design is straightforward. A good design is one in which the treatment conditions selected and manipulated by you are not confounded with extraneous subject-, environment-, or time-related variables. Conversely, a bad design is one in which treatment conditions are unknowingly confounded with one or more of these extraneous variables.

The application of any statistical test to a given set of data also is relatively simple: (1) a specific test statistic is computed from a formula, for example, chi-square, t, or F; (2) the calculated value of the test statistic is compared with the theoretical sampling distribution of the statistic; and (3) this comparison gives the likelihood (probability) of the calculated value of the test statistic occurring by chance given no expected difference among treatment conditions. With this information you decide whether a significant treatment effect occurred. Because most of you have access to computer statistical packages, computational procedures for the various test statistics and the abbreviated tables of their theoretical sampling distributions are not presented in this book. Rather, the logic of experimental design and statistical inference is emphasized and the rationale, interpretation, and application of widely used statistical procedures are presented within an experimental context.

Each of the experimental design problems is a unique research tutorial. Most of these research problems have serious design flaws, inappropriate statistical analyses, or invalid conclusions. However, in some research problems the design, the analysis, and the conclusions are all appropriate. In short, for each research design problem you must decide whether the experiment was properly conceived, correctly controlled, adequately analyzed, and correctly interpreted. Comparing your evaluations with the detailed critiques of the 100 design problems will increase your understanding of the use of the experiment as an inferential tool in biological research. The more you are exposed to both good and bad experimental designs the better your own scientific output should become.

Because the research design tutorials will serve readers with varying backgrounds in experimental design and statistical methodology, the organization of this book deviates from the organization of traditional biostatistics books (see "Structure of Book").

ACKNOWLEDGMENTS

This book evolved from my teaching of experimental design and statistical inference to biology, physiology, and other biomedical students during the last decade. After a brief review of the essentials of design and statistical inference, course participants evaluated research design problems and prepared briefs of similar problems in their research area. I am indebted to the following individuals who prepared initial briefs of some of the design problems included in this book: Bradford Addison, James Boone, Jr., Phillip Budzenski, Kathryn King, Lu-Yuan Lee, Chris Maynard, Janet Neiswander, Ivan Welsford, Thomas Wood, and Ellen Wurster. I am also grateful to many other students for their corrections and suggestions for improving the design problems and critiques.

Several colleagues read all or selected portions of the manuscript critically and made suggestions for improving the final drafts. I thank Kirk Barron, John Dose, Henry Hirsch, Douglas McMahon, David Randall, Robert Revelette, Dexter Speck, and Robert Taylor for their constructive comments. I am particularly indebted to John Haley who eliminated many statistical errors from the drafts and to Kim Ng who suggested that detailed critiques be prepared for each design problem and who provided me an academic home at La Trobe University where I converted classroom notes, handouts, and problems into a readable manuscript. I have benefited greatly from the help of these colleagues and students, and any remaining errors or shortcomings are, of course, my own.

Finally, I am grateful to Mitchell Zolman who prepared all illustrations, to Randall Wilson who helped prepare figures for typesetting, to Jennifer Raleigh who typed the original classroom material, to Anna Hopkins who typed many revisions of the manuscript, and to Maryann Rosenberg of Oxford University Press for superb copy editing.

STRUCTURE OF BOOK

In this book, you are encouraged to learn the essentials of experimental design and statistical inference by identifying design and statistical errors in research problems. To provide a common frame of reference, the essentials of design and statistical inference are presented briefly in the first three sections. Topics within each section (e.g., Section I: Experimental Design) are numbered by the conventional decimal numbering system; the number before the decimal point refers to the general topic area (e.g., 1.0 The Anatomy of an Experiment) and the number after the point refers to a specific subtopic (e.g., 1.1 Formulation of Research Question).

Most of the subtopics are concise discussions of restricted content, and the extensive cross-referencing within each subtopic provides, if desired, an in-depth discussion of closely related topics and subtopics (see "Contents"). The tables (and figures) are also numbered with the same decimal system. The first number denotes the general topic area and the second number denotes the number of the table or figure within the general topic area. Most tables and figures also include citations to relevant subtopics. This extensive cross-referencing among subtopics, tables, and figures will allow you to find quickly the answer to a specific question or to select a particular topic and, by following the citations provided within each subtopic, to read almost all of the first three sections of the book.

Topics covered in Section A: Introduction include the misuse of statistical methods in biological research (A.1, A.2), experimental design and control by randomization (A.3), improving biological research methodology (A.4, A.5, A.6), levels of analysis in biology (A.7, A.8), causality in science (A.9, A.10), the creative–conceptual phase of research (A.11), experimental design and statistical inference (A.12), and how readers with different levels of scientific training may effectively use the book (A.13).

The first section (Section I: Experimental Design) presents brief previews of the anatomy of an experiment (Chapter 1), the anatomy of a scientific paper (Chapter 2), and the evaluation of a scientific article (Chapter 3). This first section concludes with a detailed discussion of experimental design (Chapter 4). The rationale, interpretation, and application of the most commonly used statistical procedures for experimental data are given in Section II: Statistical Inference, Analysis of Variance, and Post Hoc Analysis. The assumptions, advantages, and disadvantages of various parametric and nonparametric tests are compared in Section III: Statistical Tests. In this section special ANOVA designs and analyses (Chapter 9), post hoc multiple comparison tests (Chapter 10), and nonparametric tests are also discussed (Chapter 11). The selection of statistical tests (Chapter 12) provides a summary of the first part of the book (Sections I–III).

The core of this book consists of 100 detailed briefs of biological experiments and their critiques which are presented in Section IV: Research Design Problems and Their Critiques. Critiques of the briefs include a restatement of the research hypothesis, the ANOVA table (if appropriate), and whether the inferences of the researchers are appropriate. If serious design–statistical errors in the briefs do exist, citations to relevant subtopics in the first part of the book are given (e.g., treatment conditions are confounded by time in this within-subject design, 4.16, 4.19).

Lexington, Ky.   J.F.Z.
June 1992

CONTENTS

III STATISTICAL TESTS

BIOSTATISTICS

A

Introduction

A.1 STATISTICAL BIAS

A curious attitude exists among many biological scientists regarding the statistical analysis of research data. When simple statistical tests are used, these scientists believe the research was well-designed or that the differences between the treatment groups are obviously true because their significance can be simply demonstrated. On the other hand, when more advanced statistical procedures are used to evaluate experimental outcomes these biologists tend to view the author's interpretations with skepticism. Indeed, some biologists may even distrust the use of advanced statistical procedures, like analysis of variance, and consider their use as unjustified manipulations of research data.

Popular views of statistical interpretations probably reinforce this bias of some scientists regarding the statistical analysis of experimental data. We are all familiar with the most common derogatory quotes on statistics: "There are three kinds of lies; lies, dammed lies, and statistics"; "Figures don't lie, but liars figure"; and "Statistics can prove anything." It is not surprising, therefore, that some biologists remain convinced that well-designed biological experiments do not require statistical analysis because the results will be obvious. Unfortunately, this statistical bias continues to be passed from these mentors to their students.

It is not true that statistics can be made to prove anything and reputable statisticians *do not* indulge in the unwarranted manipulation of data (see Hooke, 1983). In the past, biologists might have said that "I don't believe in statistics" or " Statistics does not make sense to me scientifically." Today, however, most biologists realize that they must use both descriptive and inferential statistics (5.1) in their data analysis and interpretation and their only choice is to use appropriate or inappropriate statistical methods.

A.2 THE MISUSE OF STATISTICAL METHODS IN BIOLOGICAL RESEARCH

Given the statistical bias among some biologists (A.1), examples of inappropriate statistical analyses are easy to find in the biological literature. Critical reviews of recent biomedical publications, for instance, have consistently found about half of the published articles used incorrect statistical methods (see Altman, 1982; Godfrey, 1986b; Glantz, 1987, pp. 6–9; Williamson, Goldschmidt, and Colton, 1986). These research papers were the ones that reviewers judged to be scientifically acceptable for publication! Many more research papers were probably rejected by reviewers for misusing elementary statistical tests of hypotheses. If valid data are analyzed improperly, the results may be invalid and the conclusions may be inappropriate. A conservative estimate is that about 25 percent of biological research is flawed because of incorrect conclusions drawn from confounded experimental designs and the misuse of statistical methods. In most of these cases, design and statistical errors generally bias the study on behalf of the treatment (see Hofacker, 1983; Williamson, Goldschmidt, and Colton, 1986).

In other cases, the experimental design may be very insensitive or the sample size may be so small that it is unlikely that a significant treatment effect could be detected. These latter problems center around the power of a given statistical test. In many publications, the power of the statistical test used is very low (1.7, 5.12, 5.15).

In short, biological scientists have been slow to adopt appropriate and sensitive statistical procedures to analyze and interpret their experimental data. The reasons for this reluctance are complex and do not just reflect an ingrained statistical bias (A.1) or a lack of familiarity with statistical methodology. Many biologists who have taken statistics courses as undergraduate or graduate students are still not sure when a t-test, a Mann-Whitney U test, a chi-square test, or an analysis of variance is the appropriate statistical test to analyze a given set of data. As a solution to this problem, a few biostatistics books have concentrated on the presentation and interpretation of statistical concepts rather than on computational techniques (e.g., Bland, 1987; Bourke, Daly, and McGilvray, 1985; Elston and Johnson, 1987; Gilbert, 1989; Glantz, 1987; Glantz and Slinker, 1990).

A.3 EXPERIMENTAL DESIGN AND CONTROL BY RANDOMIZATION

Many biologists who believe they have statistical problems actually have problems in constructing appropriate experimental designs to answer their particular research questions, that is, conceptual–design problems. *After* collecting their data, they may realize that some help is required for the analysis and interpretation of their data. Statistical consultation may then be sought but often the data are in a form that defies statistical analysis. The typical outcome is that these biologists in their self-inflicted frustation blame either statistics or the statistician for their problems. The real problem is not statistics nor the statistician but the lack of an appropriate research design.

As a field of science progresses, both the research questions and the required methodologies become more complex. In the initial phase of investigation in a scientific field like biology, the effect of a robust treatment is studied on a reliable biological response. To achieve these experimental conditions usually only a small part of the total biological system is used. Thus, a cell, a piece of tissue, a nerve, or a muscle is removed from an animal, the sample placed in an experimental chamber within which extraneous variables (e.g., O_2, pH, temperature) are precisely controlled, a specific treatment is applied, and the resulting biological response is recorded. This response outcome is normally of an all-or-none type so that any treatment effect is clearly observed by inspection of the recorded measurement. With this type of preparation, the biologist usually does two or more additional "experiments" to determine the reliability of the treatment effect. Because all extraneous variables are assumed to be precisely controlled, the researcher concludes that the biological response was caused by the specific treatment applied and *publishes the individual data collected*. Using identical procedures, similar data are obtained by another biologist and scientific knowledge in the field accumulates rapidly. This initial rapid progress is primarily because relatively large treatment effects are being studied with minimal experimental error (see 5.12, 5.13, 5.14).

In this initial phase of investigation the design of an experiment is straightforward. The most significant design requirement is the precise control of all known extraneous variables, thereby reducing experimental error (producing stable baseline and treatment records). This stability is usually achieved by standardization of the preparation and of the procedures of intervention and recording. Subsequent research questions, however, may not permit all extraneous variables to be precisely controlled, particularly when most of the total biological system is used or the measurement procedure requires a number of time-consuming and possibly error prone stages (e.g., biochemical assay of receptors). In such cases, therefore, extraneous variables must be controlled by equating (randomizing) their potential influences across the treatment groups or conditions, a procedure which increases experimental error (noise). Consequently, the design of an experiment in which extraneous influences must be controlled by a randomization procedure requires a systematic plan for data collection. This plan must ensure that the treatment conditions are not *confounded* with subject-, environment-, or time-related extraneous variables (1.2). Because it is impossible to identify all potential extraneous influences, control by randomization is an important aspect of any experimental design (1.4), even in the simple designs used in the initial investigations in a given scientific field.

The most common mistakes in the design of experiments are the failure to randomly allocate study units to the treatment conditions, neglecting to include a proper control group, and the confounding of treatment conditions (Chapter 4). The most common statistical errors are misusing elementary tests of hypotheses, lack of knowledge regarding the underlying assumptions of the statistical model used, and low or unknown power of the statistical test (Chapter 5). Fortunately, if the experiment has been designed properly, statistical errors may be identified and corrected. However, valid statistical methods cannot salvage an experiment that has serious conceptual or design problems (A.11). Unfortunately, these latter problems are easily confused with statistical procedures which may lead one to equate erroneously bad science with statistical ritualization (see Bolles, 1988).

A.4 STATISTICAL ANALYSIS: FORMULAS AND DATA CALCULATIONS

Most statistics books concentrate on data reduction methods, calculation of various statistics, mathematical derivations from various formulas, and theoretical sampling distributions of test statistics. Even in those few statistics books which emphasize experimental design, a significant portion of each is given to data manipulations and computational skills. But, the increasing availability of computer-based statistical packages has made it easy to do extensive data manipulations and to perform numerous statistical tests simply by pressing a few terminal keys (A.5). Consequently, many biologists when designing their experiments do not review the books used in their previous statistics courses. Unfortunately, researchers who do attempt to consult statistics books before collecting their experimental data become frustrated either by the different symbolic language used by various authors (see Keppel, 1982, pp. 616–617) or because most statistics books are not organized to quickly provide answers to specific questions. The usual outcome is that the statistical tests eventually used are selected more for convenience, after data are collected, rather than for their appropriateness for the proposed experimental questions.

A.5 DATA INTERPRETATION: STATISTICAL LITERACY

Various packaged computer statistical programs are now available [e.g., BMDP Statistical Software, Minitab, Statistical Analysis System (SAS), SYSTAT (see Dixon, 1983; Cody and Smith, 1987; Everitt, 1989; Ryan, Joiner, and Ryan, 1982; Wilkinson, 1990; Woodward, Elliott, Gray, and Matlock, 1988)]. Each of these statistical packages is a collection of statistical programs that do the calculations required to describe data and perform various statistical tests on the data (5.1). Some biologists, however, attempt to interpret the summary outputs from these computer packages without an understanding of either the theoretical assumptions of the particular statistical tests used or of the general calculations made to obtain the different variance estimates, mean squares, F-ratios, and so forth. The available statistical computing packages cannot choose the correct statistical test to be used, they can only compute the statistical test selected. If an inappropriate test is selected, the package will compute it (if possible) and the computer printout will present the attained significance levels even if they are incorrect. Hence, statistical tests applied indiscriminately to experimental data can produce reams of analyses and many erroneous conclusions. As Bland (1987) has commented . . . "More than once I have been approached by a researcher bearing a computer print-out two inches thick, and asking what it all means. Sadly, too often, the answer is that another tree has died in vain" (p. 3).

Unfortunately, even when examining a correct statistical treatment of their data (e.g., a two-way analysis of variance) some scientists do not fully understand the implications of significant main effects and a significant interaction (Chapter 6). Indeed, many biologists may eventually realize that *the* answer to their specific research question (given the design used) is only revealed by the simultaneous effects of two or more conditions, yet they do not know how to interpret a two-way interaction (6.13). These scientists are likely to use multiple t-test comparisons to analyze data obtained from four or more treatment conditions and their reported levels of significance would not be correct (5.19; Wallenstein, Zucker, and Fleiss, 1980). Interpretational problems for both reviewers and readers are also compounded by the editorial policy of most biology journals, which require only probability levels (e.g., $p < .05$, which reads probability is less than .05, one out of twenty) be given following statements regarding the significance of certain comparisons. Consequently, readers of these journals cannot determine whether appropriate treatment comparisons were made or what statistical tests were used for these comparisons.

A.6 IMPROVING BIOLOGICAL RESEARCH: STATISTICAL REVIEWS AND REPORTS

The ever-increasing importance and application of statistics to biological data are shown by the dramatic increase in the percentage of research reports using these quantitative procedures. Consequently, anyone who needs to read intelligently these biological studies must understand the essentials of biostatistics (see Day, Hutton, and Gardner, 1990). To improve statistical analysis in biological research, the editorial evaluation of some journals now includes a separate statistical review by a qualified statistician. This editorial policy implies, of course, that the critical peer reviews provided by experts in a given research field are not adequate. If specialists cannot evaluate the research in their own discipline then who can? As a stopgap measure, a few journals are also routinely publishing special statistical reports to educate their readership in the use of appropriate statistical methods (see Bailar and Mosteller, 1986). Also, many universities provide routine statistical consulting for their biological scientists. In short, many biologists are abdicating their responsibilities for the design and analysis of their own experiments and their evaluation of their colleagues' research to statisticians (see Miké and Stanley, 1982). If this trend continues, a research approach of questionable merit may eventually evolve. A biologist may have an idea which would be translated by a statistician into a research question and an appropriate design. The data would be collected by technicians or graduate students, and analyzed and interpreted jointly by the biologist and the statistician. The final draft of the paper would be prepared by the biologist, the statistician, and a communications officer from the university's Public Affairs department. Given the striking increase in multiple-authorship papers in the biological sciences, some research programs appear to have already reached this evolutionary stage!

A.7 LEVELS OF ANALYSIS: BIOLOGICAL MEASUREMENTS, EXPERIMENTAL DESIGN, AND STATISTICS

In biological experiments, specialized equipment and techniques are widely used to measure the functions of cells, tissues, or organ systems. The rationale for using a particular piece of equipment or a specific technique rests primarily on biophysical considerations, and scientific knowledge of a field determines whether the resulting data are valid measures of a particular function (see Scott and Waterhouse, 1986). In cardiovascular research, for example, ultrasound flow transducers, pressure transducers, catheters, ultrasound piezoelectric crystals, and bipolar electrodes may be used in chronically instrumented dogs to measure cardiovascular function. From these dogs, heart rate, coronary flow, coronary vascular resistance, and left ventricular pressure may be spectrally analyzed and calculations made of the power spectral densities of each variable and of the cross-correlation functions between variables. With a high speed computer, digital subtraction angiography may provide enhanced visualization of myocardial structure and perfusion. As sophisticated as these methods are, cardiovascular physiologists, like all biological scientists, must be aware of methodological limitations (accuracy, sensitivity, effective range, possible artifacts), and must ascertain whether the final calculated values are valid measures of biological processes.

Much of biological research is devoted to the development of reliable and sensitive techniques which provide accurate and valid measurements of biological processes (see Wise, 1990). Measurement error must be considered by every scientist. An *accurate* measure can be defined as one which is *precise* and *unbiased*. Assuming that a true value exists, an accurate measurement would vary very little (precise) around the true value (unbiased). If a measurement is not precise, the averaged value of repeated measurements will reduce the imprecision. If a measurement is biased, the only way to correct this problem is to adjust the observed value or more commonly to check and recalibrate the measuring equipment. A *valid* measure is one which actually reflects the biological process that the scientist wants to study. Experimental design and statistics play very limited roles in the researcher's decisions in the development of accurate and valid measurements of biological processes.

Once instrumentation, quantification, and measurement problems have been solved, this methodology becomes available for experimental studies. At this stage of analysis, experimental design and statistical analysis would play critical roles in the conclusions that may be made by the researcher. Depending upon the research question, either a between-subject, a within-subject, or a mixed factorial design would be selected (Chapter 4). Subsequent statistical analysis would determine whether the differences among the treatment groups or conditions were significantly greater than chance expectations (Chapter 5). *Note, at this experimental stage of analysis, neither the design used nor the statistical analysis will affect the accuracy or validity of the biological measurements.* Rather, from a design–statistics perspective the numerical observations (data) are neutral.

An experimental design is a plan to assure that treatment conditions are not confounded with either subject-, environment-, or time-related nuisance variables; whereas statistical analysis is concerned with the scale of measurement, whether the data collected violate assumptions of the selected statistical model, and the probability of random occurrence of the observed treatment differences (A.12). Hence, if the measurements do not reflect true functional processes, the experimental design and statistical analysis may be correct but the conclusions of the researcher would be wrong. For example, in adult male rats significant differences in the width of synaptic clefts [measured by electron micrographs (EMs)] may be found between neocortical and hippocampal tissue samples. The experimental design (e.g., counterbalancing tissue removal, "blind" histological and EM procedures, "blind" measurements of synaptic cleft widths, and so forth) may have controlled for all potential confoundings and an appropriate statistical procedure (e.g., within-subject analysis) used to determine statistical significance levels. Yet, a possible conclusion of the researcher ". . . synaptic cleft widths in the hippocampus are significantly greater than those in the neocortex" may not be correct. Actual differences in synaptic cleft widths in the two brain samples may have existed in the EMs but these differences may have been produced artificially by the histological procedure (e.g., because more lipid may exist in the membranes of hippocampal neurons the reagents produced a greater shrinkage of these cells resulting in a greater distance between pre- and post-synaptic membranes). In this case, the histological procedures would not provide valid measures of cleft widths in vivo.

In this book, we will assume that accurate and valid data are collected and will concentrate on problems of experimental design and statistical interpretation. But, we must realize that an appropriate experimental design and proper statistical methods will not ensure correct scientific conclusions if the data collected are inaccurate or invalid. Hence, to ensure correct conclusions from an experimental study, the biologist must be concerned with three distinct levels of analysis—specifically, (1) accurate and valid data collection, (2) appropriate experimental design, and (3) correct statistical analysis and interpretation. Interestingly, most biologists would be appalled with the suggestion that someone else assume the responsibility for determining whether their data are accurate and valid measures of biological processes. Yet, they appear content to have a statistician determine whether their experimental designs or statistical analyses and interpretations are appropriate (A.6).

A.8 BIOLOGICAL MODELING: FITTING BIOLOGICAL MODELS TO DATA

Biologists are more familiar with biological (mathematical) modeling of experimental data than with the probabilistic framework that is required in the statistical interpretation of experimental outcomes (A.10). In the specialized field of biological modeling, a conceptual model is defined as a set of related ideas or concepts intended to explain the functions of a particular biological system (Yates, 1978). A mathematical model is some form of differential, algebraic, or Boolean equation or formula intended to relate the variables in such a system. There is nothing new about using mathematical models to describe various aspects of living systems (see Siebert, 1978). But, even today some experimentalists argue that any form of mathematical modeling in biology is premature. The most common criticisms of biological modeling are that most models are difficult to comprehend and use arbitrary assumptions which produce subjective conclusions about isolated, artificial systems (see A.10). Other biologists, however, argue that only mathematics provides a language disciplined and comprehensive enough to allow careful, complete, and objective descriptions of a model, a hypothesis, or a theory. Criticisms of biological modeling are thought by these biologists to be true only for bad modeling in which the model and its validation are both poorly documented (see DiStefano and Landow, 1984; Gar-

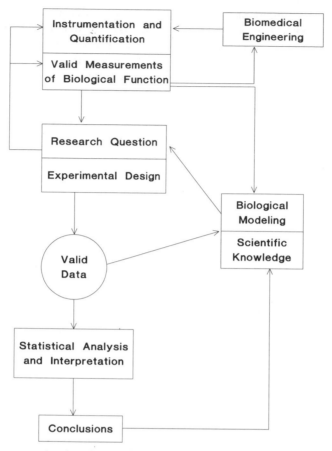

Figure A.1   Levels of analysis in biological research (A.7).

finkel and Fegley, 1984; Landow and DiStefano, 1984). At present, most biological research is guided by loosely interwoven conceptual models. Whether in
the near future these conceptual models will be replaced by formal, quantitative
models is debatable (see Rideout, 1991).

A good biological model, however, will not emerge from confounded experimental data. Hence, this book focuses on experimental design and statistical
inference so that the biological data collected and interpreted will be suitable for
subsequent model development. The reciprocal relationships among instrumentation, valid measurements, modeling, experimental design, valid data, and
statistical analysis and interpretation must be considered in any scientific study
(see Figure A.1).

A.9 CAUSALITY IN SCIENCE

The aim of scientific studies is to make causal statements, that is, A causes B.
The issue of cause and effect is still debated vigorously among philosophers of

science. There are many principles or canons that are used widely to identify causality—the most common of which are the method of agreement and the method of difference. In the method of agreement, several instances of an event (e.g., B) are studied to determine if there is a common element (e.g., A). In the method of difference, two situations are examined that are alike in all ways except one. If different effects are observed, these effects are ascribed to the factor (e.g., A) that was *not* common to the two situations.

In science both the method of agreement and the method of difference are used. The method of agreement is exemplified by correlational analysis which determines whether two variables are related (4.1). This type of study is used to generate hypotheses to be tested by the method of difference, which is best exemplified by an experiment (4.1). In the biological sciences, a linear causality approach has been used successfully. But, with the numerous positive and negative feedback cycles that operate in most biological systems, a linear causality approach has certain limitations in understanding normal biological functioning (A.10).

A.10 CYCLES OF CAUSALITY IN BIOLOGY

In linear causality every phenomenon is assumed to have a single (unique) cause and in a complex system a chain of cause and effect precedes every event; that is, the cause of Z is Y and the cause of Y is X, and so forth,

$$\cdots X \rightarrow Y \rightarrow Z \qquad \text{(linear causation)}.$$

In living systems, however, positive and negative feedback cycles are interwoven among all elements so that the effects produced by changes in one element (A) affect another element (B) which affects another element (C) which in turn affects the first element (A),

$$\cdots A \rightarrow B \rightarrow C \qquad \text{(cycle of causation)}.$$

The chains of cause and effect in a living system are circular and the influence of these *cycles of causation* radiates to all elements in the living system (see Figure A.2). Positive feedback cycles result in the growth of the system's response as small effects in such cycles are transformed into larger ones, and these into still larger ones, and so forth. In contrast, negative feedback cycles (stabilizing cycles) contribute to the great stability of living systems. Given this stability (even during ontogeny) positive feedback cycles are eventually counterbalanced by stabilizing negative feedback cycles.

In any experiment it is impossible to measure all the adjustments that may occur when a living system is perturbed by a treatment condition; consequently, most biological experiments focus on relatively simple, isolated cycles of causality. But cycles of causality must be considered when attempting to understand complex normal biological functioning. This integrative knowledge can generate significant research questions which may be evaluated experimentally (con-

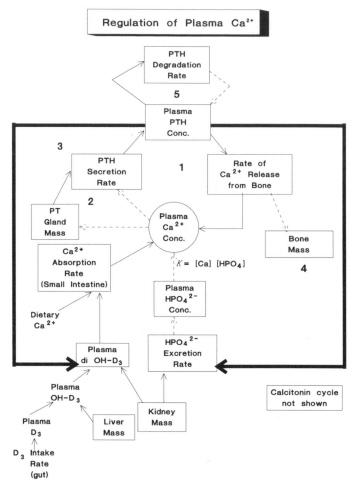

Figure A.2 An example of cycles of causality in biology: Regulation of plasma Ca^{2+}. Solid lines are positive cycles and dashed lines are negative cycles (A.10). Five distinct cycles (1,2,...,5) are presented in this example. (From Engelberg, 1983.)

ceptual–design phase, A.11). As Sokal and Rohlf (1981, p. 6) have stated . . . "In biology most phenomena are affected by many causal factors, uncontrollable in their variation and often unidentifiable. Statistics is needed to measure such variable phenomena with a predictable error and to ascertain the reality of minute but important differences." Biological phenomena may be fundamentally deterministic. Only the number of interwoven cycles of causality and our inability to control all of them may make biological phenomena appear probabilistic. On the other hand, biological processes may truly be probabilistic. Whichever of these alternatives is correct the fact remains that the experimental data recorded by the biologist can only be evaluated within a probabilistic framework.

A.11 CREATIVE–CONCEPTUAL PHASE OF RESEARCH

The creative–conceptual phase of research involves observation, insight, and ideas. To be creative a person is advised to look at facts in a new way, express ambiguities openly, and be spontaneous, imaginative and flexible. To achieve this creative state, the person is told to let the right hemisphere of the brain roam freely so new relationships among separate events are visualized. How we perceive, learn, think, and create are important questions. But, so far, answers to these questions are not known.

The formation of ingenious research questions (1.1) is a creative process and cannot be taught. The logic of experimental design and statistical inference, however, can be learned. This does not imply that the mechanical application of a hard and fast set of rules will determine whether an experiment is properly conceived, correctly controlled, adequately analyzed, and properly interpreted. But a critical perception can be cultivated so that important, and hopefully ingenious, research hypotheses are more likely to be evaluated in well-designed experiments. In short, any idea may be evaluated in either a well-designed or a poorly designed experiment. Hence, do not expect an ingenious idea to be accepted when evaluated in a poorly designed experiment nor a trivial idea to become important when evaluated in a well-designed experiment.

A.12 EXPERIMENTAL DESIGN AND STATISTICAL INFERENCE: AN OVERVIEW

Biological scientists are concerned primarily with designing and interpreting their own experiments as well as evaluating critically their colleagues' articles and papers. But, biologists have been reluctant to use sensitive statistical procedures to analyze and interpret their experimental data (A.1–A.4). To increase the statistical literacy of biologists (A.5) universities are providing statistical consultation and some journals are publishing special statistical reports (A.6).

The experiment is the inferential tool in biological research in which conclusions are made about large groups (populations) from data obtained from smaller groups (samples). A liaison exists between experimental design and statistical inference which, if properly exploited, will increase the likelihood of making correct decisions. A well-designed experiment is one in which the treatment conditions are not confounded by subject-, environment-, or time-related extraneous variables, *and* the statistical methodology selected makes the two statistical errors of inference (1.7) as small as possible for the data to be collected and the comparisons to be made. Hence, in their research, biologists strive to translate important questions into appropriate treatment conditions, to obtain accurate and valid measures of important biological processes, to perform well-designed experiments which provide unequivocal data, and to integrate their data with current knowledge. In these endeavors the biologist must consider the different levels of analysis in biology (A.7, A.8), causality in science (A.9, A.10), and the creative–conceptual phase of research (A.11).

A.13 USERS OF BOOK

This book is intended primarily for researchers in the biological sciences who design experiments and interpret the results from their own and other's experiments (see "Preface"). The essentials of experimental design and statistical inference are taught by encouraging you to identify design and statistical errors in 100 research problems (see "Structure of Book").

The research tutorial organization of the book with its extensive cross-referencing among related subtopics will be useful to biologists who are beginning their research training. These individuals will benefit from reading the first part of the book and reviewing this material by comparing their evaluations of the research design problems with the critiques presented. Biologists with biostatistics training will benefit from the cross-referencing of subtopics on the underlying principles of experimental design and statistical inference. Answers to common design and statistical questions may be found quickly without the necessity of learning a unique symbolic language (A.4). Experienced researchers, therefore, may want to start by identifying design and statistical errors in the research design problems and reviewing relevant subtopics only when their evaluations disagree with those of the critiques. Health-related professionals who must evaluate the biological research literature will find the book a valuable guide to specific experimental designs and statistical procedures. The rules for reconstruction of analysis of variance (ANOVA) tables will help all readers identify the treatment comparisons being made in research reports (6.3, 6.4, 6.5, 6.6).

The importance of both research design and statistical inference in understanding biological phenomena cannot be overemphasized. This book, however, is not meant to, and cannot, replace traditional biostatistics books or the need for statistical consultation. Indeed, the problem tutorials in this book should be studied in conjunction with the more advanced discussions of statistical application found in research oriented books (e.g. Bourke, Daly, and McGilvray, 1985; Elston and Johnson, 1987; Everitt, 1989; Glantz and Slinker, 1990; Keppel, 1991; Sokal and Rohlf, 1981). The more you know of statistical theory and its application to biological phenomena the better your end product will be. As Glantz (1987) has adeptly advised ". . . if you decide to contribute to the fund of scientific and clinical knowledge, take the time and care to do it right" (p. 351).

I
EXPERIMENTAL DESIGN

1

The Anatomy of an Experiment

1.1 FORMULATION OF RESEARCH QUESTION

An experiment begins with the formulation of one or multiple *research hypotheses*. These hypotheses may be deductions from previous research in a field, derivations from theoretical models, hunches, or speculations. The formulation of important research questions is a creative process (the creative–conceptual phase of research, A.11). Eventually the proposed research questions must be translated into appropriate *treatment conditions* (1.2) so that accurate and valid measurements of appropriate biological responses can be obtained (A.7). If the treatment conditions cannot be specified or if the measurements cannot be made, the research questions must be either reformulated (conceptual–design phase of research) or new techniques must be developed before the original research questions can be answered (A.7). The importance of a significant research question that can be translated into appropriate treatment conditions cannot be overemphasized. Too often, technical expertise determines the research questions asked.

1.2 RESEARCH HYPOTHESES

In many cases biologists are interested in answering more than one question in their experiments. Therefore, these multiple research hypotheses must be translated into a set of treatment conditions. The particular treatment conditions used must be capable of evaluating each of the proposed research questions (1.1).

In the typical experiment, there are three classes of variables—*independent, dependent,* and *extraneous* (or *nuisance*) variables. The *independent* variable is the variable the scientist manipulates (the treatment) to determine its effect on some biological response (the *dependent* variable). Independent variables are often referred to as manipulated variables, treatments, conditions, or factors. *Nuisance* variables are potential independent variables which could exert a systematic influence on the manipulated treatment conditions. The separation of these systematic influences from the selected independent variables is an important part of the experimental design. Hence, in planning experiments a major task of the biologist is to select procedures that control nuisance or extraneous variables.

If treatment and nuisance variables are systematically related (*confounded*) then the treatment condition is not an adequate test of the research hypothesis.

In a well-designed experiment the only difference between the experimental (treatment) and control groups should be the variable selected and manipulated by the researcher. The ability to formulate specific research questions into precise treatment conditions and to identify and control potential confoundings is what distinguishes the expert from the novice in a given research discipline. In a poorly designed experiment, the research hypothesis may not be related to the chosen treatment condition (1.1) or the treatment condition may be confounded with systematically varying nuisance variables. For instance, in an experiment studying the chronic effects of a drug, environment-related confounds would include such blunders as housing one group of animals (experimental) in a different room from the control animals or unintentionally handling one group of animals more than another group.

1.3 SAMPLE AND POPULATION: STATISTICAL GENERALIZATION

When a research hypothesis is being translated into an appropriate treatment regimen (1.2), the animals selected for the experiment (the sample) and the generalization of the conclusions from the research data must be considered. The primary aim of experimental research is to draw conclusions (inferences) that pertain to a larger group (*population*) than the limited one from which data have been collected (*sample*). Hence, experimental conclusions (inferences) are made about a group (population) based upon limited data (sample).

A *population* is a complete set of animals or measurements sharing one or more common observable characteristic. The population of interest may be heart rates in rats, temperatures of hamsters, blood pressures of dogs, cholesterol levels of women, or blood samples or tissue specimens from a particular species. A given population may be considered to be made up of individual study units. In statistics, a population is the group of all study units about which an experiment may provide information. A distinction between the *target population* and the *study population* is often made (Elston and Johnson, 1987; Marks, 1982a). The target population is the whole group of study units to which we want to generalize our experimental conclusions. The study population is the group of study units to which we can *statistically generalize* our experimental conclusions if a *random sample* has been selected and used (4.6, 4.25, 4.27).

A *sample* is a subset of the specified population, that is, a sample is some fraction of the study units from the study population. *Random sampling* requires the specification of a study population along with the assurance that each member of the study population has an equally likely chance of being selected for the experiment. If these requirements are met, the conclusions of an experiment with a random sample can be generalized to (assumed to be true for) the specified study population (*statistical generalization*). Suppose, for example, a random sample of 90-day-old male rats from the Sprague-Dawley colony of a university (the study population) was selected for an experiment on cardiovascular functioning and cholesterol levels. Random sampling would permit the outcome of this particular rat experiment to be generalized to this university's Sprague-Dawley 90-day-old male rats *but* not to all 90-day-old male Sprague-Dawley rats.

Other assumptions are necessary if inferences from this particular experimental study are applicable to all Sprague-Dawley male rats (1.8). Rats in this university colony may be infected with a mild virus, housed under fluorescent lights, or weaned at 18 rather than 21 days of life. Any one of these conditions could make this rat colony significantly different from other colonies of Sprague-Dawley rats. Indeed, in most experiments the sample used is not a random sample of the total population of interest (the target population) and *statistical generalization* permits conclusions to be inferred only for the specified study population (1.8, 4.6). Hence, other *nonstatistical* considerations are necessary to determine whether experimental outcomes should be generalized beyond the normally restricted study population (1.8, 4.6, 4.27).

1.4 RANDOM ASSIGNMENT OF ANIMALS TO TREATMENT CONDITIONS

Random sampling from a specified study population permits inferences from the experimental data to be generalized to the study population (1.3). In contrast, the *random assignment* (allocation) of animals to treatment conditions is a method to control for potential extraneous influences that may vary systematically (be confounded) with the treatment conditions (A.3, 1.2). Thus, the random sampling of animals and the random assigning of animals to treatment conditions are different elements in any experimental plan.

There are basically two ways to control for extraneous (nuisance) variables (1.2). The first way to reduce experimental variability (noise) is to hold constant during the experiment as many environmental and biological variables as possible (A.3). To control for experimental noise, the general health of an animal may be monitored continuously and treatment conditions applied only within certain narrow physiological ranges or a preparation may be held at a constant temperature and pH, and so forth. This method of control is familiar to most biologists because it is the traditional experimental procedure to control for (reduce) unwanted variability (noise).

A major source of uncontrolled variability present in any experiment, however, is the different magnitudes of the biological responses of animals. As examples, body weights, heart rates, and respiratory rates are not identical even among male animals of the same age and strain; consequently, a specific treatment will not produce exactly the same response magnitude in all animals. Variability in a population of animals is a very familiar concept to biologists. As biological differences among animals may affect treatment outcomes, these animal-related influences must be controlled in any experiment. But, all potential extraneous variables associated with animals selected randomly cannot be identified and held constant in any experiment (traditional control procedure). Therefore, the random assignment of animals to treatment conditions is used to make it unlikely that any one of these extraneous variables will be confounded (vary systematically) with treatment conditions (4.7, 4.8). The differences between random sampling (1.4) and random assignment of animals are presented in Table 1.1.

Table 1.1   Differences Between Random Sampling and Random Assignment of Animals

Random sampling of animals (4.6)[a]	Random assignment (allocation) of animals to treatment conditions (4.7, 4.8)[a]
A. Identification of target population (1.3).	A. Each animal of study sample (1.3) has an equally likely chance of being assigned to any of the treatment conditions (1.4).
B. Identification of study population (1.3).	
C. Each animal in study population has an equally likely chance of being selected for the experiment (1.3).	
	B. Controls for subject confounding with treatment conditions (1.5, 4.11).
D. Statistical generalization (1.3, 4.25): Inferences from random sample of experiment to study population.	C. Distinguishes between experimental and classification studies (4.1, 4.2, 4.4).
E. Scientific generalization (1.8, 4.25, 4.27): Inferences from sample to target population.	D. The method of random allocation (assignment of animals to treatment conditions) may be done with a random numbers table.

[a]See this book section.

1.5 EXPERIMENTAL DESIGN: BETWEEN- AND WITHIN-SUBJECT DESIGNS AND MIXED FACTORIAL DESIGNS

An experiment consists of a well-conceived plan for data collection, analysis, and interpretation. Consequently, the experimental plan should include the statistical methods that will be used to analyze the data and permit valid conclusions or inferences to be drawn from them. Fortunately, an isomorphism exists among many of the experimental designs used by biologists and the mathematical models developed by statisticians (1.7). Hence, you can take advantage of these statistical models to analyze your experimental data so that quantitative (probability) statements about current and future findings can be made (5.7, 5.16).

The type of experimental design chosen by you, however, imposes restrictions on the conclusions that may be drawn from the experimental outcomes. Too often, experiments are started, some data collected, and concerns then arise regarding how the data will be evaluated. Because some biologists regard data collected from each animal as an experiment, the experimental protocol (4.5) may be changed slightly for each animal. In such cases, valid statistical models may not be available to make inferences from this "individual-sample" data. Most likely, only a small portion of the data may be properly analyzed with most of the data becoming scientific folklore; that is, "I know there is a significant treatment effect, but I can't test it! Damn statistics!" In other cases, researchers may select a statistical model that is inappropriate for a particular experimental design. These experimental data are most likely to appear in those journals that require only probability levels be reported (e.g., statements regarding the significance of certain comparisons, A.5).

Experimental designs may be classified into two general types: *between-subject* or *within-subject*. In a *between-subject* design, animals or their parts (organs, tissues, cells) are randomly assigned to the various treatment conditions (1.4). A different group of animals is given each of the treatment conditions. In the simplest between-subject design, there would be a treatment group of animals and a control group of animals. Because any differences in biological responses observed among the treatment conditions are based on different groups of randomly assigned animals, this type of design is also known as a *completely randomized design*. In between-subject designs, the number of independent measurements is equal to the total number of animals used in the experiment (4.9). Likewise, the total number of observations (i.e., data points) is equal to the total number of animals used (Figures 1.1 and 1.2).

In the other basic experimental design (*within-subject*) each animal serves in all the treatment conditions. This design is also known as a *repeated-measures* design because the same biological measurement (e.g., blood pressure) is taken more than once from each animal. Thus any treatment effects (e.g., drug and vehicle control conditions) are evaluated from differences within the single group of animals used in the experiment. In a within-subject design the number

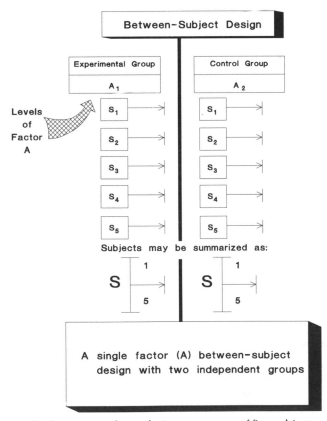

Figure 1.1 In this between-subject design one group of five subjects receives the treatment and the other group of five subjects serves as a control (1.5, 4.10, Figure 1.10).

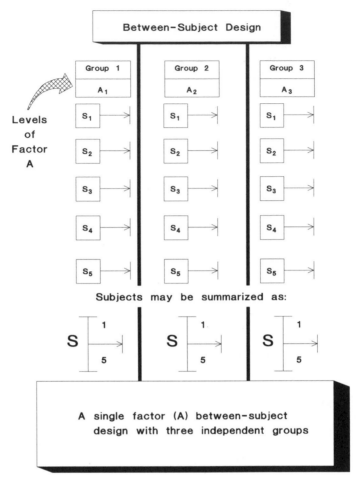

Figure 1.2 In this between-subject design the magnitude (levels) of a single treatment (Factor A) is normally manipulated. Each different (independent) group of five subjects receives a different level of the treatment (1.5, 4.10).

of independent measurements is also equal to the total number of animals (4.9), and each animal has the same number of repeated (correlated) measures taken (Figures 1.3 and 1.4). In summary, the total number of observations in a within-subject design is equal to the total number of subjects (independent observations) multiplied ($\times$) by the number of repeated measures taken from each subject (e.g., 5 animals $\times$ 3 measures per animal = 15 total observations).

There are a variety of permutations of these simple between-subject and within-subject designs (Figures 1.5 and 1.6). In a *between-subject factorial design*, for instance, different groups of subjects are used to study the effects of more than one independent (treatment) variable in the same experiment (4.13). A *mixed factorial design*, as the name implies, is a mixture of between- and

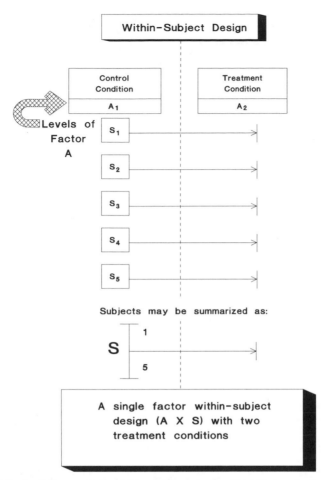

Figure 1.3 In this complete within-subject design (2 X 5) the single group of five subjects receives both levels of Factor A, normally the two levels are a control condition and a treatment condition (1.5, 4.16). The within-subject factor is enclosed in parentheses with subjects (A X S) to identify dependent (correlated) measurements (4.9, 9.2, 9.5).

within-subject components (see Figures 1.7, 1.8 and 1.9) and is one of the most common designs used in biological research (4.21).

1.6 STATISTICAL HYPOTHESES: NULL HYPOTHESIS AND ALTERNATIVE HYPOTHESIS

A research hypothesis, even when precisely and correctly translated into treatment conditions, cannot be tested directly (1.2). The only way to provide support for the research hypothesis is to reject the *null hypothesis* (H_0). This statis-

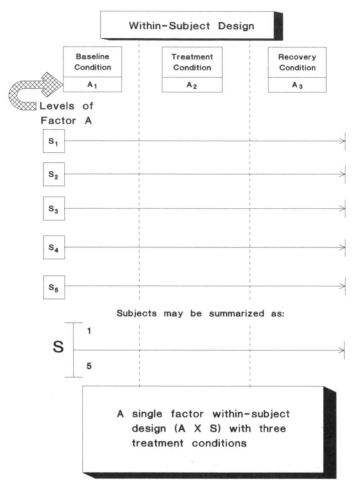

Figure 1.4 In this complete within-subject design (3 × 5) the single group of five subjects receives all three levels of Factor A (1.5, 4.16). The within-subject factor is enclosed in parentheses with subjects (A × S) to identify dependent (correlated) measurements (4.9, 9.2, 9.5).

tical hypothesis is that the experimental treatment has no effect on the dependent variable being measured and may be stated as H_0: treatment mean equals (=) control mean. Hence, an experiment cannot prove that the research hypothesis is correct but can only result in a rejection of the null hypothesis with a *specified* degree of confidence (1.7). If the null hypothesis is rejected then the alternative statistical hypothesis is asserted which is H_i: treatment mean does not equal (≠) control mean. Concluding that the alternative statistical hypothesis is probably correct—that the two study populations means are not equal (1.3)— does *not* also indicate that the research hypothesis is correct (5.5, 5.10). Before this latter assumption may be considered, the research hypothesis (1.1) must

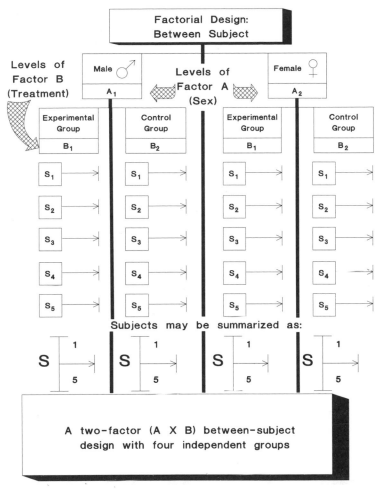

Figure 1.5 In this 2 × 2 between-subject factorial design there are two levels of each of the two factors, A and B (4.13). An independent (different) group of subjects is used for each of the four unique treatment conditions, A_1B_1, A_1B_2, A_2B_1, and A_2B_2.

have been precisely and correctly translated into treatment conditions (1.2) and potential confoundings must have been controlled in the design of the experiment (4.23).

1.7 STATISTICAL ANALYSIS AND INTERPRETATION: DECISION RULES, ERRORS OF INFERENCE AND POWER

All statistical methods are based on an abstraction (a mathematical model) which may approximate some real-world phenomenon (empirical events). The

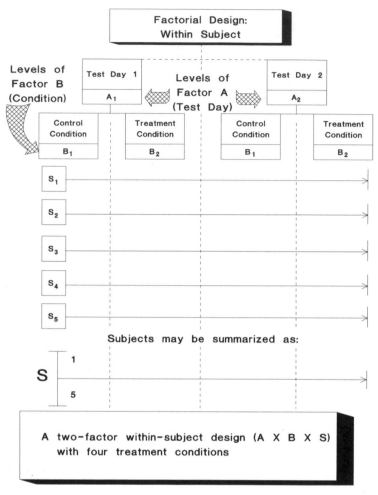

Figure 1.6 In this 2 × 2 within-subject factorial design there are two levels of each of the two factors, A and B (4.13). A single group of five subjects is given each of the four unique treatment conditions, A_1B_1, A_1B_2, A_2B_1, and A_2B_2. Within-subject factors are enclosed in parentheses with subjects (A × B × S) to identify dependent (correlated) measurements (4.9, 9.2, 9.5).

statistical model is neither right nor wrong; rather, the model is either appropriate or inappropriate for a given set of data (5.7). If the approximation between the model and empirical events is good, a useful, sometimes powerful, inferential tool is available to the researcher. But, if the approximation is poor, the researcher may easily draw erroneous conclusions from the data. Hence, experimental design and statistical analysis must be complementary for the researcher to draw valid inferences from biological data.

The logic of a statistical test is to assume that the *null hypothesis* is correct (1.6) and to generate a theoretical sampling distribution based on this assumption

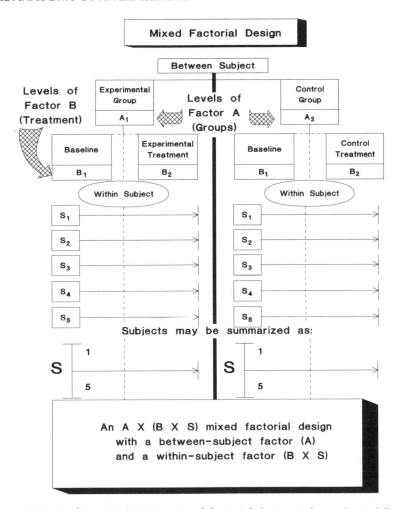

Figure 1.7 In this 2 × (2 × 5) mixed factorial design independent (different) groups of five subjects are used for the two levels of the between-subject component, A_1 and A_2. Repeated (dependent) measurements on the same subject are the levels of the within-subject component, B_1 and B_2 (1.5, 4.10, 4.13, 4.16). The within-subject factor is enclosed in parentheses with subjects (B × S) to identify dependent (correlated) measurements (4.9, 9.2, 9.5).

(5.7). Experimental data are compared with this sampling distribution to decide whether the null hypothesis (H_0) should be rejected. If the distribution of the experimental data is similar to the distribution generated by this statistical (null) hypothesis, there is no basis for rejecting the null hypothesis. But if the experimental data deviates greatly from the null hypothesis, the null hypothesis is rejected and the *alternative statistical hypothesis* is asserted (1.6). "Deviated greatly" is *defined arbitrarily* as a value of a statistic (e.g., t or F) which would occur on the basis of chance only a small proportion of the time, for example, 1

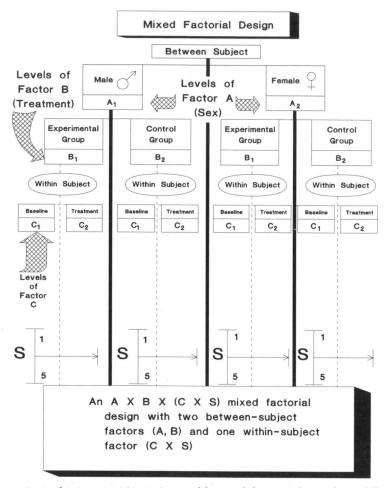

Figure 1.8 In this 2 × 2 × (2 × 5) mixed factorial design independent (different) groups of five subjects are used for each of the four unique group conditions, A_1B_1, A_1B_2, A_2B_1, and A_2B_2. Repeated (dependent) measurements on the same subject are the levels of the within-subject component, C_1 and C_2 (1.5, 4.10, 4.16). The within-subject factor is enclosed in parentheses with subjects (C × S) to identify dependent (correlated) measurements (4.9, 9.2, 9.5).

time in 20 ($p < .05$). Theoretically, a researcher may choose any significance level ($p < .05$ or $p < .01$, the latter means that probability of occurrence is less than 1 in 100 if H_0 is true) to reject the null hypothesis as long as the choice is made *before* data are collected (5.8).

This statistical hypothesis testing, however, does not guarantee that a correct inference will be drawn. Errors of inference can be made, and they are of two types. The first error, *Type I*, occurs when the null hypothesis is rejected for the sample data but is true in the population. The second error, *Type II*, occurs when the null hypothesis is accepted for the sample data but is false in the population

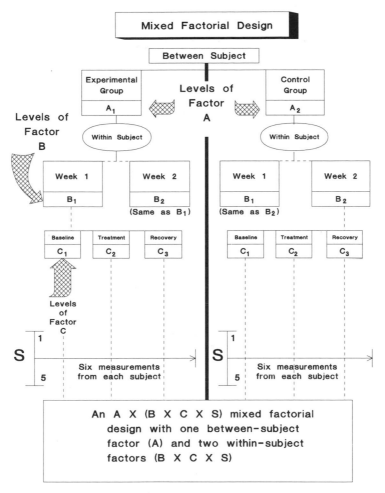

Figure 1.9   In this 2 × (2 × 3 × 5) mixed factorial design independent (different) groups of five subjects are used for the two levels of the between-subject component, A_1 and A_2. Repeated (dependent) measurements on the same subject are the six unique condition combinations, B_1C_1, B_1C_2, B_1C_3, B_2C_1, B_2C_2, and B_2C_3. Within-subject factors are enclosed in parentheses with subjects (B × C × S) to identify dependent (correlated) measurements (1.5, 4.10, 4.13, 4.16, 9.2, 9.5).

(5.10). The size of the Type I error can be directly controlled by selection of the significance level; that is, with a significance level of $p < .001$, the null hypothesis would not be rejected falsely as readily as when a significance level of $p < .05$ was used (5.11). However, decreasing Type I errors by this method would result in more Type II errors being made, that is, accepting the null hypothesis when it is false. In this latter case, the sensitivity of the statistical test would not be very great. *The smaller the Type II error, the greater the power and the greater the sensitivity of the test.* The power (or sensitivity) of a statistical test is defined in

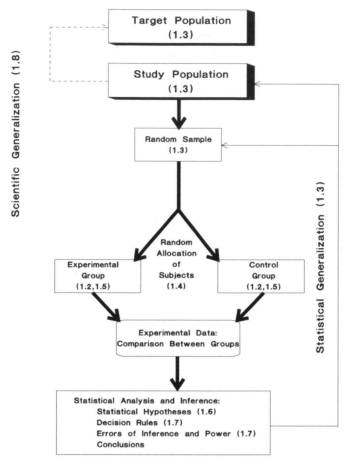

Figure 1.10 The basic skeleton of a typical between-group experiment with a control group and an experimental group (See Figure 1.1).

terms of the probability of making a Type II error, namely, power = 1—Type II error. Power, therefore, refers to the probability of *rejecting* the null hypothesis when an alternative hypothesis is *true* (5.12, 5.13).

Ideally, to minimize errors of inference a researcher would like to choose a significance level of .001 or lower and have the power of the test be .90 or higher (5.12). Unfortunately, this idealized state of affairs does not exist with small sample sizes, and each researcher must decide whether to accept a lower Type I or II error of inference. Usually, biologists have been less concerned with Type II errors. They set their significance levels to control Type I errors and let the power of their tests be what it may (5.11). Type II errors, however, may be decreased by increasing sample size (number of animals in each treatment group) and by reducing error variance through the design of a more precisely controlled experiment (5.12). The logic of experimental and statistical hypothesis testing is summarized in Figures 1.10, 1.11, and 1.12.

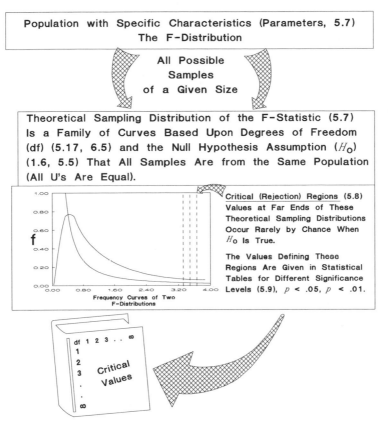

Figure 1.11 Schema of how theoretical sampling distributions of a test statistic (e.g., F-statistic) are used to establish critical regions for significance levels of statistical tests (e.g., analysis of variance, 6.0).

1.8 SCIENTIFIC GENERALIZATION

The results of an experiment with a random sample can be generalized to the study population (1.3). Yet, in most experiments the sample used is not a random sample of the population of interest (target population). Usually, the study population from which the sample was drawn is very restricted (e.g., the Sprague-Dawley rat colony of a university). How then can you generalize your results beyond the single experiment or the restricted study population? The extension of experimental results beyond the explicit limits of statistical generalization is based upon *scientific generalization*. Scientific or *nonstatistical generalization* depends on knowledge of a particular research area. The appropriateness of any scientific generalization is determined by the adequacy of the animal model used, the state of development of the research area, and, most important, the extent to which past extrapolations have been successful (4.25, 4.27).

The distinction between statistical generalization and nonstatistical (scientific) generalization has been adeptly made by Cornfield and Tukey (1956):

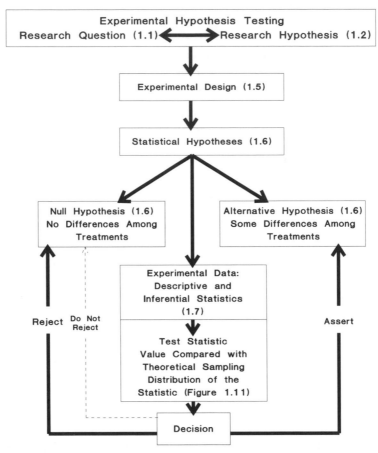

Figure 1.12 A flowchart diagramming the relationship between experimental and statistical hypothesis testing.

In almost any practical situation where analytical statistics is applied, the inference from the observations to the real conclusion has two parts, only the first of which is statistical. A genetic experiment on *Drosophila* will usually involve flies of a certain race of a certain species. The statistically based conclusions cannot extend beyond this race, yet the geneticist will usually, and often wisely, extend the conclusion to (*a*) the whole species, (*b*) all Drosophila, or (*c*) a larger group of insects. This wider extension may be implicit or explicit, but it is almost always present (pp. 912–913).

2

The Anatomy of a Scientific Paper

2.1 ABSTRACT

The abstract of a scientific paper presents a summary of the article; it describes concisely the research problem and hypotheses, the cells, tissues, organs or animals used (number, age, sex and species), the experimental methods, the findings (including statistical tests and significance levels), and the conclusions and implications of the findings. In short, an informative abstract will briefly state the problem, the methods used to study the problem, relevant data, and major conclusions. Abstracts are usually strictly limited to a specified number of words; consequently, both brevity and clarity are essential (see Cremmins, 1982).

2.2 INTRODUCTION: BACKGROUND AND SIGNIFICANCE

The introduction of a scientific article presents the specific problem under study and describes the general research strategy. Previous research *pertinent* to the specific problem is evaluated critically and the logical continuity between previous work and the present work is usually emphasized. An exhaustive historical review *is not* required; rather the background review should emphasize pertinent findings, relevant methodological issues, and major conclusions. Many introductions provide too much tangentially relevant and even totally irrelevant material. Authors of a scientific paper do not need to document their knowledge of the research area, although degree candidates may be required to do so in their theses.

After the research problem is introduced along with relevant background information, the significance and rationale of the intended research are usually presented. At this stage, a brief statement of the research hypotheses gives clarity to the paper (1.2). If the relation of the research hypotheses and experimental design to the research problem can now be explicitly made, the reader will understand the purpose and theoretical implications of the study (1.1). Sometimes, very brief previews of the principal results and major conclusions are given to guide the reader through the paper (see Katz, 1985).

2.3 METHODS

The Methods section describes in detail how the study was conducted. This section provides a concise description of the animals or preparations used and the techniques and procedures which were applied so that the methodology of the study can be reproduced by colleagues. Some journals require labeled subsections (e.g., Animals, Materials, Procedures) to organize this specific information; whereas, other journals permit authors to organize their own Methods sections. When animals are used, the genus, species, and strain number are reported as well as the number of animals and the animals' sex, age, weight, and physiological condition. All *essential* details of the animals' treatment and handling are also presented. The description of materials or techniques used are given in sufficient detail (supplies, model numbers, drugs) so that the same items and techniques could be employed in a replication study (7.3). The experimental procedure summarizes each step in the execution of the research and includes the formation of the groups and specific experimental manipulations. Randomization, counterbalancing, and other control features of the experimental design, as well as statistical methods, are described explicitly (4.20). In summary, the Methods section indicates what was done and how it was done clearly enough so that the experiment could be reproduced by other scientists (7.3, 7.4).

2.4 RESULTS

The Results section summarizes the data obtained and the statistical treatment of the data. The major results or findings are usually presented first followed by appropriate data analysis to justify the statements made. Typically, detailed data are presented in tables or figures including descriptive statistics of central tendency and variability of individual group data (5.1). When reporting inferential statistics (e.g., t-tests, F-tests, chi-squares) the magnitude or value of the test, the direction of the effect, the degrees of freedom (5.17), and the significance (probability) level (5.9) should be given. Too often, only probability levels ($p < .05$) follow major conclusions reported and the reader must guess what test was used, what groups were compared, and how many animals were used in the comparison. Nonsignificant results and trends obtained with small samples usually are uninterpretable (6.20); hence, they should be presented briefly without elaboration.

2.5 DISCUSSION

The Discussion section evaluates the major findings and interprets their implications as they relate to the research hypotheses and the research problem (2.2). The theoretical consequences of the results and the validity of the conclusions inferred from the data are usually emphasized. Similarities and differences between reported results and those of others are clarified briefly. However, an extensive discussion of possible reasons for different experimental outcomes or negative results should be avoided. Inconclusive interpretations and implications only distract from the actual contributions of the study. Any speculations on the scientific generalization of the conclusions are given concisely at the end of the Discussion section. Numerous manuals and books are available which inform scientists how to effectively communicate their research to others (e.g., Day, 1988; Huth, 1982; Luey, 1987; Wilkerson, 1991).

3

Evaluation of a Scientific Article

3.1 THE REVIEWER'S TASK

The task of a reviewer of a scientific paper is to identify quickly whether an experimental study is *properly conceived, correctly controlled, adequately analyzed, correctly interpreted, and concisely presented.* If the author of the paper has followed the guidelines presented in Chapter 2, "The Anatomy of a Scientific Paper," the task of the reviewer is relatively easy. Unfortunately, with many articles the reviewer must evaluate the research done in spite of the author's organization and presentation. The reviewer must decide, given the research hypothesis, the experimental plan, and the data analysis, whether the author's conclusions should be accepted or rejected (see Section IV, "Research Design Problems and Their Critiques").

3.2 EVALUATING A SCIENTIFIC ARTICLE

The proliferation of research has made it difficult for most of us to keep pace with current developments in our research disciplines. General abstract services and specialized computer searches do help identify quickly those articles that may be of interest to us. These individual papers must then be reviewed to evaluate whether the research reported is both valid and pertinent to one's research interests. Because about one-half of the articles in biological journals have been found to contain elementary statistical errors and many others may have serious confounding problems (A.2), we must develop quick methods to separate the acceptable from the unacceptable reports. Figure 3.1 presents an idealized schema of an experimental paper and lists a series of significant questions that may be asked (also see Bourke, Daly, and McGilvray, 1985, pp. 238–258; Elston and Johnson, 1987, pp. 246–250; Scott and Waterhouse, 1986, pp. 3–19). For any paper you should be able to reconstruct the experimental design used, the experimental protocol for animals in the different groups (4.5), and the analysis of variance model used (when appropriate) to determine significance levels (6.3).

3.3 RESEARCH PROBLEM AND SCIENTIFIC GENERALIZATION

Answers to the series of questions proposed in Figure 3.1 will help determine whether the experiment was properly conceived, correctly controlled, ade-

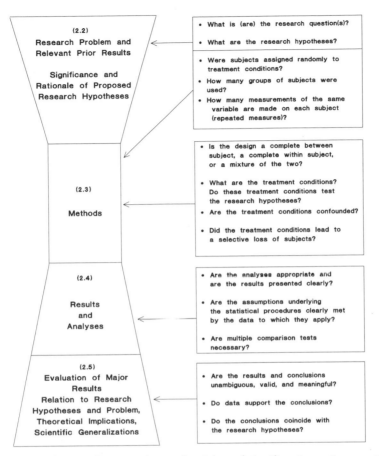

Figure 3.1 Schema of an experimental article and significant questions pertinent to sections of the article. The typical latitude the scientist has within each of the sections is represented by the width of the section in the schema.

quately analyzed, and correctly interpreted. However, the research problem chosen may be trivial; consequently, only limited scientific information may be obtained from the experiment. Many so-called "parametric" studies using the standard paradigm of a given experimental discipline are candidates for this trivial category (A.11). On the other hand, important research questions often are asked that cannot be answered with available methods (1.1). To propose important research questions and expect valid answers to emerge mysteriously from inappropriate methodology hinders scientific progress much more than pedestrian questions asked within the context of a well-conceived experimental plan. In the former case, subsequent experiments of colleagues may be based upon the reported invalid data and conclusions (7.3, 7.4). In the latter case, the data and conclusions are usually valid but often are ignored because they add so little to scientific knowledge (see Figure A.1).

Experimental Design

4.1 CORRELATIONAL VERSUS EXPERIMENTAL STUDY

A correlational study determines whether two or more variables are significantly related to each other. A correlation establishes the degree to which two variables vary together, but does not establish that changes in one variable *cause* changes in another (A.9, A.10). The Pearson-correlation coefficient r is thus a statistical association between two naturally occurring (random) variables and a causal inference cannot be made (5.27). For example, a significant negative correlation between the number of telephones installed in the United States and the general physical fitness level of young adults can be demonstrated. Does this negative correlation imply that if telephones were eliminated an increase in general physical fitness in young adults would occur? No, of course not! Most young adults, rather than walking or running to deliver important messages, would probably drive their cars. Hopefully, no biologist would attempt to draw causal inferences from this type of correlational data. But, suppose in a group of runners a significant negative correlation was found between the number of fast-twitch–slow-fatiguable (FTSF) muscle cells in the athletes' legs and 880-yard run times, that is, the greater the number of FTSF muscle cells the lower 880-yard run times. As an exercise physiologist would you be tempted to conclude that an increase in FTSF muscle fibers in the athletes' legs *produces or leads to or results in* (*causes*!) lower time in the 880-yard run? Remember, not all variables that are associated are causally related!

4.2 CLASSIFICATION VARIABLES

Experiments are frequently found that include the systematic variation of characteristics which are *intrinsic* to the subjects studied. The effects of exercise on heart rate may be studied, for example, by measuring heart rates in men who are classified as being inactive, joggers, or marathon runners. These data may be reported as if they were the results of an experiment but the groups (inactive individuals, joggers, and runners) were created by selecting subjects on the *classification dimension* to be included in the study. In this study, to vary physical activity subjects were segregated (assigned) to the three groups *on the basis of their own activity*. But these types of manipulation do not constitute a true experiment because the administration of the "treatments" is obviously *not* under the control of the researcher. Similar studies are often called *quasi-experimental designs*. In a quasi-experimental design, intact groups are assigned to the treatment conditions. These groups normally differ systematically on a number of characteristics which may be relevant to treatment outcomes. As might be expected, increasing the group size will have no systematic effect on preexisting differences. Statistical procedures used to evaluate the results of experiments, in which individual animals are randomly allocated to the treatment conditions (A.3, 4.4), are not appropriate for quasi-experimental designs. Nor can analysis of covariance (6.18) be used to statistically control for preexisting group differences because this method requires that the animals be randomly assigned to the treatment conditions (Table 1.1).

In an experiment the independent variable is the only feature of the situation that is allowed to vary systematically from condition to condition (Chapter 1, 4.4). It is this characteristic of an experiment that permits the inference that a particular manipulation caused systematic differences in the biological responses observed among the different groups. When a classification variable is used to create treatment groups, subjects normally differ systematically from group to group with respect to characteristics other than the classification variable, that is, the classification variable is confounded with other variables (1.2). Indeed, classification variables are always subject-confounded (4.11). For example, men who are inactive, joggers, or runners probably differ in their ages, in their diets, their responses to stress, their self-esteem, their body weights, and so forth. Because these confounded variables cannot be controlled by the researcher, making cause-and-effect conclusions are impossible when only classification variables are used in a study.

In reality, a classification study is a correlation study (4.1) with the classification variable simply another dimension that is observed and recorded in addition to the dependent variable. Sometimes classification variables are introduced in conjunction with independent variables that are manipulated by the researcher (see Figure 1.8). These latter designs can produce a more sensitive context in which to study the effects of independent variables across different kinds of groups. Such combined designs permit you to examine the treatment effects separately for each classification group (e.g., strain, age or sex), and to determine whether the treatment effects change or remain the same for the different groups of subjects (4.13). In general, however, when *only* classification variables are used to separate animals into two or more groups you should be wary of explicit or implicit cause-and-effect inferences. Whenever the animals are not assigned randomly to the treatment conditions (1.4), assume a correlation study has been done. With classification variables, extrapolation of the obtained results must be made carefully. Classification studies are common in the biomedical research literature (4.3) and frequently become "real" experiments when reported in the popular press (4.4).

4.3 CASE–CONTROL (RETROSPECTIVE) STUDIES, COHORT (PROSPECTIVE) STUDIES AND RANDOMIZED CLINICAL TRIALS

Most correlation (or classification) studies (4.1, 4.2) can be identified quickly by determining whether data are collected on already-existing subject groupings (*retrospective study*) or whether subjects are selected for some characteristic (such as health status) and then are followed into the future (*prospective study*). Retrospective studies begin with subjects who have already developed a certain disorder (case) and subjects who have not developed the disorder (control); consequently, these types of studies are often called *case–control* studies. Prospective studies begin *before* the people have developed a disorder of interest (e.g., cancer) and follow them forward in time to determine who subsequently will develop the disorder. Prospective studies also are called *cohort* studies. A cohort is defined as a group of individuals who share a common experience (e.g., smokers compared with nonsmokers).

In a retrospective study medical records of patients with oral cancer may be examined to determine whether they differ from control patients (without oral cancer) in their smoking and drinking habits. If a higher incidence of alcohol consumption occurs in the oral cancer patients, these two variables are correlated (4.1, 4.2). However, drinking alcohol cannot be assumed to cause oral cancer because classification groups are always subject-confounded groups (4.11). Subject-related confounding means that the groups differ on many other variables (extraneous variables), some of which may be causally linked to oral cancer.

Similar interpretative problems occur in prospective studies. Suppose a group of alcohol drinkers took a behavioral modification course in which one-half of the subjects quit drinking. For the next five years the drinkers and nondrinkers were examined yearly for oral cancer and during this period the nondrinkers had significantly fewer incidences of oral cancer than did the drinkers. Would it be appropriate to conclude that drinking alcohol causes oral cancer? No, this conclusion would be suspect because the subjects who stopped drinking after their behavioral modification course were *obviously different* from those who could not stop drinking. In this case, individuals *by their own choice* divided themselves into the two classification groups (4.2). The only conclusion possible would be that individuals who could stop drinking have fewer incidences of oral cancer than those who continued to drink. Prospective studies must assume that the groups differ only in one common experience (are matched on all other relevant variables), an assumption that may or may not be true.

Although inferences from either retrospective or prospective studies are normally limited, these types of studies are not useless. These studies can identify variables that are related and which *could be* causally linked to one another; consequently, they often lead to hypotheses that can be experimentally tested (4.1). The question that usually separates an experiment from a classification study is "Were the subjects randomly assigned to the treatment conditions?" If the answer to this question is yes then an experimental study is being performed; if the answer is no then a classification study has been done and the treatment conditions will be confounded with extraneous variables that are subject-related (4.2).

If a biologist used two pure strains of mice and assigned a random sample from one strain to the experimental condition and a random sample from the other strain to the control condition, would it be appropriate to conclude any significant group difference was produced by the treatment applied? No, it would not be appropriate because treatment conditions are confounded with the strain of mice used. If the biologist matched individual mice in the two strains on sex, age, and body weight and then assigned the matched sample from one strain to the experimental condition and the matched sample of the other strain to the control condition, would it *now* be appropriate to conclude with these matched samples that a significant effect was produced (caused) by the treatment applied? No, it still would not be appropriate because the treatment conditions are still confounded with the strain of mice used. Similarly, in retrospective and prospective studies treatment conditions *are always* confounded with subject-related variables because these studies use classification variables (4.1, 4.2).

Prospective and retrospective designs along with the cross-sectional design and the experimental (randomized) clinical trial are the four main study designs used in medical research (see Hulley and Cummings, 1988). Unfortunately, applied clinical research is hazardous and Sackett (1979) has identified 56 sources of potential bias in medical research. Vaisrub (1985) lists about 20 insolvable biomedical design problems. In a shorter list, Morgan (1986) presents the seven deadly scientific sins of clinical studies which are (1) insufficient information on the patient population which would be necessary for replication (2.3), (2) sample size is too small (5.13, 5.15), (3) biased sample (4.11, 4.12), (4) confounding factors (4.15, 4.19, 4.23), (5) vague classifications (e.g., improved, no change) which indicate problems of measurement (5.3), (6) not evaluating the original hypothesis (1.2), and (7) number problems which include numerical errors, failures of subgroup totals to add up to the grand total, missing values in long-term measurements (6.19), and so forth. Michael, Boyce, and Wilcox (1984) in their book *Biomedical Bestiary: An Epidemiologic Guide to Flaws and Fallacies in the Medical Literature* illustrate many problems which reside in medical research reports. Other discussions of confounding bias may be found in books and articles that focus on medical statistics (see Armitage and Berry, 1987; Bailar and Mosteller, 1986; Bland, 1987; Bourke, Daly, and McGilvray, 1985; Gehlbach, 1988; Murphy, 1985; Schlesselman, 1982).

Epidemiological studies of infectious disease have achieved some outstanding health accomplishments (see Feinstein, 1988). Many other epidemiological studies, however, have been the subject of major uncertainties and controversies (Feinstein, 1988; Mayer, Horwitz, and Feinstein, 1988). These latter studies have attempted to establish cause-and-effect relationships between substances used in daily life (such as coffee, alcohol, and chronic pharmaceutical treatments) and cancer or other major diseases. The difficulty is that statistical rather than experimental control must be used to "equate" treatment groups in these studies (see 6.19). Hence, many epidemiological studies, particularly those dealing with "menace" substances in daily life, are flawed and their conclusions based upon scientifically inadequate data (Feinstein, 1988).

Randomized controlled clinical trials in humans are accepted as the "gold standard" for establishing cause-and-effect relations but these trials normally are used only to evaluate short-term effects of pharmaceutical or surgical treatments. Randomized clinical trials are not normally feasible or ethical for evaluating either the long-term effects of medical intervention or of "menace" substances found in daily life. The experimental (randomized) clinical trial requires

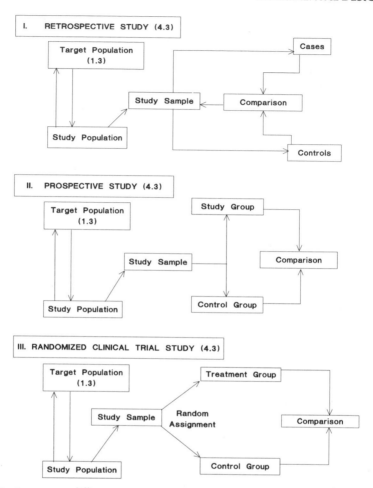

Figure 4.1 Important differences among retrospective, prospective, and random-ized clinical trial studies. Only in the randomized clinical trial are subjects ran-domly assigned to the different treatment conditions.

specialized methodology and control to obtain appropriate inferences and a bio-statistician should be included in the research team (Miké and Stanley, 1982). The differences among a retrospective study, a prospective study, and a random-ized clinical trial study are summarized in Figure 4.1. Elwood (1988) presents a critical appraisal of potential cause-effect relations in the four main study designs used in medical research (also see Riegelman and Hirsch, 1989).

4.4 AN EXPERIMENT: INDEPENDENT AND DEPENDENT VARIABLES

In an experiment, the independent variable is the variable the scientist manip-ulates (the treatment) to determine its effect on a particular biological response (the dependent variable). More than one independent variable (treatments, conditions) may be manipulated and the biologist may want to study their individual effects only or both their individual and joint effects on the dependent variable (see Marks, 1982a,b).

In many studies in biology, the effects of the treatment conditions are commonly determined on more than one dependent variable. Each dependent variable may be viewed as a separate experiment. When many different dependent measurements are made, this presents a problem for statistical interpretation (5.19, 10.1). Renal physiologists, for example, are notorious for recording many basic measurements and for calculating derived measures (e.g., ratios) from some of these basic measurements (5.25). If statistical comparisons were made between two groups (treatment and control) on 20 separate dependent variables, then at least one significant difference would be expected to occur by chance (assuming that a significance level of $p < .05$ is used, 5.9).

Many measurements are usually recorded to monitor the general well-being of the animal during the experiment. For some of these dependent measurements significant differences between the groups are not expected. Hence, the experimenter may decide to focus on those dependent measures in which a difference is predicted or expected given the specific treatment condition (6.10). However, interpretation problems may occur if the treatment condition also produces a significant effect on a dependent variable used to monitor the general physical health of the animal. A significant change in a general health measurement may produce a significant change in kidney function data (5.25). For example, a difference in blood pressure may produce a significant change in kidney clearance rate supposedly caused by a certain treatment. Rather than rely on a creative discussion (2.5) to salvage this or a similar pattern of results (which may only be caused by chance) a more reasonable alternative is to replicate the experiment (7.3, 7.4) to determine whether both blood pressure and kidney clearance rate are affected reliably by the treatment condition (6.10).

On the other hand, nonsignificant differences between treatment and control groups on general health measurements must be interpreted with caution because the power of the statistical test (5.12) has to be considered. Given the small sample size common in biological experiments in which many dependent measurements are recorded, the power of the statistical test probably is not very high (5.13). Also, although the treatment may not produce significant differences between the experimental and control groups on many of the dependent variables measuring physical well-being, a synergistic effect of some of these nonsignificant variables may be responsible for significant treatment effects on the important dependent variables (A.9, A.10). Finally, a difference in a response outcome, even if significant, does not mean that the sensitivity (accuracy) is the same for all the response outcomes in the experiment (A.7). Different biological responses will have different experimental errors (variability in measurement or in subjects). This is important to remember because to conserve animal resources, many different measurements typically are taken from preparations requiring time-consuming instrumentation procedures.

4.5 EXPERIMENTAL DESIGN AND EXPERIMENTAL PROTOCOL

For any given research question, the experimental design should be a well-conceived plan for data collection, analysis, and interpretation which will permit, if the research question has been translated into appropriate treatment conditions (1.1, 1.2), a tentative answer to the proposed research question. A well-conceived plan assures that the treatment condition is not confounded with nuisance variables (either subject-, environment-, or time-related) so that the only difference between the treatment group and the control group is the variable (treatment) manipulated (4.15, 4.19, 4.23). Hence, the experimental plan (design) should be regarded as the "blueprint" for the construction of the experiment. In a between-subject design using two groups of animals, the blueprint indicates that the only difference between the two groups of randomly assigned subjects is the treatment condition (1.5).

In contrast, the *experimental protocol* is the detailed description of all events that an animal experiences during the experiment. In a sense, the experimental protocol describes each nail driven, each board cut, and so forth during the experiment. Note that the experimental design describes what should be the only difference (treatment) between the two groups; whereas, the experimental protocol describes in detail all the conditions experienced by the animals in the two groups.

When asked to describe their experimental design many biologists respond by giving their detailed experimental protocol. In contrast, the statement ". . . the effects of anoxia on brainstem dopamine levels in young dogs was studied using a two-group between-subject design" immediately informs the reviewer that the only difference between the two separate groups of young dogs should be the anoxia treatment. With this knowledge, the reviewer can read the experimental protocol for a detailed description of the experiences all the young dogs shared, the random assignment procedure, and the treatment condition. Hence, once the experimental design is known, the reviewer can determine quickly from the experimental protocol whether all animals were treated identically except for the treatment variable.

In many biological studies, the experimental protocol is changed slightly for various "control groups" of animals. Thus, data may be available from eight experimental animals and eight control animals, but four of the control animals (control A) were treated differently from the other four control animals (control B). In this situation, comparisons between the eight experimental animals and the four animals of control A and the eight experimental animals and the four animals of control B could be made. However, the power of the statistical test would probably not be very great given the small sample size for each of the control groups (5.12). In some cases, all control animals may be incorporated into an overall control group (A + B). For this combined control group, because all control animals were not treated alike, an increase in within subject variance would be expected (1.7, 5.16). This increase in experimental noise (error) would make it more difficult to detect any significant treatment difference between the experimental and control animals. Good statistical reasons also exist for maintaining a balanced design (5.23).

4.6 RANDOM SAMPLING: STATISTICAL GENERALIZATION

Very few animal experiments use a random sample of the population of interest (target population, 1.3); consequently, reliance only on statistical generalization would limit the conclusion of the experiment to a very restricted population (the study population). Most of us obtain our experimental animals (samples) either directly from commercial suppliers (who will provide different species and strains of animals at a requested weight, age, and sex) or from our university's animal care division in which small animals may be bred and larger mammals (dogs, cats) obtained from licensed suppliers. Statistical generalization requires that the sample is drawn randomly from the total population of interest. However, typical animal procurement procedures do not provide random samples. Fortunately, obtaining a truely random sample of the target population is not critical in most biological experiments (1.3, 4.27, 6.21).

In many biomedical studies, restrictions on random sampling of patient populations do produce interpretation problems. In market research, survey research and political polling, the population of interest can be defined, located, and an appropriate random sample taken. In clinical research, however, the sample generally must be drawn from patients and volunteers at medical centers who are willing to participate in the study. This sampling restriction makes inferences from the clinical study to the population of interest (all people with the disorder) prone to error (4.3). Relatively few patients are admitted to medical research centers, and these patients are not representative of the population as a whole or even the population of people with a specific disorder. Conclusions of a biomedical study, therefore, cannot be generalized indiscriminately because patients treated at academic medical centers do not represent the true spectrum of illness in the community. Referrals to academic medical centers normally imply that these patients require very specialized care.

Medical center patients are a very selected population of hospitalized patients; they are either physician-selected (referred) or self-selected patients. Hence, even though these patients may be assigned randomly to a treatment and a control group (random clinical trial), the characteristics of the patient study population (1.3) may restrict the statistical generalization of the results of the clinical study. Indeed, correlational analysis among various diseases and symptoms may reflect the characteristics of the patients that are hospitalized in academic medical centers, rather than a true association among the diseases. This phenomenon is so common it is given a special name: *Berkson's fallacy* (Walter, 1980).

4.7 RANDOM ASSIGNMENT OF ANIMALS TO TREATMENTS

To reach a meaningful conclusion regarding the efficacy of a particular treatment, data from animals that receive the treatment must be compared with data from animals in a control group that are identical to the treatment group in all respects except for the treatment received (4.4, 4.5). Yet animals vary on many biological characteristics, which makes it impossible to select groups that are identical in all respects. To have the animals assigned to an experiment as alike as possible the researcher will usually restrict the kind of animals selected. Thus, adult female rats of a particular strain, 90 days old, and weighing between 160 and 180 grams may be selected for a particular experiment. This animal restriction would normally reduce subject variability, a reduction that has important implications for subsequent statistical analysis (5.16). But even with these precautions, significant variability still will remain among the female rats selected for the experiment.

Because animals cannot be matched on all potential biological differences, subject-related variability must be controlled by ensuring that the normal biological differences among animals are not allowed to vary systematically with the manipulated treatment conditions. The only way to achieve this aim is to randomly assign animals to the various treatment conditions. The random assignment procedure chosen must ensure that each animal has an equal chance to be assigned to each of the treatment conditions. Any animal whose biological characteristics could enhance the treatment effect on the biological response being studied must have an equal chance of being assigned to the experimental or control condition. Notice that random assignment of animals to the various treatment groups *does not ensure* that the animals in the two groups will be identical. With very large samples, random assignment procedures will result in no significant initial differences between the animals in the groups. But with relatively small sample sizes, more animals with biological characteristics that enhance (or depress) the treatment condition may, by chance, be assigned to the treatment condition (4.8). For this reason, significance tables of all statistical tests show that the smaller the sample size, the larger the difference between the treatment means must be to assert significance (5.9).

4.8 MATCHING OF ANIMALS: RANDOMIZATION OF BLOCKS

With relatively large sample sizes (30 or more subjects in each group) individual animals may be assigned randomly to the treatment and control groups (4.7) and initial differences between the groups will be extremely unlikely. With small sample sizes, which are very common in biological research, the random assignment of individual animals to the different treatment groups may produce serious problems. By chance, with the random assignment of a limited number of animals, most of the heaviest animals, or most of those with the lowest heart rates, or most of those with faster kidney clearance rates may end up more frequently in either the experimental or the control group. This initial difference in the two groups of animals indicates treatment conditions will be confounded with subject-related variables. Consequently, the experiment would be flawed before treatment conditions were introduced (but see 6.18).

If an unbiased coin were flipped only 10 times, it is not unlikely that 7 or more heads (or tails) would occur by chance. However, if the same coin were flipped

100 times it is very unlikely that 70 or more heads (or tails) would occur by chance. The same principle applies to small and large sample sizes in biological research. With small samples the random assignment of animals to treatment conditions is more likely to result in an initial difference in subject-related variables among treatment groups than if large samples are used. Indeed, with a sufficiently large number of animals the randomization of animals in the assignment to conditions will ensure that the treatment conditions are not confounded with subject-related variables.

With small sample sizes it is wise, if possible, to match animals on relevant characteristics. In a two-group experiment in which heart rate was to be the dependent variable, blocks of two matched animals with similar heart rate could be formed, and one of the animals within each block randomly assigned to the treatment condition with the other matched animal placed in the control condition. This matching procedure ensures that the two groups of animals would have similar means and variances for the dependent variable (heart rate) before the application of the treatment conditions. Three or four animals could also constitute a block of matched animals (for three or four treatment conditions), but it is advisable to use the smallest possible block. Indeed, it is often difficult to form well-matched blocks of animals for an experiment with a large number of treatment conditions; therefore, in these cases, the normal randomization of animals to treatments is the best choice (4.7). Detailed information on the blocking of experimental units may be found in Mead (1988).

4.9 INDEPENDENT OBSERVATIONS

In many experiments, the effects of a given treatment on a number of biological responses may be determined (4.4). Each of the biological responses would normally require a separate statistical analysis (but see 6.17). For example, the effects of a beta-receptor blocking drug on heart rate, cardiac output, and blood pressure might be determined in 10 experimental (drug) and 10 control (vehicle) animals. In such a study three separate statistical tests would normally be done— one for heart rate differences, another for differences in cardiac output, and the last for blood pressure differences. For each of these analyses, there would be 20 independent observations (i.e., the number of animals used) and 19 degrees of freedom (5.17). Even though three measures are taken from each animal and they may be related within each animal, they are usually analyzed separately. The reason for separate analysis is simple—heart rate, cardiac output, and blood pressure are expressed in different units (but see 6.17). Hence, this type of experimental design is a simple two group between-subject design (4.10) and *not* a within-subject design (4.16). Only one measure for each of the three different biological responses was taken from each animal; consequently, for each separate analysis there would be 20 independent observations.

But, what if these three biological responses were measured once from each animal before the treatment condition was introduced and measured again 10 minutes after the drug (experimental group) or vehicle (control group) was given? In this case, *a within-subject component (i.e., the same biological response was measured twice in each animal)* would be added to the between-subject component. This data would be analyzed by three separate mixed factorial designs (4.21). But, the number of independent observations for each of these three analyses would still be 20 (the number of animals in the experiment). The total degrees of freedom, however, would be increased to 39 because two measurements of the same biological response would have been taken from each of the 20 animals (5.17, 6.5).

An important point to remember is that *in any experiment the total number of independent observations is equal to the total number of animals (or preparations) used.* In between-subject designs the total number of degrees of freedom (5.17) is one less than the total number of animals used in the experiment. To draw correct inferences from the statistical analysis of between-subject designs appropriate total degrees of freedom must be used to calculate mean squares (6.4), F-ratios (5.18), and significance levels (5.9).

Suppose an experiment was reported with two groups of eight animals each and a t-test (5.18) with 24 degrees of freedom was used to determine if a significant difference existed between the two groups. A between-subject design with 16 independent observations and 24 total degrees of freedom—how could this outcome occur? Unfortunately, this occurrence is very common in biology. In these situations, a few of the animals were good preparations, and more than one measurement was obtained and reported from these "good" animals. But these extra measurements are not independent observations; rather, they are correlated observations from the same animal (9.2, 9.5). Similarly, a neurophysiologist may report data from 29 respiratory neurons in the medulla from six control cats and 18 respiratory neurons from the same location in eight experimental cats. In the result section the neurophysiologist may report that the respiratory neurons in the medulla of experimental cats had significantly higher frequencies of action potentials compared with those of control cats, $t(45) = 7.52, p < .01$. But the correct degrees of freedom in this experiment are 12 (5.17). Obviously, the neurophysiologist regarded each neuron as an independent observation and violated an important assumption of the parametric t-test (5.16).

Although the neurophysiologist may argue that recordings from different neurons from the same animal are independent observations, this argument is not convincing. Many subject-related variables are confounded with any good experimental preparation (general health of the animal, tolerance to the anesthetic used, surgical trauma, modulatory effects of circulating hormones, peptides, or amino acids and so forth). Whatever the reasons may be for obtaining more neuron recordings from some animals than others, animals with multiple measurements contribute more observations to the total sample. Unfortunately, these animals do not provide a representative sample of even the restricted population of laboratory-obtained animals (4.6). More important, the statistical model used to evaluate data from between-subject designs requires that each individual data point represent an independent observation (5.21).

In neurophysiological studies, units (neurons) are often treated as independent observations; consequently, when between-subject designs (4.10) and their statistical analyses are reported, the wise reviewer will identify quickly the number of independent observations (animals) in the experiment. At the other extreme, some neurophysiologists do not use statistical methods to analyze their data even when two or more treatment conditions are used in the study. Rather, these neurophysiologists present representative records from one or two animals in the various groups. In these cases, the wise reviewer may conclude that the records presented are very interesting and then ponder whether other animals treated similarly would show the same outcomes as the representative animals *selected* by the neurophysiologist.

Neurophysiologists are not the only biologists that confuse independent observations and the number of animals in an experiment. Biologists who take cells or tissues from a few animals for use in subsequent experimentation also have potential problems with their statistical analysis and inference. For example, 40 kidney tubules may be harvested from four rats. These 40 kidney tubules may be randomly assigned to a treatment (drug) and a control (vehicle) condition, and the reported statistical analysis based upon a between-subject design with 39 total degrees of freedom. But, 40 independent observations were not obtained in the study—only 4 independent observations (animals) were available.

The renal physiologist by assuming that each tubule (nephron) harvested from the kidney of a single rat may be treated as an independent observation is also using questionable scientific reasoning and violating statistical assumptions. Because of genetic, developmental, dietary, and environmental conditions it is reasonable to expect that the nephrons from one rat would be more similar to each other than to the nephrons removed from another rat (9.2, 9.5). If biological variability and nutritional–environmental experiences produce different initial clearance or absorption rates in different rats, then nephrons taken from the same rat would be correlated, these nephrons would not be independent, and the three or four rats normally used would not provide a representative sample of independent observations.

It would be a tragic waste of animal resources to sample only one or two cells or nephrons from 10 to 12 animals for a single experiment. And, this is a common argument from biologists who use tissue samples from animals. As a solution, renal physiologists could harvest as many tubules from each animal as possible, and then randomly assign tubules within each block to three or more *independent experiments*. Each block of tubules, therefore, represents the material from one animal (9.4). Some of the tubules in each block could be randomly assigned to the treatment conditions within a single experiment, and the rest used in other independent experiments. Also in some experiments, two tubules from each animal could be used in each treatment condition, and then an estimate of the sensitivity of the measurement technique could be obtained. Because each tubule from each animal should produce about the same treatment effect (assuming that tubules are about the same in each animal), differences between the tubules within a given treatment condition will provide an estimate of the variability of the measurement procedures. On the other hand, if two or more tubules are used from the same animal within a given treatment condition, the *averaged value* of the tubules from each animal could be used for subsequent statistical analysis. An averaged value (mean) would provide a more accurate estimate of any treatment effect for each animal (A.7). The adaptation of procedures such as these would provide a more representative sample for each experiment, provide a more accurate measure of any treatment effect within each experiment, permit valid statistical analysis of the data, and conserve valuable animal resources.

4.10 BETWEEN-SUBJECT DESIGNS

In a *between-subject* design, animals are randomly assigned individually or within the restriction of matched blocks to the various treatment conditions (4.8). In the simplest between-subject design (single-factor) there would be a treatment group of animals and a control group of animals (see Table 4.1). Because any differences in biological responses observed among the treatment conditions are based on different groups of randomly assigned subjects this type of design is also known as a *completely randomized design*. In between-subject designs, the number of biological measurements (the number of independent measures) is equal to the number of subjects (4.9). That is, even though many different biological measures may be taken from each animal (e.g., heart rate, stroke volume, blood pressure), each separate analysis of variance (5.18, 6.1) uses only one measurement (e.g., blood pressure) from each animal.

Table 4.1   Two-Group Between-Subject Design and ANOVA Table

Experimental design: A × S[a]	
A_1 Group I (treatment)	A_2 Group II (control)
S_1	S_1
S_2	S_2
S_3	S_3
.	.
.	.
.	.
$\underline{S_N}$	$\underline{S_N}$
$N = 12$	$N = 12$

Total number of animals = 24
Total number of independent observations = 24
Total degrees of freedom = 23

Analysis of variance (ANOVA) table (6.3)[b]		
Source (6.4)[b]	df (6.5)[b]	F-ratio (5.18)[b]
Between-Subject (Group) A	1	(Group, A) / (Error, S/A)
Within-Subject (Error) S/A	$\underline{22}$	
Total	23	

[a]Factor S represents subjects and is not normally presented when describing between-subject designs (6.2).
[b]See this book section.

Usually, equal numbers of animals are randomly assigned to each of the two treatment conditions. With about the same number of animals in each group, between-subject designs are relatively free from restrictive statistical assumptions. Essentially, t- and F-ratios (5.18) from between-subject designs are very robust (5.23) which indicates that assumptions regarding normality of the sampled populations and equality of variances within the treatment populations are not as critical as they may be for other types of designs (4.18, 8.1).

The main disadvantages of between-subject designs are the large number of animals required, particularly if more than two treatment conditions are used (4.13, 4.14), and the relative lack of sensitivity in detecting treatment effects when they exist. This latter disadvantage is concerned specifically with the power of the statistical test used (5.12). The error term for a between-subject design is based on the variability of animals given the same experimental treatment and estimates of animal variability in each of the different groups are combined to form the within-group mean square (5.16). The major source of error variance in biological research is the individual differences among animals; hence, this variability becomes a significant portion of the error variance.

In some cases, two experimental groups and one control group (or vice versa) may be used in a three group between-subject design (see Table 4.2). Note in a two group between-subject design, a significant F-ratio or t-value indicates a significant difference between the means of the two groups (see Table 4.1). But in a three (or more)-group between-subject design (single factor), the F-ratio indi-

Table 4.2 Three-Group Between-Subject Design and ANOVA Table

Experimental design: A $\times$ S[a]		
A_1 Group I (treatment 1)	A_2 Group II (treatment 2)	A_3 Group III (control)
S_1	S_1	S_1
S_2	S_2	S_2
S_3	S_3	S_3
.	.	.
.	.	.
.	.	.
S_N	S_N	S_N
$N = 12$	$N = 12$	$N = 12$

Total number of animals = 36
Total number of independent observations = 36
Total degrees of freedom = 35

Analysis of variance (ANOVA) table (6.3)[b]		
Source (6.4)[b]	df (6.5)[b]	F-ratio (5.18)[b]
Between-Subject (Group) A	2	(Group, A) / (Error, S/A)
Within-Subject (Error) S/A	33	
Total	35	

[a]Factor S represents subjects and is not normally presented when describing between-subject designs (6.2).
[b]See this book section.

Table 4.3 Four-Group Between-Subject Design and
ANOVA Table

Experimental design: A $\times$ S [a]			
Group I (dose 1)	Group II (dose 2)	Group III (dose 3)	Group IV (dose 4)
S_1	S_1	S_1	S_1
S_2	S_2	S_2	S_2
S_3	S_3	S_3	S_3
.	.	.	.
.	.	.	.
.	.	.	.
S_N	S_N	S_N	S_N
$N = 12$	$N = 12$	$N = 12$	$N = 12$

Total number of animals = 48
Total number of independent observations = 48
Total degrees of freedom = 47

Analysis of variance (ANOVA) table (6.3)[b]		
Source (6.4)[b]	df (6.5)[b]	F-ratio (5.18)[b]
Between-Subject (Group) A	3	(Group, A) / (Error, S/A)
Within-Subject (Error) S/A	44	
Total	47	

[a]Factor S represents subjects and is not normally presented when describing between-subject designs (6.2).
[b]See this book section.

cates significant differences *among* the means of the various groups (see Tables 4.2 and 4.3). A multiple comparison procedure (6.8, 10.0), such as the Newman-Keuls test (10.3), is then used to determine significant differences between pairs of groups (i.e., group 1 versus group 2, group 2 versus group 3, group 1 versus group 3). Many biologists continue to make individual t-test comparisons when three or more groups are used in a between-subject design (5.19). Usually, normal t-value probabilities are used for these multiple comparisons. Using this multiple t-test procedure the null hypothesis is more likely to be rejected when it should *not* be rejected, a Type I error (6.8). In three-group between-subject designs in which one control group and two experimental groups are used, you may only be interested in comparisons between the control group and experimental group 1 and the control group and experimental group 2. In these three group situations in which it may not make biological sense to compare experimental group 1 with experimental group 2, Dunnett's test (10.6) may be used to determine statistical significance.

4.11 CONFOUNDING: ANIMAL SELECTION

With between-subject designs the most important consideration is to ensure that animals are randomly assigned to the treatment conditions (4.7, 4.8). Any systematic bias in the assignment of animals to the treatment conditions could result in the treatment conditions becoming confounded with subject-related differences (1.4). Hence, subject bias has to be controlled by random assignment of animals to the treatment conditions (see Table 1.1).

4.12 CONFOUNDING: TREATMENT AND ANIMAL LOSS

Most experiments are planned with an equal number of animals in each treatment condition, which gives equal weight in the statistical analysis to all groups in the experiment. Unequal sample sizes in an experiment are common because of the inadvertent loss of data in some of the experimental conditions. The death or illness of animals produces unequal sample sizes as does occasional technical problems either in the recording of biological responses or in subsequent analyses of fluid, cell, or tissue samples. For any biological experiment it is of critical importance to evaluate the implications of significant losses of animals or samples. The random assignment of animals to treatment conditions controls for subject-related confounding of the treatment conditions (4.11). If the loss of animals is because of experimental procedures then a loss of randomness occurs and the experiment becomes flawed.

In many biological experiments, surgical, instrumentation, and recording procedures all must work properly to collect accurate and valid data (A.7). Hence, as the complexity of obtaining the required measurement increases, preparation failures also tend to occur more frequently. We are all familiar with both the exuberant biologist whose preparation for the day was excellent and the agitated biologist who was unable to collect data from a bad preparation. If good and bad preparations are related to treatment conditions (e.g., more good preparations are associated with the control procedure), randomness is lost and a systematic bias is added to any differences among the conditions, which cannot be separated from any significant treatment effect. If the preparation of animals in the experimental group produces more stress than control preparations, this stress may result in more animal loss in the experimental group. In such an experiment only the strongest and healthiest animals would survive the preparation procedures and an obvious confounding of subject differences and treatment conditions would occur. The more difficult preparation group would contain a larger proportion of the "fittest" animals than would the control group in which all animals survived.

Replacing the bad preparations in the experimental condition with new animals drawn from the same population *will not* solve this treatment-selection problem. The replacement subjects will not "match" the ones that were lost, that is, the more susceptible animals. Of the replacement animals, again only the healthiest may survive the experimental procedure. Even if the biologist's skills improved so that all replacement animals do survive, a disproportional number of the stronger and healthier animals still would be in the experimental group. Unfortunately, many biologists are not aware of this subject-treatment confounding problem, and continue to replace animals in their experimental group until a sufficient number is obtained to match the number in the control group.

Selective loss of subjects is also a serious problem when classification variables (4.2) are used to separate groups (e.g., young and mature or old and mature).

Even though one-half of the animals in each age group may be randomly assigned to control and experimental groups, the selective loss of subjects (or the difficulty in obtaining good preparations for any of the age groups) would produce a confounding of subject-treatment effects. In an experiment with classification variables (self-selection, 4.2) and the selective loss of animals caused by treatments, any conclusions are best considered to be in double jeopardy.

The loss of subjects in an experiment may present serious interpretation problems. Consequently, biologists must first convince themselves, and eventually others, that subject loss did not produce a significant treatment bias.

4.13 FACTORIAL DESIGNS

In a single-factor between-subject design (4.10), the effect of a single independent (manipulated) variable is measured on one or more biological responses. Normally, two groups, an experimental and a control, are used in a single-factor design (see Table 4.1), but three or more groups can be used providing the levels of a single variable are manipulated (see Tables 4.2 and 4.3). For example, the effects of different dosage levels of a given drug (0, 1 mg/kg, 2 mg/kg, and 4 mg/kg) could be studied using a single-factor between-subject design with different groups of animals. The four groups would be classified as four levels of factor A (A_1, A_2, A_3, and A_4). Essentially, *in a single-factor study all variables except the manipulated variable are maintained at the same level in all the different treatment groups.*

In contrast, *in a factorial experimental design the effects of one independent variable in conjunction with one or more other independent variables are studied.* In a factorial design every level of every variable (factor) is paired with every level of every other variable (factor). Hence, in a factorial design the effects of one of the studied variables may augment, cancel out, or function independently of the effects of another variable. Factorial designs may be used to study the effects of an unlimited number of variables and their interactions, but in practice the most common factorial design in biological research focuses on only two variables (a two-way factorial design). These variables could be levels of two manipulated independent variables (e.g., factor A being exercised or normal and factor B being drug doses), but in many cases one of the variables is a classification (4.2) variable (male and female; young and old) and the other is levels of a manipulated variable (drug doses).

Suppose a biologist expected that a new beta-blocking drug would produce different effects on heart rate depending on the sex of the animal. Also, the biologist may postulate that a sex difference on heart rate would occur at some drug doses but not at others. In other words, an *interaction* between sex and drug dose was expected (6.12). To test this expectation, a factorial design could be used to study the effects of four doses of the beta-blocking drug (factor B) on heart rates of male and female dogs (factor A). In this two-way factorial study a total of 4 × 2, or 8 different, treatment groups would be required. Thus, in a factorial design the number of treatment combinations is equal to the product of the number of categories or levels of each variable. The usual procedure in describing a factorial design is to label the factor with the fewest levels as factor A, the factor with the next fewest levels as factor B and so forth. In some cases, however, the logic of the particular design makes it appropriate to change this classification order. Note the 2 (sex) × 4 (drug doses) factorial design could be treated as two separate independent experiments. The biologist could first study the effects of the four drug doses on heart rate in females (a single-factor between-subject design, 4.10) and then do an identical study with males (another single-factor between-subject design). With 12 animals in each group a total of 96 animals would be used in these two single-factor studies. With only female dogs the first experiment would include the groups and analysis given in Table 4.3, and the F-ratio would indicate whether significant differences among the four treatment groups of female dogs existed. If the F-ratio was significant, a multiple comparison test (6.8, Chapter 10) would then be used to determine significant differences among all the possible between-group comparisons.

In the second experiment, the same treatment conditions, procedures, and statistical analysis would be used to evaluate the effects of the four dosage levels on heart rate in male dogs. But, in these two separate experiments what if both F-ratios were statistically significant (5.9, 5.16)? What could the biologist conclude given this outcome regarding sex differences in drug responses? Indeed, what could the biologist conclude if a significant F-ratio was found for females but not for the males as the pattern of group means in Figure 4.2 might produce?

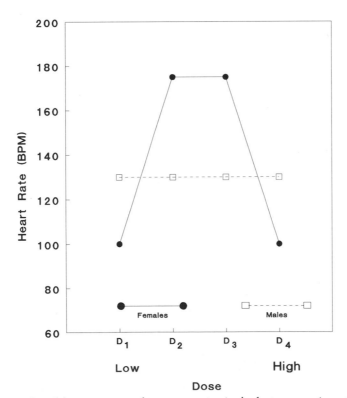

Figure 4.2 Possible outcomes of two separate single-factor experiments (Figure 1.2) studying the effects of the same drug doses on the heart rates of male dogs (Experiment 1) and female dogs (Experiment 2).

What comparisons would the biologist need to make to determine whether the group means among the male and female dogs differed significantly?

A factorial experiment provides a solution to this interpretation problem. What the biologist wants to know is whether a significant interaction occurs between sex and drug dosage level and this information is not given by two separate single-factor between-subject designs. To answer the proposed question the two single-factor between-subject designs must be combined into a factorial design with two factors. Factor A would have two levels, male (A_1) and female (A_2), and factor B would have four levels (drug doses B_1, B_2, B_3, and B_4). This type of arrangement is referred to as a 2×4 factorial design (Table 4.4). Notice that this 2×4 factorial design provides more information than the two single-factor between-subject designs, namely whether a significant interaction exists between the two factors (sex and drug doses). For example, in this factorial design, the overall effect of one variable (e.g., sex) is averaged over all levels of the other variable (drug doses) and this *main effect* (sex) compares for differences between the mean heart rate from all males and the mean heart rate from all females. Likewise, the overall effects of drug doses are averaged over the two sexes, and the second *main effect* (drug) compares heart rate differences among

Table 4.4 A 2 (Sex) × 4 (Dose) Factorial Design and ANOVA Table

Experimental design: A × B × S[a]							
Level of factor A (sex)							
A_1 (male)				A_2 (female)			
B_1	B_2	B_3	B_4	B_1	B_2	B_3	B_4
(1)	(2)	(3)	(4)	(1)	(2)	(3)	(4)
S_1	S_1	S_1	S_1	S_1	S_1	S_1	S_1
S_2	S_2	S_2	S_2	S_2	S_2	S_2	S_2
S_3	S_3	S_3	S_3	S_3	S_3	S_3	S_3
.	.	.	.	.	.	.	.
.	.	.	.	.	.	.	.
.	.	.	.	.	.	.	.
S_N	S_N	S_N	S_N	S_N	S_N	S_N	S_N

(Levels of factor B (dose) labels the rows)

$N = 12$
Total number of animals = 96
Total number of independent observations = 96
Total degrees of freedom = 95

Analysis of variance (ANOVA) table (6.3)[b]		
Source (6.4)[b]	df (6.5)[b]	F-ratio (5.18)[b]
A (Sex)	1	A / S/AB (Error)
B (Dose Level)	3	B / S/AB (Error)
A (Sex) × B (Dose Level)	3	A × B / S/AB (Error)
S/AB (Error)	88	
Total	95	

[a]Factor S represents subjects and is not normally presented when describing between-subject designs (6.2).
[b]See this book section.

the four means of the drug doses. Hence, by averaging across one factor, the main effects convert part of the factorial design into a single-factor between-subject design (6.13, Table 6.13). But, the factorial design also determines whether a significant interaction exists between the two independent variables, that is, between sex and drug doses (Tables 4.4, 6.14 and 6.15). When a significant two-way (A × B) interaction is present (6.13), the averaged main effects are not that important because the effects of one independent variable (sex) must be qualified by a consideration of the levels of the other independent variable (dosage level).

If the biologist had done two separate experiments, using female dogs first and then males, the data collected could be analyzed using a factorial design. However, a major interpretative problem would be the possible confounding of the sex condition with variables that may change systematically with time (4.19). These time-related changes could be in injection procedures, daily preparation of the drug, drug efficacy, environmental temperature, and so forth. Hence, even though an appropriate statistical test could analyze data collected sequentially from two groups, statistical inferences may be biased because of the potential time-confounding problem (4.19). A diagram of the A (sex) × B (dose) factorial design is presented in Figure 4.3.

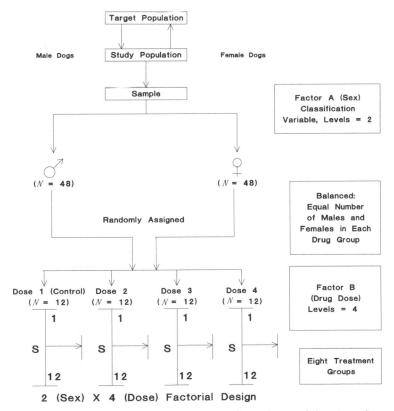

Figure 4.3 A diagram of an A × B between-subject factorial design with two levels of factor A (male and female dogs) and four levels of factor B (different doses). Eight independent groups are required for this 2 × 4 between-subject factorial design (4.13, Figure 1.5, Table 4.4).

4.14 FACTORIAL DESIGNS: ADVANTAGES AND DISADVANTAGES

The major advantages of using a factorial design are economy, experimental control, and generality of results. Because the main effects in a factorial design are averaged estimates (4.13) fewer subjects are necessary in each group than if two single-factor experiments were done. For example, with only six animals in each group of the 2 (sex) by 4 (dosage level) factorial design discussed previously (4.13), the averaged main effects would be based upon the same number of animals (s = 12) as may be used in a single-factor experiment (Table 4.3). Hence, the factorial experiment can produce these estimates much more economically by using only half the number of animals required in two separate single-factor experiments.

Another common use of factorial designs is to control within-subject variability by using categories of animals as a factor (see Table 4.4). An undesirable alternative to the factorial design represented in Table 4.4 would be to randomly assign an equal number of male and female dogs to the four dose levels (4.13) and evaluate group differences in a single-factor between-subject design. In this case, the error term (within-subject variability) would include the variability due to animals of the same sex, to measurement error, to sex difference, and to any interaction between sex and dose level (6.12). Essentially, the variability of animals treated alike (within-subject variability) will be smaller with a restricted group of animals (only males, only young males, or only old males) than with unrestricted groups of animals (males and females or young, mature, and old animals). But, one problem with restricting the age or sex of the animals used is that the results of the experiment will be limited in generality. If only young female rats are used, the results of the experiment could only be generalized to the population of young female rats (4.6).

Using a factorial design and separating female animals into young, adult, and old animals would reduce within-subject variability (more than if animals of the total age range were randomized across treatment conditions) and also permit a reasonable generalization of the data. Generalization of data is increased because the inferences may be extended to all those levels used in the factorial design and to any interactive effects among the factors studied. In a sense, a more realistic effect of the treatment conditions is obtained with a factorial design because changes in endogenous or exogenous factors do not normally produce their effects in isolation (i.e., all other biological processes being constant, A.10).

The disadvantages of factorial designs are their relative insensitivity to treatment effects (common to all between-subject designs, 4.10) and the likelihood of too much complexity. Complexity occurs both in the number of independent groups that may be used and the difficulty in interpreting higher-order interactions (6.14, 6.15). As indicated, a 2×4 factorial design requires 8 different treatment groups, a 3×4 factorial design would require 12 groups, and a 4×4 factorial design would require 16 groups.

With three or more factors, the number of groups also increases dramatically. For a $4 \times 4 \times 4$ factorial design a total of 64 groups would be required. With a limited sample population, as is common in most biological research, three-factor between-subject experiments are not usually feasible. For example, with a rather large sample population of 54 animals and a $2 \times 3 \times 3$ factorial design only 3 animals could be assigned to the required 18 different treatment conditions. In this situation, the accuracy of the means of each of the unique treatment combinations (based upon only three values) would not be very high (A.7). In addition, the interpretation of significant two-way and higher-order interactions must be considered (6.12, 6.15).

4.15 CONFOUNDING IN FACTORIAL DESIGNS

Potential confoundings in factorial designs are the same as in single-factor between-subject designs; hence, potential confounds are any systematic bias in the assignment of animals to the various treatment conditions (4.11) and any subject-treatment bias caused by the selective loss of animals in any given treatment condition (4.12). Environment– or time-related confoundings are possible in between-subject designs (1.2, 4.19) but these confounds are usually easy to identify and avoid.

4.16 WITHIN-SUBJECT DESIGNS

In between-subject designs, animals are assigned randomly to the different conditions in the experiment and are given only one of the treatments (4.10). Therefore, these designs are also called completely randomized designs. In between-subject or completely randomized designs, all the sources of variability extracted in the analysis of variance (ANOVA) *represent differences between subjects* (Tables 4.1, 4.2, 4.3, and 4.4).

In a single-factor *within-subject design* every animal receives all the treatment conditions (crossover design). Given this type of design, some of the sources of variance isolated in the statistical analysis will reflect differences within each subject; consequently, these designs are called within-subject designs. These designs are also referred to as repeated measures designs emphasizing that *repeated measurements of the same biological response are taken from each animal* and *treatment effects are associated with differences observed within subjects*.

For comparison, a single-factor between-subject design and a single-factor within-subject design are presented in Table 4.5. In the ANOVA of a single-factor between-subject design, the group source is used to estimate the effects of the different treatment conditions (along with experimental error), and the within-subject error (S/A) is used to estimate the degree to which experimental error is responsible for the differences observed among the treatment means (Table 4.5). This (S/A) error term, however, overestimates experimental error in a within-subject design (6.6). Chance differences between the treatment conditions produced by the random assignment of animals to treatment conditions (in a between-subject design) are absent in a within-subject design because the same animals are used in all treatment conditions. To obtain an appropriate error term in a single-factor within-subject design, the extent to which animals are

Table 4.5 Between-Subject and Within-Subject Single-Factor Designs

Between-subject design: A × S[a]			Within-subject design (A × S)		
A_1	A_2	A_3	A_1	A_2	A_3
Treatment 1	Treatment 2	Treatment 3	Treatment 1	Treatment 2	Treatment 3
S_1	S_1	S_1	S_1		
S_2	S_2	S_2	S_2		
S_3	S_3	S_3	S_3		
.	.	.	.		
.	.	.	.		
.	.	.	.		
S_N	S_N	S_N	S_N		
$N = 12$	$N = 12$	$N = 12$	$N = 12$		
Total number of animals = 36			Total number of animals = 12		
Total number of independent observations = 36			Total number of independent observations = 12		
Total degrees of freedom = 35			Total degrees of freedom = 35		

ANOVA (6.3)[b]			ANOVA (6.3)[b]		
Source (6.4)	df (6.5)	F-ratio (5.18)	Source (6.4)	df (6.5)	F-ratio (5.18)
Between Subject Group (A)	2	A / S/A	Treatment (A)	2	A / A × S
S/A (Error)	33		Subject (S)	11	
Total	35		A × S (Error)	22	
			Total	35	

[a]Factor S represents subjects and is not normally presented when describing between-subject designs (6.2).
[b]See this book section.

consistent across the treatment conditions *is subtracted* from the total estimate of experimental error. Consequently, the resulting error term (A × S in Table 4.5) estimates the degree to which chance factors are responsible for the observed differences among the treatment conditions in a single-factor within-subject design (6.6).

4.17 WITHIN-SUBJECT DESIGNS: ADVANTAGES

Because physiological measurements often require extensive preparation of animals, repeated measures (within-subject) designs are very common in biological research (9.2, 9.3, 9.4, 9.5). Unfortunately, many biologists confuse within- and between- subject designs (4.10) and do inappropriate statistical analyses of their within-subject data (4.16). Within-subject designs are usually more efficient and sensitive when compared with equivalent between-subject designs. The reason is that within-subject designs reduce the amount of error variance (experimental error) in experiments (4.16). Any reduction in error variance will result in an increase in the magnitude of the F-ratio (5.16) which increases the likelihood of rejecting the null hypothesis (1.6, 5.5).

The primary source of error variance in most experiments is the biological variability among animals; consequently, using the same animal in all the treatment conditions will reduce error variance. This reduction in error variance represents a direct increase in economy and power (5.13). This advantage is very significant for biological research in which small sample sizes are used because of the difficulty in preparing animals for physiological recordings.

4.18 WITHIN-SUBJECT DESIGNS: DISADVANTAGES

The major experimental problem with within-subject designs is the possible influences of residual biological effects from previous treatments combining with a subsequent treatment condition. In some experiments, these *general carry-over* effects may be reduced by allowing sufficient time to pass between successive treatments. In many biological experiments, the animal's responses are required to return to control (baseline) levels before another treatment condition is given. Even with this precaution, latent effects may occur when the effects of a previous treatment appear to have disappeared (a return to control levels) but are activated when a subsequent treatment is given. Fatigue of a response system or deterioration of the preparation or habituation (learning) are always potential problems in biological research using a repeated-measures design. The counterbalancing of treatment conditions (4.20) is a common method to control for some of these general carry-over effects.

A second problem with within-subject designs is the possibility of *differential carry-over* effects which counterbalancing will not control. Differential carry-over effects are quite specific as the earlier administration of one treatment (A) may affect a subsequent treatment (B), but giving treatment B first may not affect the following treatment (A). Certain drugs or surgical procedures, for example, if given first will affect the biological responses of the animal so that baseline levels (control) are markedly affected.

The third problem with within-subject designs is statistical. The statistical model justifying the analysis of a repeated-measures design is very restrictive; that is, the individual measurements are supposed to have certain mathematical properties (5.21). Thus, within-subject analysis of variance tests may not be very robust (5.23), and violations of the underlying mathematical assumptions regarding distribution and variance characteristics may cause significant problems in subsequent statistical inference (9.6).

4.19 CONFOUNDING IN WITHIN-SUBJECT DESIGNS: TIME AND CARRY-OVER EFFECTS

The two major sources of confounding in within-subject designs are variables associated with the passage of time and differential carry-over effects of one treatment to another (4.18). Fatigue of a specific biological response system or general deterioration of the preparation may be controlled by ensuring the equal occurrence of each treatment condition at each time period during the experi-

Table 4.6 Counterbalancing of Treatment Conditions
(Within-Subject Design)

Block 1	S_1	(TO_1)	Treatment 1, Treatment 2, Treatment 3
	S_2	(TO_2)	Treatment 2, Treatment 3, Treatment 1
	S_3	(TO_3)	Treatment 3, Treatment 1, Treatment 2
Block 2	S_4	(TO_2)	. . .
	S_5	(TO_3)	. . .
	S_6	(TO_1)	. . .
Block N	S_{N-2}	(TO_3)	Treatment 3, Treatment 1, Treatment 2
	S_{N-1}	(TO_1)	Treatment 1, Treatment 2, Treatment 3
	S_N	(TO_2)	Treatment 2, Treatment 3, Treatment 1

Animals in each matched block should be randomly assigned to the three treatment orders. S = subject, TO = treatment order

ment. For example, with three treatment conditions a different testing order would be used for the first three animals as shown in Table 4.6. Although this cyclic Latin square design does not vary the order of conditions (i.e., treatment 3 always follows treatment 2), more desirable arrangements (e.g., diagram balanced in which each condition precedes and follows all other conditions once) are impossible to construct with small samples and, therefore, have limited applicability in biological research.

A counterbalancing procedure, however, will not protect against substantial response fatigue or deterioration of a preparation. Both of these events would increase significantly experimental error and make a Type II error more probable (5.10). In these situations, the experimental protocols (4.5) must be changed to eliminate these time-dependent problems. An examination of individual data (e.g., comparing treatment 1 effects in the first position with its effects in the last position) may identify any general time-dependent carry-over problems across animals. Similarly, differential carry-over effects may be identified by an examination of individual measurements. With large sample sizes, statistical procedures are available to determine whether significant carry-over effects occurred in an experiment. But with the small sample size typically used in biological research, the power of these tests would normally be so low as to be meaningless (5.12). Consequently, researchers must examine their individual measures and judge whether significant time-dependent confounding appears likely. If time-dependent confounding is likely, experimental protocols should be modified.

4.20 RANDOMIZATION OR COUNTERBALANCING OF TREATMENT CONDITIONS

With the small samples used in biological research, the counterbalancing of treatment conditions is a better alternative than randomization of treatment conditions (4.19). By chance, with small samples a given treatment may be assigned randomly more often to the first (or last) treatment order than the other treatments (4.7, 4.8).

4.21 MIXED FACTORIAL DESIGNS

The mixed factorial design represents a combination of between- subject (4.10) and within-subject (4.16) designs. In a mixed two factorial experiment (A, B) independent groups are the levels of one factor (factor A), and repeated measures are the levels of the other factor (factor B). For example, male dogs could be assigned randomly to an exercised (experimental) or an unexercised (control) group, and this between-subject condition would be factor A. The exercise regimen could be 1 hour on an inclined treadmill for five days a week. Once a week, both the exercised and control dogs could be given an exercise stress test (on one of the rest days for the trained animals) and various biological response measurements taken (multiple dependent measures). These training and test procedures could be continued for eight weeks and the repeated measures condition (stress test) would be factor B. A representation of this type of mixed factorial design is presented in Table 4.7. This mixed factorial design would be referred to as a 2 (group) $\times$ 8 (stress test) factorial design with repeated measures on the last factor. A shorthand description of this mixed factorial design would be an A $\times$ (B $\times$ S) or a 2 $\times$ (8 $\times$ 8) which indicates that factor A is the between-subject

Table 4.7 Mixed Factorial Design: A $\times$ (B $\times$ S)

Levels of factor A	(B_1) Test 1	(B_2) Test 2	(B_3) Test 3	(B_4) Test 4	(B_5) Test 5	(B_6) Test 6	(B_7) Test 7	(B_8) Test 8
			Levels of factor B Stress test performance					

A_1
Exercised ($N = 8$)

S_1 ⟶ S_1
S_2 ⟶ S_2
.
.
.
S_N ⟶ S_N

A_2
Not exercised ($N = 8$)

S_1 ⟶ S_1
S_2 ⟶ S_2
.
.
.
S_N ⟶ S_N

Total number of animals = 16
Total number of independent observations = 16
Total degrees of freedom = 127

component (in this case two independent groups) and factor B is the within-subject component by its association in parentheses with subjects (B × S), in this case 8 correlated measures of the same response from each of the 8 dogs. A diagram of this A × (B × S) mixed factorial design is presented in Figure 4.4.

The design represented in Table 4.7 would be rather easy to analyze and interpret because only a two-way interaction is possible (Tables 4.8 and 6.13). But, suppose that during each stress testing session three measures of a single biological response (e.g., heart rate) were taken from each animal, the first before the stress period (baseline), the second during the stress period (active), and the third after the stress period (recovery). Because the same three measurements were taken from each animal in the two groups, differences in baseline, stress, and recovery heart rates between the two groups of animals across the eight stress test sessions could be determined. Long-term exercise might be expected to change

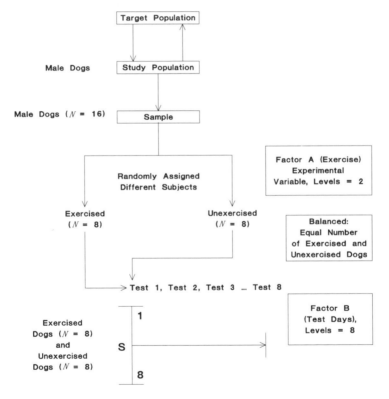

2 (Exercise) X (8, Test Day X 8, Subject)
Mixed Factorial Design

Figure 4.4   A diagram of an A × (B × S) mixed factorial design (4.10, 4.13, 4.16, 4.21, Figure 1.7). In this 2 × (8 × 8) mixed factorial design, two independent groups of dogs (factor A, exercised and unexercised) are tested for eight days (factor B, test day). Eight repeated (correlated) measurements are taken from each of the eight dogs (× S) in the two groups (9.2, Table 4.7).

Table 4.8 Analysis of Variance (ANOVA) Table (6.3) for
A × (B × S) Design (Table 4.7)

Source (6.4)[a]	df (6.5)[a]	F-ratio (5.18)[a]
A (Group)	1	A (Group) / S/A (Error)
S/A (Error)	14	
B (Weeks)	7	B (Weeks) / B × S/A (Error)
A × B (Group × Weeks)	7	A × B / B × S/A (Error)
B × S/A (Error)	98	
Total	127	

[a]See this book section.

baseline and recovery heart rates. A representation of this mixed factorial design is presented in Table 4.9 and its ANOVA table given in Table 4.10. Note that this factorial design would be referred to as a 2 (group) × 8 (stress test) × 3 (measurements) factorial design *with repeated measures on the last two factors.* The shorthand description of this mixed factorial design would be an A × (B × C × S) or a 2 × (8 × 3 × 8). A diagram of this mixed factorial design is presented in Figure 4.5.

A comparison of the ANOVA tables for the two mixed factorial designs (see Tables 4.8 and 4.10) indicates clearly that as more within-subject factors are

Table 4.9 Mixed Factorial Design: A × (B × C × S)

			Levels of factor B: Stress test performance				
(B₁)	(B₂)	(B₃)	(B₄)	(B₅)	(B₆)	(B₇)	(B₈)
Test 1	Test 2	Test 3	Test 4	Test 5	Test 6	Test 7	Test 8
			Levels of factor C				
C₁C₂C₃	C₁C₂C₃	C₁C₂C₃	C₁C₂C₃	C₁C₂C₃	C₁C₂C₃	C₁C₂C₃	C₁C₂C₃
BAR[a]	BAR	BAR	BAR	BAR	BAR	BAR	BAR

Levels of factor A
A_1, exercised ($N = 8$)
S_1 ————————————————————→S_1
S_2 ————————————————————→S_2
.
.
.
S_N ————————————————————→S_N

A_2, not exercised ($N = 8$)
S_1 ————————————————————→S_1
S_2 ————————————————————→S_2
.
.
.
S_N ————————————————————→S_N

[a]B = baseline value, A = active value, and R = recovery values; total number of animals = 16; total number of independent observations = 16; total degrees of freedom = 383

Table 4.10 Analysis of Variance (ANOVA) Table for A $\times$ (B $\times$ C $\times$ S) Design (6.3,[a] Table 4.9)

Source (6.4)[a]	df (6.5)[a]	F-ratio (5.18)[a]
A (Group)	1	A / S/A
S/A (Error)	14	
B (Weeks)	7	B / B $\times$ S/A
A $\times$ B (Group $\times$ Weeks)	7	A $\times$ B / B $\times$ S/A
B $\times$ S/A (Error)	98	
C (Measurements)	2	C / C $\times$ S/A
A $\times$ C (Group $\times$ Measurements)	2	A $\times$ C / C $\times$ S/A
C $\times$ S/A (Error)	28	
B $\times$ C (Weeks $\times$ Measurements)	14	B $\times$ C / B $\times$ C $\times$ S/A
A $\times$ B $\times$ C (Group $\times$ Weeks $\times$ Measurements)	14	A $\times$ B $\times$ C / B $\times$ C $\times$ S/A
B $\times$ C $\times$ S/A (Error)	196	
Total	383	

[a]See this book section.

added in any experiment, the statistical analysis and subsequent interpretation become more complex. In the 2 $\times$ (8 $\times$ S) factorial design (Table 4.8) there are one between-subject (group) comparison with a single between-subject error term, one within-subject comparison (weeks) and a two-way interaction (Group $\times$ Weeks). These latter two comparisons both use the same within-subject error term. With the addition of another within-subject factor, 2 $\times$ (8 $\times$ 3 $\times$ S), how-ever, there are one between-subject (group) comparison with a single between-subject error term, two within-subject comparisons, three two-way interactions, one three-way interaction, and three different within-subject error terms (Tables 4.9 and 4.10). Hence, with additional within-subject factors or between-subject factors, the statistical analysis and interpretation become more complex because of both the number and type of interactions that must be considered and the selection of the appropriate error term for each of the comparisons (6.3, 6.4, 6.6, 6.13, 6.14).

4.22 MIXED FACTORIAL DESIGNS: ADVANTAGES AND DISADVANTAGES

Mixed factorial designs, comprising both between-subject (4.10) and within-subject (4.16) components, have an admixture of the advantages and disadvan-tages of these two components (4.14, 4.17, 4.18). The type of mixed factorial design used will determine its particular advantages and disadvantages when compared with equivalent between-subject or within-subject designs. *In general*, however, the advantages and disadvantages of a mixed factorial design will be skewed toward those of the within-subject component (4.17 4.18). Mixed fac-torial designs are commonly used in biological research.

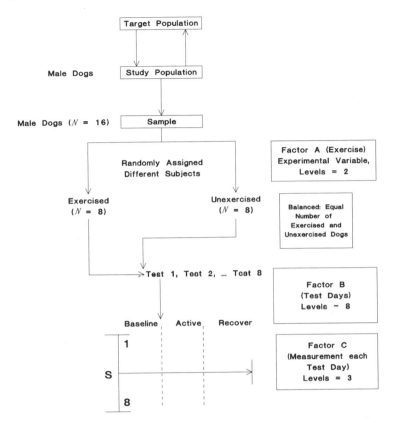

2 (Exercise) X (8, Test Day X 3, Measurement X 8, Subject)
Mixed Factorial Design

Figure 4.5 A diagram of an A × (B × C × S) mixed factorial design (4.10, 4.13, 4.16, 4.21, Figure 1.9). In this 2 × (8 × 3 × 8) mixed factorial design two independent groups of dogs (factor A, exercised and unexercised) are tested for eight days (factor B, test day) and three measurements are taken from each dog (factor C, measurement) on each test day. Twenty-four repeated (correlated) measurements are taken from each of the eight dogs (× S) in the two groups (9.2). These repeated measurements can be separated into two within-subject factors, B and C (Table 4.9).

4.23 CONFOUNDING IN MIXED FACTORIAL DESIGNS

Confounding problems in mixed factorial designs are identical to those considered for between-subject and within-subject designs. Thus, animal selection (4.11) and animal loss produced by treatments (4.12) must be considered (between-subject component) along with any time or carry-over effects (4.19) associated with repeated measurements (within-subject component). Potential environment- or time-related confoundings in the between-subject component must also be considered. Potential confoundings in various experimental

Table 4.11 Potential Confoundings in Between-Subject, Within-Subject, and Mixed Factorial Designs

Between-Subject Design (4.10, 4.13)[a]
A. Selective bias in assignment of subjects (4.11)
B. Selective loss of subjects because of treatment conditions (4.12)
C. Treatment condition associated with another potential independent variable (1.2)

Within-Subject Design (4.16)[a]
A. General carry-over effects across treatments (4.18)
B. Differential carry-over effects from one treatment to another (4.19)
C. Time-related effects (4.19)
D. Treatment condition associated with another potential independent variable (1.2)

Mixed Factorial (4.21)[a]
A. Between-subject component: Animal selection (4.11) and treatment-animal loss (4.12)
B. Within-subject component: Time-related (4.19) and carry-over effects (4.19) associated with repeated measurements
C. Treatment condition associated with another potential independent variable (1.2)

[a]See this book section.

designs are summarized in Table 4.11. Several significant questions whose answers may be used to evaluate an experimental report are listed for experimental design and protocol in Table 4.12 and for statistical analysis and interpretation in Table 4.13. Different notations for between-subject (4.10), within-subject (4.16), and mixed factorial (4.21) are listed in Table 4.14.

Table 4.12 Experimental Design: Structure and Significant Questions

Research question and experimental design	Valid data
1. Translation of research question into specific treatment conditions (1.1)[a]	1. Blind control procedures (4.26)
2. Population-random sample (1.3)	2. Valid measures of biological function (A.7)
3. Selection of design: Between-subject, within-subject, or mixed factorial (1.5)	
4. Assignment of animals to groups (1.4)	
5. Control of potential confounding problems (Table 4.11)	

Assignment: confounding	Assessment: measurement
1. Is there a selection bias? (4.7)	1. Is the biological measurement appropriate for research question? (A.7)
2. Did treatment conditions produce a selective loss of subjects? (4.12)	2. Is the biological measurement precise, unbiased, and valid? (A.7)
3. Are the treatment conditions confounded (environment- or time-related)? (Table 4.11)	3. Is the biological measurement affected by the process of observation? (A.7, 4.26)
4. Are classification variables used in experimental design? (4.2)	4. How many animals are used? How many measurements per animal? How many total observations? (4.9)

[a]See this book section.

Table 4.13 Statistical Analysis, Interpretation, and Generalization for an
Experimental Design (Table 4.12)

Statistical analysis and inference	Generalization

1. Statistical hypotheses (5.5)[a]
   Null (H_0): $\mu_1 = \mu_2$
   Alternative (H_i): $\mu_1 \neq \mu_2$
2. Decision rules, errors of inference,
   power (1.7, 5.10, 5.12)
3. Selection of statistical tests (Chapter 12)
	1. Statistical generalization (1.3)
	2. Scientific generalization (1.8, 6.21)

Analysis and interpretation	Conclusions and discussion

1. Are Type I and Type II errors (power)
   considered? (5.10, 5.12)
2. Are assumptions of statistical test met
   by data (scale of measurement,
   normality, variability)? (5.3)
3. Do data and analysis support the
   interpretation?
	1. Do the data support the conclusions?
	2. Do the conclusions coincide with
	   research hypothesis?
	3. What are the restrictions in data?
	4. Are statistical differences biologically
	   meaningful? (6.21)

[a]See this book section.

4.24 OVERDESIGNING OF EXPERIMENTS

As the number of control groups increases in a single-factor between-subject design (4.10) so does the likelihood of the F-ratio being nonsignificant (5.16). The omnibus (overall) F-ratio determines whether a significant difference exists among the treatment group means. This F-ratio is a conservative test when many means are included because a very large difference between means is required to attain significance and reject the null hypothesis, H_0 (6.8). Essen-

Table 4.14 Notations for Experimental Designs (1.5)[a]

Between-Subject Designs (4.10)[b]
   A $\times$ S single-factor, *one-way analysis of variance, completely randomized design, t-test* (special case of single-factor ANOVA with only two groups, 5.18).

   A $\times$ B $\times$ S—two factors, A $\times$ B $\times$ C $\times$ S—three factors.

   Factorial design (4.13), *two-way analysis of variance with replication, completely randomized factorial design.*

Within-Subject Designs (4.16)
   (A $\times$ S) single-factor, *complete repeated-measures design, change-over design, crossover design, paired t-test* (special case of single-factor within-subject design with only two treatment conditions), *randomized blocks factorial design* (A $\times$ B $\times$ S).

Mixed Factorial Design (4.21)
   Combination of between-subject (4.10) and within-subject (4.16) factors, e.g., A $\times$ (B $\times$ S) is a mixed factorial design with repeated measures on the last factor, *split-plot design.*

[a]See Tables 6.1–6.11 for a listing of these designs with various factors.
[b]Factor S represents subjects and is not normally presented when describing between-subject designs. When factor S is enclosed in parentheses with other factors this notation indicates repeated measures on those factors enclosed with S.

tially, the more nondifferences (controls) that are built into an experiment, the smaller the overall treatment effect will become (5.16). Hence, as the number of control groups increases (and no significant differences are expected among these groups), the less likely the overall F-ratio will be significant. In this case, a nonsignificant F-ratio indicates that all control groups performed as expected. Therefore, control groups or conditions should not be added indiscriminately to an experiment (6.20). In any experiment with three or more control groups their expected outcomes should produce meaningful comparisons as determined by the research hypotheses. If several treatment-control comparisons are crucial for evaluating the research hypotheses, a planned comparison approach should be used (6.10).

As additional factors are added in a mixed factorial design, statistical analysis and interpretation also become more complex primarily because of the increase in the number of interactions that may be significant (4.21). In most situations significant two-way interactions can usually be interpreted, and in some situations significant three-way interactions can be interpreted (6.14). However, in biological research four-way interactions ($A \times B \times C \times D$) are usually impossible to interpret. Consequently, in biological research most experimental designs that may reveal significant four-way interactions should not be used (6.15). Remember all the important questions in a research area cannot be answered in a single experiment.

4.25 EXPERIMENTS AND SCIENTIFIC GENERALIZATION

Because random samples are not used in biological research, a statistical basis does not exist for generalizing the results of any given experiment to the target population (4.6). Based upon only statistical considerations, the generalization of the collected data from a given experiment to the target population requires random sampling.

Nonstatistical generalization, or *scientific generalization*, depends instead upon knowledge of a particular research area. In most experimental fields, therefore, the generalization of data collected from a particular strain or species (under certain specified conditions) to other species and situations is based primarily on scientific knowledge (1.8). The extent of this knowledge in any given research area and whether extrapolations from previous experiments have been successful will determine the appropriateness of certain generalizations.

Fortunately, in biological research the number of strains and species commonly used has not been as restrictive as in many experimental disciplines. Scientific generalization depends on accumulated data collected from related studies that vary in a number of different ways. The greater the variation among experiments in which outcomes remain the same, the greater the generalization provided to other situations and settings. When only a few species are used in a specific field, researchers tend to reduce variation from study to study, to duplicate procedures, to use the same manipulations, that is, to standardize the apparent nonessential features of an experiment. But a balance between standardization (which limits generalization) and variation among experiments (which

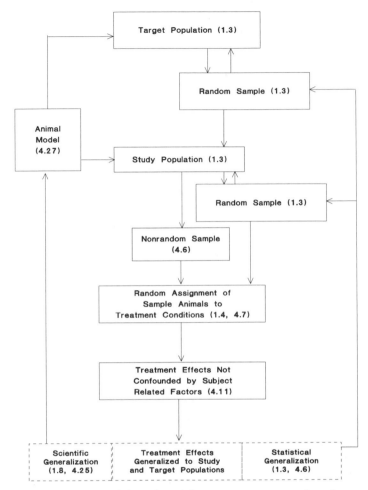

Figure 4.6 A summary of the relationships among target and study populations, random sampling and random assignment of animals, and statistical and scientific generalizations.

increases generalization) must be achieved. Some of the important relationships among target and study populations (1.3), random sampling and random assignment of animals (4.6, 4.7, 4.8), and statistical and scientific generalizations (4.27) are summarized in Figure 4.6.

4.26 "BLIND" CONTROL PROCEDURES

Most biological studies that depend on quantitative measurements of prior treatment conditions can be improved by using some form of "blind" control procedure when the measurements are taken. For example, a biologist may want to determine the effects of different doses of testosterone on protein synthesis in a particular hypothalamic region. In this experiment, different groups of randomly assigned animals might first be injected with varying doses of testosterone (e.g., three hormone and one vehicle control group), the animals sacrificed, and chemical analysis performed on dissected hypothalamic tissue. After the animals were injected, each animal could be given a code number (e.g., 1, 2, 3, and 4) so that the treatment (drug) history of the animal was unknown to those individuals conducting the subsequent dissection and chemical analysis. This coding procedure is an example of a *single blind* control procedure. Also, the drugs to be injected could be prepared by another individual, assigned a code number, and given to the individual injecting the animals. This procedure would control for any handling or injection differences among the four groups and if combined with a coding of the animals after injection (before tissue removal and chemical analysis) would be an example of a *double blind* control procedure. The individual injecting the animals would not know what drugs or doses were being given and those doing the subsequent surgical preparation and chemical analysis would be unaware of the prior treatment history of the animals. In some cases, blind control procedures are not practical, but in many situations these procedures can be incorporated easily into the experimental protocol. The use of blind control procedures does not imply that biologists are basically dishonest; rather, these control procedures eliminate any subtle researcher influences from affecting systematically any of the different treatment conditions. The limitations of using a blind control procedure are that many individuals must be involved in the study and the code sheet must not be misplaced during the experiment!

4.27 ANIMAL MODELS AND SCIENTIFIC GENERALIZATION

Many scientists do research with animals in an attempt to understand human biology. These biologists are interested in generalizing their data to humans. The choice of the species of animal used for a given research project will then depend upon how closely this species (study population) resembles humans (target population) on the measure of interest (1.8). In one sense, it is impossible to generalize data obtained from one animal species to another but as biological scientists we must.

In some cases, the nature of the problem will determine the species to be used (see Calabrese, 1983). In other cases, a biological model must be selected based upon ethical, theoretical, and practical considerations (see Scott and Waterhouse, 1986). In modern biology the study of specific biological systems plays a central role (see Botstein and Fink, 1988; Dawid and Sargent, 1988; Jaenisch, 1988; Kenyon, 1988; King, Yarbrough, Anderson, Gordon, and Gould, 1988; Magasanik, 1988; Rubin, 1988; Varmus, 1988). The heated debate over animal use in research to benefit people has led to an evaluation of some alternative methods to animal research, experimentation, and testing (e.g, see Follath, 1988). These alternatives are useful in some types of research and they can often supplement work with live animals (Lembeck, 1989). But the fact is that virtually all medical knowledge and treatment has involved research with animals. The reason is relatively simple. Procedures and compounds must eventually be tested on living systems made up of interrelated organs and organ systems (A.10) before they can be used with people. If the study of the complex interactions among the cells, tissues, and organs in human beings is to continue then research with living animals will also have to continue (Cohen, 1986; Nicholl and Russell, 1990). Both in vitro and in vivo preparations will continue to be important in understanding biological systems (4.28).

4.28 IN VIVO AND IN VITRO PREPARATIONS

Experimental preparations may be divided into two major classes: in vivo and in vitro. Both types of experimental preparations are necessary for the study of biological systems (see Scott and Waterhouse, 1986, pp. 8–18). In vivo preparations are those using intact animals and *in vitro* preparations are those that use cells, tissues, or isolated organs taken from the animal (4.27). Each type of preparation provides unique information and each of the two experimental preparations has its own advantages and disadvantages (see Table 4.15). When both types of preparations are used to focus on a general research problem, the infor-

Table 4.15 Advantages and Disadvantages of in Vivo and in Vitro Preparations[a]

Type of preparation	Advantages	Disadvantages
In vivo	1. Processes studied while all cycles of causation are able to function (A.7).[b] 2. Compensatory mechanisms initiated by significant treatment effect may be studied. 3. Generalization of treatment effects to target population greater than with other procedures.	1. Difficult to obtain accurate and valid measurements of physiological processes (A.7). 2. Difficult to separate initial treatment effect and subsequent compensatory responses. 3. Complexity of responses (interactions among cycles) makes causal interpretations difficult.
In vitro	1. Accurate and valid measurements of physiological process can be obtained (A.7). 2. Treatment effects easier to manipulate, control, and isolate. 3. Complexity of treatment response greatly reduced and causal inferences easier to make.	1. Normality of preparations when studied in abnormal environment (removal of organ, tissue, or cells from body) difficult to determine. 2. Deterioration of preparation when supportive environment removed (homeostatic control processes eliminated). 3. Isolated procedures reduce complexity and make it difficult to extrapolate results to intact, target population (1.3).

[a]Adapted from Scott and Waterhouse (1986, pp. 12–18).
[b]See this book section.

mation obtained is usually complementary and the advantages of each preparation are maximized.

4.29 INTERNAL AND EXTERNAL VALIDITY

The best experimental studies have both high internal and external validity. High internal validity of an experiment indicates that the treatment conditions used are not confounded by extraneous subject-, environment- or time-related variables (4.4, 4.11, 4.12, 4.15, 4.19, 4.23, 4.26). The external validity of an experiment assesses the extent to which specific experimental results can be extrapolated to the population of interest. Many factors are involved in determining the external validity of any experimental result. Some of these factors are the study population, the sampling procedure, the animal model used, the type of preparation used, and the population of interest (1.8, 4.6, 4.25, 4.27, 6.21).

II

STATISTICAL INFERENCE, ANALYSIS OF VARIANCE, AND POST HOC ANALYSIS

5

Statistical Inference

5.1 DESCRIPTIVE AND INFERENTIAL STATISTICS

Statistics is involved in the collection, organization, and interpretation of data. The two major categories of statistics are *descriptive* and *inferential* statistics. *Descriptive statistics* are concerned with the enumeration, organization, and graphical representation of data (data reduction). In an experimental report, descriptive statistics are used to summarize the data obtained from the treatment groups by presenting measures of central tendency and variability in either tables or figures. Guidelines for the effective presentation of data in tables and figures have been summarized in a number of articles and books (e.g., see Bourke, Daly, and McGilvray, 1985, pp. 1–18; Cleveland and McGill, 1984; Elston and Johnson, 1987, pp. 32–40; Schmidt, 1983; Tufte, 1983, 1990; Wainer, 1984).

One useful measure for summarizing the data is to define a *measure of central location* (tendency) of which the most common are the *arithmetic mean*, the *median*, and the *mode*.

- The arithmetic mean is the sum of all the observations divided by the number of observations.
- The median is the value of the middle observation (or the mean of the value of the two middle observations) when the observations are arranged in numerical order.
- The mode is the most common value—the value of the greatest number of observations in a sample.

The mean is influenced by extreme scores and its value may not actually exist in the sample (e.g., an average of 1.8 children per household). The mean can enter into algebraic equations and in estimation its unbiasedness and efficiency are important advantages. The median and mode are not affected by extreme scores, but the mode may not be representative of a set of observations. When the distribution is symmetric the mean and median will be equal, and only when the distribution is symmetric and unimodal will all three of these central location measures be the same. When the mean is greater than the median, the sample distribution is skewed to the right. When the mean is smaller than the median the sample distribution is skewed to the left. A unimodal, symmetric distribution is called a normal distribution. A bimodal distribution refers to any distribution which has two predominant peaks, whether or not these peaks are of exactly the same height (equal number of observations).

In addition to some measure of central location, the spread (dispersion) of the observations in a sample provides another useful summary statistic. Many samples can be adequately described by a measure of central location and a measure of spread. The most common measures of variability (dispersion) are the *range*, the *interquartile range*, the *variance*, and the *standard deviation*.

- The range is the difference between the largest and smallest observation in the sample.
- The interquartile range is the difference between the value of the 75th percentile minus the value of the 25th percentile.
- The variance (s^2) is the average of the sum of the squared deviations from the mean of the sample divided by the degrees of freedom (5.17).
- The standard deviation (s or SD) is the positive square root of the variance; that is,

$$s = \sqrt{s^2}$$

The range is the easiest measure of dispersion to compute and understand but its total reliance on extreme values is a serious disadvantage. The interquartile range is sometimes used to circumvent the effect of extreme values on the range. Range statistics are not used much in inferential statistics, however, they are the easiest method of providing some information about dispersion.

The variance and standard deviation are very sensitive to extreme observations. These measures of dispersion, however, provide unbiased and efficient estimators of population parameters and play a very important role in inferential statistics (5.2).

Another measure of spread is provided by the *coefficient of variation* which is the standard deviation (5.2) expressed as a proportion or percentage of the mean of the sample. The coefficient of variation is a dimensionless measure and provides a useful descriptive index of the variability relative to the mean.

Inferential statistics are concerned with reaching conclusions from incomplete information (sample data), that is, generalizing from known sample characterics to parameters of the population of interest (the target population 1.3). Classical statistical inference involves *estimation* and *hypothesis testing*. In estimation, the unknown parameter of a study population is estimated from a statistic computed from the data of a sample drawn randomly from the study population. The *unbiasedness* and *efficiency* of an estimator are of particular importance to statisticians. An estimator (statistic) whose expected value equals the parameter to be estimated is called an *unbiased estimator*. For example, the expected value of the sample mean is equal to u, the population mean. The efficiency of an estimator is a relative term and indicates that one statistic is more accurate than all other statistics as an estimate of a particular parameter. The fact that sample means cluster more closely around μ (the mean of the population from which the samples were drawn) than do sample medians indicates that the mean is the more efficient estimator of μ. The unbiasedness and efficiency of the mean and standard deviation of a sample make these two sample statistics very important in inferential statistics (5.2).

Standard errors (5.2) are the statistics which measure the reliability of estimates, and confidence limits provide boundaries to these estimates of population parameters. Confidence intervals (limits) provide indexes of the relative precision with which the sample treatment means are measured. Hypothesis testing determines whether differences exist in the parameters of two or more populations. For this latter task theoretical probability distributions of various statistics (5.7) are used to determine the likelihood (probability, 5.6) of certain numerical outcomes in experimental data. Inferential statistics are used to determine whether the null hypothesis (5.5) should be rejected at a given level of significance (5.8, 5.9).

In summary, both descriptive and inferential statistical procedures are used in most experimental reports. Descriptive statistics present the characteristics of the sample treatment conditions, and inferential statistics provide the rationale for assuming that significant treatment conditions exist. In some papers the identification of associations (relationships) between and among sets of data may be studied (5.26, 5.27).

5.2 STANDARD DEVIATION AND STANDARD ERROR OF THE MEAN

The *standard deviation* (SD) and the *standard error of the mean* (SEM) are often confused in descriptive statistics (5.1). Most biologists summarize their data with the *standard error of the mean* because it is always smaller than the standard deviation; consequently, the data plotted look better (less variable). The standard deviation quantifies the variability in the sample data such that about 68 percent of the data obtained (assuming a normally distributed population, 5.1) will fall within one standard deviation from the mean, and about 95 percent of the data obtained within two standard deviations from the mean. Reviewers are usually interested in evaluating the data obtained in the experiment, and the best way to convey this information is to present the mean and its standard deviation for each treatment condition.

The *standard error of the mean* (SEM) quantifies the precision with which the sample mean *estimates* the population mean (5.1). The SEM is, therefore, the standard deviation of the sampling distribution of the mean and is calculated as:

$$\text{SEM} = \frac{\text{SD}}{\sqrt{n}}$$

If the standard error of the mean is confused with the standard deviation, the range of the sample values would be incorrectly assumed to be very narrow. Therefore, if the SEM is given in a report the number of animals in the sample *must* also be given so that the SD can be calculated to determine the variability in the sample data.

5.3 SCALES OF MEASUREMENT

To use appropriate statistical procedures to analyze data the experimental design (Chapter 4), the statistical model (5.7) and the measurement scale used to record the data must all be considered. The four basic types of scales of measurement are *nominal, ordinal, interval,* and *ratio.*

Nominal scaling involves classifying (labeling) animals, objects, or events in terms of attributes they share. When numbers are assigned to these classes, they do not possess quantitative properties nor do they show sequential order. Proportions or percentages are the statistics most often used with nominal scales. For example, in each treatment condition the number of animals with a specific attribute (infected) could be counted and a percentage computed. *Ordinal* scaling, like nominal scaling, involves classifying things in terms of attributes they share but the categories are ordered (ranked) along some continuum. In this case, the severity of infection for each animal could be ranked from 0 (none) to 5 (highest) based on the "redness" of the infection site. These ordered relationships are expressed by the algebra of inequalities with their respective symbols of $>$ (greater than) and $<$ (less than). Hence, qualitative measurements result in discrete, or categorical, data in which order is present (ordinal scaling) or not present (nominal scaling).

Both *interval* and *ratio* scales are quantitative: the values of the variable can be *meaningfully* added, subtracted, and multiplied. Equal differences in scale values are equal throughout the scale. The only difference between interval and ratio scales involves the value of zero. In ratio scales a zero implies an absence of the quality being measured, whereas in interval scales placement of zero is arbitrary.

A conservative rule is that a biological variable may be considered on a lower scale of measurement for analysis purposes but may not be considered on a higher scale. The types of biological variables can be ranked by the amount of information that an individual measurement provides:

$$\text{Nominal} < \text{ordinal} < \text{discrete} < \text{continuous}$$

When choosing a statistical analysis, a discrete or continuous variable may be evaluated by an "ordinal scale" test. But, a biological variable should not frequently or freely be treated on a lower scale of measurement: *the measurement should be treated on the highest scale possible to maximize the information obtained.*

Opinions vary as to the importance of scales of measurement and some statistics books only briefly cover the topic whereas others use these scales of measurement for their general organization (see Gaito, 1980; Howell, 1987, for brief reviews of this general issue and for additional references). Numbers may be assigned to ordinal data and these numbers may be added, subtracted, multiplied, and divided (i.e., a statistical test performed on the data). *The important question is whether these statistical results bear any meaningful relationship to the empirical objects or events measured.* As Howell (1987) has concluded "Our statistical tests can only apply to the numbers that we obtain, and the validity of statements about the objects or events that we think we are measuring hinges primarily on our knowledge of these objects or events and not on the scale of measurement" (p. 10).

5.4 THE PROBLEM OF UNCERTAINTY

Research and the subsequent statistical analysis and interpretation of data always take place in the context of uncertainty. In an experimental study, a research hypothesis is formulated, specific treatment conditions are given which reflect the critical elements of the research hypothesis, a design is used which eliminates systematic confounding, statistical analysis is done, inferences are drawn from this analysis, and finally the new information is integrated with existing knowledge and theory (Chapters 1 and 2). The uncertainty involved in experimental research and its accompanying statistical analysis and interpretation occurs because the research hypothesis cannot be tested directly, and the two statistical hypotheses which are tested cannot be proved or disproved (1.7, 5.5).

5.5 DECISION RULES FOR UNCERTAINTY: NULL AND ALTERNATIVE HYPOTHESES

To evaluate statistically a research hypothesis, the biologist forms two mutually exclusive and exhaustive hypotheses, called the *null hypothesis* and the *alternative hypothesis* (1.6). These statistical hypotheses refer to the hypothetical outcome of the experiment as though it was administered to an infinitely large number of subjects. The null hypothesis states some expectation about the parameters of the treatment populations in this hypothetical situation. The null hypothesis is stated in the negative form (hence the use of the term null). The null hypothesis specifies that no differences exist among the treatment population means, that is, the population means (μ's) are equal. In symbols, the null hypothesis (H_o) is given as

$$H_0: \quad \mu_1 = \mu_2 = \mu_3 = \mu_i$$

or more simply as

$$H_0: \quad \text{all } \mu_i\text{'s are equal (identical).}$$

The other statistical hypothesis, referred to as the alternative hypothesis (H_i), specifies all the possible ways that a set of population treatment means could differ. In symbols, H_i is given as

$$H_i: \quad \mu_1 \neq \mu_2 \neq \mu_3 \neq \mu_i$$

or more simply as

$$H_i: \quad \text{not all } \mu_i\text{'s are equal.}$$

In summary, because the H_0 and H_i are mutually exclusive, both cannot be correct. Also, because they are exhaustive, one of them must be correct. But, neither the null hypothesis nor the alternative hypothesis can be proved directly. Using descriptive statistical methods (5.1) you can calculate the means and variances of the treatment groups (samples) in your experiment but still you would not know the true values of the population treatment means. Inferential statistics, based upon probability theory (5.6) and the sampling distribution of an appropriate test statistic (5.7), permit you to determine the likelihood that the differences between (or among) the observed treatment means of the samples would have occurred by chance (i.e., do not reflect true differences in the populations).

5.6 PROBABILITY

An exact definition of the term *probability* is difficult to give but two general definitions of probability are commonly used. Each of the definitions focuses on a different aspect of the concept of probability. The *theoretical (mathematical) definition* of probability and the *frequency (empirical) definition* of probability are explained in most biostatistics books (e.g., see Elston and Johnson, 1987, pp. 60–83). Theoretical probabilities are those which can be determined with a good degree of confidence purely on formal or logical grounds. The foundations of the mathematical theory of probability are based on basic rules and axioms. These axioms are used to generate probability distributions and these distributions are the cornerstones of statistical inferences (5.7).

Probabilities are usually expressed as proportions with values varying between 0 and 1. A 0 probability indicates that it is impossible for some event to occur and a probability of 1.00 indicates that the event will always occur. Mathematical models in statistics are based upon the theoretical approach to probability which assumes that in a conceptual (theoretical) experiment the probabilities of all possible outcomes are known and that all trials are theoretically perfect. Theoretically perfect means, as an example, that if a hypothetical coin is tossed, it must come up heads or tails and not stand on its end. Using this approach probabilities are fixed and unvarying and are used to calculate the theoretical sampling distributions of various statistics (5.7). Hence, probability theory forms the basis for all statistical procedures.

5.7 SAMPLING DISTRIBUTIONS OF STATISTICS

The sampling distribution of a statistic is the basic concept underlying all statistical tests. Essentially, a sampling distribution shows what values would be expected for a particular statistic under certain specified conditions (assumptions). Using the mathematical (axiomatic) approach to probability (5.6) the sampling distribution of a statistic is the theoretical (expected) distribution of the statistic if *all possible samples of a given size* were drawn from a population (Figure 1.11). Various theoretical probability distributions have been developed by mathematical statisticians and some of these theoretical distributions are applicable to experimental events (1.7, 5.21). These theoretical distributions are neither right nor wrong; rather, they may be useful or not useful for understanding certain empirical events. For example, the normal probability model deals with continuous random variables that are distributed in a symmetrical bell-shaped fashion (5.1).

If certain assumptions can be made regarding the distributions, variances, and measures of the samples used to calculate the test statistic, then a given theoretical probability distribution may be used to determine the likelihood of a range of numerical outcomes of the statistic in an experimental situation (Figure 1.11). The theoretical probability distribution of a statistic (e.g., F) is actually a family of curves determined by the number of degrees of freedom (5.17) associated with the numerator and denominator mean squares in the F-ratio (5.16). Moreover, the theoretical distribution is the sampling distribution of the statistic when the population means are equal, that is, when the null hypothesis is true (5.5). Theoretical probability distributions and their underlying assumptions are the foundations on which inferential statistics are built, and this is the rationale for their emphasis in most statistics books.

In summary, statisticians are concerned with the generation of theoretical probability distributions, their underlying assumptions, their relation to empirical events, and alternative approaches to statistical inference (see Oakes, 1986). Debates among statisticians, therefore, focus primarily on these types of problems. Fortunately, biologists can use many of the available statistical models without fully understanding the derivations of their sampling distributions. But, it should be evident that probability theory underlies the entire structure of statistical inference (5.6).

5.8 CRITICAL REGIONS

The logic of statistical inference requires the biologist to decide whether the differences between the experimental sample means could have occurred by chance. If the treatment differences were unlikely to occur by chance, the biologist rejects the null hypothesis of equality of population means (5.5), and asserts the alternative hypothesis. Thus, if the sampling distribution of a statistic (5.7) shows that a given outcome occurs rarely by chance, the researcher assumes that a similar rate of occurrence in an experimental study may be attributed to nonchance factors, that is, to a significant treatment effect.

The *critical regions* are the far ends of the theoretical sampling distribution of a statistic. This critical region is also called the *rejection region* because if the value of the test statistic falls in this region, designated as alpha (α), the null hypothesis is rejected (Figure 1.11). In contrast, the region of the theoretical sampling distribution not included in α (i.e., $1.00 - \alpha$) is called the *acceptance region*. Whenever a test statistic falls in this region, no basis exists for rejecting the null hypothesis because this value of the test statistic might be expected to occur by chance. The tables found in the appendices of traditional statistics books list the values of common test statistics (t, F, chi square) that would be expected to occur by chance in the far ends of the theoretical sampling distributions of these statistics (5.9, Figure 1.11).

5.9 SIGNIFICANCE LEVELS (ALPHA)

Most biologists are willing to reject the null hypothesis (H_0) and assert the alternative statistical hypothesis (H_i) if the calculated value of the statistic (e.g., t, F, chi-square) would have occurred, by chance, only 5 out of 100 times (5.5, 5.6, 5.7, 5.8). Hence, if the obtained value of the specific statistic would have occurred, by chance alone, in the sampling distribution of the statistic 5 percent or less of the time, H_0 is rejected and H_i is asserted. But, if the probability is greater than 5 percent, H_0 is not rejected. The Greek letter alpha (α) is used to designate the significance level and when the 5 percent significance level is used, $\alpha = .05$. When the null hypothesis is rejected, the statement that ". . . the probability is less than 5 percent" is given by the symbols: $p < .05$. Why is the .05 level of significance used as the decision point to reject the null hypothesis? Why not a .06 level of significance? Actually, the .05 level of significance is used because of tradition. R. A. Fisher, the founder of modern statistical methods, chose this value and other scientists have accepted this choice. Of course, no biologist should *forcefully* assert either the null or alternative hypothesis if a .06 level of significance is obtained (see 6.20, Figures 1.11 and 1.12).

The .01 significance level is a more conservative criterion for rejecting H_0 because the obtained value of the statistic must occur, by chance, only 1 percent of the time or less in the sampling distribution of the appropriate statistic to warrant rejecting H_0. This conservative approach to rejecting H_0 ($p < .01$ must occur) is usually adopted when making a Type I error is more serious than making a Type II error (5.10).

The yes-no decision format of significance levels (alpha) in null hypothesis testing (5.8) has produced considerable controversy (see Oakes, 1986). The fixation of searching for significance (6.20) assumes that a mechanical and objective set of rules will produce clear-cut yes-no decisions. Unfortunately this outcome does not occur. Cohen (1990) commenting on the .05 significance level states that ". . . In governing decisions about the status of null hypotheses, it came to determine decisions about the acceptance of doctoral dissertations and the granting of research funding, and about publications, promotion, and whether to have a baby just now. Its arbitrary unreasonable tyranny has led to data fudging of varying degrees of subtlety from grossly altering data to dropping cases where there 'must have been' errors" (p. 1307). In a shorter critique, Rosnow and Rosenthal (1989) state ". . . surely, God loved the .06 nearly as much as the .05" (p. 1277).

In planning your research you must make many informal judgments such as the size of the expected treatment effects and the risks acceptable for the two types of errors in statistical inference (5.10). From these judgments, an estimate of the power and the sample size required for the research study can then be made (5.12, 5.13, 5.15). The amount of expected experimental error can usually be estimated from previous research. With all of this information you can "decide" whether the research as conceived is worthwhile. Only you can make *this* decision!

5.10 TYPE I AND TYPE II ERRORS

The two types of statistical decisions or inferences that can be made are probabilistic (5.6). The null hypothesis is rejected when the probability is low that the observed event occurred by chance (5.9). The alternative hypothesis is asserted when the chance probability under the sampling distribution is not sufficiently low (5.5). There is the possibility of error with each of these statistical decisions: the null hypothesis may be rejected when it is actually true, that is, the alternative hypothesis may be asserted when it is actually false (Type I error) or the null hypothesis may *not* be rejected when it is actually false, that is, the alternative hypothesis may *not* be asserted when it is actually true (*Type II error*, see Table 5.1).

5.11 CONTROL OF TYPE I ERROR

You can reduce the likelihood of rejecting the null hypothesis when it is actually true (Type I error, 5.10) by selecting a more conservative level of α, that is, decrease the length of the rejection region (5.8) by decreasing α from .05 to .01 or even .001. The lower the level of α, the lower the probability of a Type I error. But, the lower the level of α, the greater the likelihood that a Type II (β) error will be made (5.10, Table 5.1).

5.12 TYPE II ERROR AND POWER

Type II error is when the null hypothesis (H_0) is false but is not rejected (Table 5.1). Type II error is a much more frequent error than Type I, and until recently Type II errors were not given much attention in biological research. The probability of making a Type I error is given by the α level established for rejecting the null hypothesis (5.11). The β probability or the probability of making a Type

Table 5.1 Type I and Type II Errors in Relation to Population Characteristics and the Researcher's Decision

Decision made by researcher from sample data	True nature of population	
	H_0 is true (5.5)[a] (all μ_i's are equal)	H_0 is false (5.5) (all μ_i's are not equal)
Does not reject H_0	Correct decision ($p = 1 - \alpha$)	Type II error (5.10) ($p = \beta$)
Rejects H_0	Type 1 error (5.10) ($p = \alpha$)	Correct decision, ($p = 1 - \beta$)

Type 1 error is the rejection of a *true* null hypothesis (Table 5.2).
Type II error is the acceptance of a *false* null hypothesis (Table 5.2).
Power is the probability of rejecting H_0 when H_0 is false ($p = 1 - \beta$).

[a]See this book section.

II error, however, must be calculated. Once β is calculated the probability of failing to reject the null hypothesis when it is actually false is known. By subtracting β from one $(1 - \beta)$, the power of the statistical test is known. *Power is defined as the probability of rejecting H_0 when H_0 is false.* In summary, a Type II error (β) is an error caused by the failure to reject the null hypothesis when the alternative hypothesis is true. Power refers to the converse side of Type II error $(1.0 - \beta)$, the probability of rejecting the null hypothesis when the alternative hypothesis is true. Any decrease in Type II error, therefore, results in an increase in power. Most biologists assume that Type I errors are more serious than Type II errors. Consequently, a power of about .80 would be a reasonable value for biological research (5.14). Hence, a 4 to 1 ratio of Type II to Type I error is a reasonable target. If α is set at .05 and power at .80, β would be .20. The ratio of Type II to Type I error would be .20/.05 or 4 to 1 (see Tables 5.2 and 5.3).

5.13 CONTROL OF TYPE II ERROR AND INCREASING POWER

The magnitude of Type II error is controlled indirectly through a variety of procedures. Type II error can be reduced by (*a*) decreasing the amount of experimental error (5.16), (*b*) increasing the number of subjects assigned to the treatment conditions, (*c*) increasing the expected magnitude of the effects by increasing the differences between treatments, and (*d*) using a more sensitive experimental design. As would be expected, these procedures also increase the power of the statistical test. Another logical way to increase the power of a test would be to increase the probability of a Type I error, setting the significance level at .10 rather than .05, which would decrease Type II error. But very rarely will the α level be set at any value greater than .05. Without a rationale for determining the relative seriousness of the two type of errors, many biologists arbitrarily accept an α level of .05 and allow Type II error (and power) to be what it has to be with the given experimental procedures (5.9). But as Keppel (1991) has stated "Low power is poor science—we waste time, energy, and resources whenever we conduct an experiment that has a low probability of producing a significant result" (p. 73).

Table 5.2 The Two Errors of Inference (Type I and II) and Their Control

Error	Description	Control (5.11, 5.13)
Type I	The H_0 is rejected when it is true for the study population. (The H_i is asserted when it is false for the study population.)	The setting of α (i.e., decreasing α from $p < .05$ to $p < .01$.)
Type II	The H_0 is not rejected when it is false for the study population. (The H_i is *not* asserted when it is true for the study population.)	Increase the number of subjects; increase the size of the treatment effects; use a more sensitive design.

The relation between the two types of errors of inference: As the α level selected by the researcher is decreased (from $p < .05$ to $p < .01$) to decrease the size of Type I error, the likelihood of making a Type II error is increased (5.4, 5.5, 5.10).

Table 5.3   Type II Error and Power in Hypothesis Testing

The power of a statistical test = 1.00 − Type II error (β) (Tables 5.1 and 5.2).[a]

Power is defined as the probability of correctly rejecting a false H_0 [i.e., the probability of rejecting the null hypothesis (H_0) when the H_0 is false and the alternative hypothesis (H_i) is correct, 5.5, 5.12].

A decrease in Type II error (see Table 5.2) results in an increase in power (5.13).

The general aim in hypothesis testing is to use statistical tests that make the two errors of inference (Type I, α and Type II, β) as small as possible (see Table 5.2). Hence, an ideal statistical outcome would be one in which the magnitude of a type I error is set at $p < .001$, the power of the test is in the high 90's, and a small sample size is used (5.14, 6.20).

[a]See this book section.

5.14   THE IDEAL STATISTICAL TEST

The general aim in hypothesis testing is to use statistical tests that make the two errors of inference (Type I, α and Type II, β) as small as possible (5.5, 5.10). Hence, an ideal statistical test would be one in which the magnitude of a Type I error is set at $p < .01$ or even $p < .001$ and the power of the test is in the 90's or higher. One of the difficulties in attempting to reduce simultaneously Type I and Type II errors in most biological research is that the sample size would have to be extremely large (see 6.20). In general, to increase power from .80 to .90 a dramatic increase in the sample size is required (5.15). Consequently, with the small sample sizes common in most biological studies a p value of .05 and power in the 80's may be the best that can be achieved. And this ideal state would only occur when experimental error is very low and the differences among treatments are very large (5.13).

5.15   POWER AND DETERMINATION OF SAMPLE SIZE

The larger the sample size used, the greater the power of the statistical test and the more sensitive the experiment would be in detecting treatment differences in the populations (5.12, 5.13). Statistical procedures are available for calculating the number of animals that should be used in an experiment (see Cohen, 1988). These estimate procedures require you to know (estimate) certain values (e.g., probable treatment effect, population error variance) *before* the experiment is started. Essentially, you must estimate the expected treatment effect, estimate the population error variance, select an appropriate level of power, select a sample size, substitute these values in a formula, and then refer to power function curves which determine the power for the initially chosen sample size. If the power is too low, the sample size selected is increased, and this iterative estimation procedure is repeated. Consequently, most researchers do not calculate sample sizes for their experiments. Rather, based upon their knowledge of their scientific discipline they assume that a particular treatment effect should be observed with a particular sample size.

When power calculations are done manually they are computationally intensive, which makes them tedious and vulnerable to error. Specialized PC programs are available to make objective decisions about appropriate sample size (see Borenstein and Cohen, 1988; Dallal, 1988). One such program, called Numberator, has been developed at Drexel University (Dubin and Herr, 1986). To use this program, you must provide answers to the following questions: (1) How many groups of subjects are to be used? (2) What is the smallest difference between means that should be detected? (3) What is the expected variability of the data? (4) What should be the value of Type I error, that is, $\alpha = .05, .01$, etc? (5) How much Type II error can be tolerated? If a significant difference exists [see (2)] is a 70, 80, or 90 percent chance of detecting it required (i.e., a Type II error of .30, .20, or .10, respectively)?

If reasonable guesses (answers) to these five questions can be provided, the Numberator program will permit one value of n at a time to be tried to determine the lowest number that will satisfy the conditions of the formula used in the computer program. The use of computer programs to calculate sample size will increase in the near future. The judicious use of these procedures would eliminate any excessive use of laboratory animals for a given experiment (4.27), a very rare event in biological research. However, it is scientifically indefensible to perform an experiment that will likely fail to yield useful results because of an uncontrolled Type II error (Altman, 1980a,b). Using a sample size that is too small can obfuscate the conclusion drawn from any experiment (5.10, 5.12).

A determination of power after an experiment is conducted can provide very useful information regarding the importance of nonsignificant findings (6.20). Most of the answers to the questions that are required for using the power formula are now known. If using the minimum treatment effect that would be of interest the calculated power is very low, another study with a more sensitive experimental design (increase in sample size, reduction of experimental error) would be worthwhile. However, if power is relatively high, another experiment with a more sensitive design would not be worthwhile. In short, if sample sizes are too small or measurements too crude the chance of detecting any differences among the treatments in the sample groups is minimal even when a large difference exists among the populations.

5.16 LOGIC OF HYPOTHESIS TESTING

In parametric statistical tests (Chapter 8) the statistical value used to decide whether the null hypothesis should be rejected (5.5, 5.8) is a ratio of two separate estimates of experimental error. Experimental error consists of all uncontrolled sources of variability in an experiment. Hence, experimental error reflects the operation of unaccounted for or randomly varying nuisance variables (1.2).

One estimate of experimental error is based upon the variability of subjects treated alike, that is, within the same treatment level. The variability of subjects within each of the treatment levels is pooled and an averaged estimate of experimental error is obtained. This estimate of experimental error is designated as *within-group variability* (differences among subjects treated alike).

The other experimental error estimate is based upon the fact that differences among the sample means will also include all the sources of unsystematic variability which contributed to the differences among subjects within a given treatment condition. But, this treatment-group variability (the variability among the treatment means) also reflects any effects of the treatments. Hence, treatment group variability equals (treatment effects) + (experimental error) and is usually referred to as *between-group variability* (5.17, 5.18).

A ratio of these two measures of variability—differences among the treatment means and differences among subjects treated alike—provides an index of any treatment effect, that is,

$$\frac{\text{Differences among treatments}}{\text{Differences among subjects treated alike}} = \frac{\text{treatment group variability}}{\text{within-group variability}}$$

$$= \frac{\text{treatment effects} + \text{experimental error}}{\text{experimental error}}$$

If the null hypothesis (5.5) is true (i.e., no treatment effect, all u_i's are equal), the average value of this ratio would be expected to be approximately 1.0 (assuming that the experiment was repeated many times with new samples of subjects drawn from the same population). Thus,

$$\frac{[(\text{Treatment effects} (= 0)] + (\text{experimental error})}{\text{Experimental error}} = 1.0$$

However, if the null hypothesis is false (i.e., a treatment effect exists, all u_i's are not equal) an additional component is added in the numerator which reflects the treatment effect. Thus,

$$\frac{[(\text{Treatment effects} (> 0)] + (\text{experimental error})}{\text{Experimental error}} > 1.0$$

Hence, in this case, if the experiment were repeated again and again, the averaged value of this ratio would be expected to be greater than (>) 1.0. The larger the treatment effect, the higher the value of this ratio. And, the higher the value of this ratio, the smaller is the likelihood that it could have occurred by chance. The theoretical sampling distribution of the statistic (5.7) provides the necessary information for determining the probability (5.6) of obtaining a particular value of this ratio given the sample sizes used in the experiment (5.17).

5.17 DEGREES OF FREEDOM (df)

In an analysis of variance (ANOVA, Chapter 6) the between-group variance estimate (treatment group variability, 5.16) and the within-group variance estimate (5.16) are called mean squares. The general formula for a mean square (MS) is

$$MS = \frac{ss}{df}$$

where df refers to the number of *degrees of freedom* associated with the sum of squares (ss).

Practically every application of probability theory to statistical analysis is related to degrees of freedom rather than to the total number of values in the data under analysis. Most biologists, unfamiliar with statistical theory and the rationale for degrees of freedom, are satisfied with knowing the correct formulas to calculate degrees of freedom (see 6.5). Essentially, the concept of *degrees of freedom refers to the number of values in a data set free to vary when restrictions are placed on the data.* One degree of freedom is lost with each additional restriction. As an example, with any four numbers whose sum is 15 which is one restriction on the data set (i.e., the sum of the numbers must equal 15), there are 3 degrees of freedom. In this case, only three numbers have the freedom to vary, the fourth number is fixed because the sum of all four numbers must be 15.

In statistics, the general rule for computing the df for any sum of squares is

$$df = \text{number of independent} - \text{number of population}$$
$$\text{observations} \qquad \text{estimates}$$

or, stated another way, df is the number of independent pieces of information remaining following the estimation of population parameters (see 6.5 for the formulas for partitioning the total degrees of freedom in experiments).

5.18 THE F-RATIO (AND t-TEST)

The analysis of variance (ANOVA, Chapter 6) technique provides the rationale for comparing any number of levels of a single variable (single factor between-subject designs, 4.10), the joint effects of two or more variables (factorial designs, 4.13), repeated measures on the same subject (within-subject designs, 4.16), and mixed (between and within) factorial designs (4.21). In these cases, the test statistic is the F-ratio, which consists of a between-group or a between-treatment variance estimate divided by a within-group variance estimate (5.16).

The ANOVA technique (Chapter 6) is a general statistical analysis involving the comparison of variances reflecting different sources of variability, and the F-ratio is a statistic relating systematic variance (treatment effect) to nonsystematic variance (error). The F-test can also be used to analyze a two-group experiment. Normally, another statistical test (Student t-test or just t-test) is used to analyze the results of two-group studies (5.19). The t-test, however, is only a special case of the F-test. If both a t-test and an F-test were performed on the same data from a two-group experiment, exactly the same information would be obtained. The reason the results would be identical is that the two statistical tests are algebraically equivalent when only two groups are used; that is,

$$F = (t)^2 \qquad \text{and} \qquad t = \sqrt{F}.$$

Consequently, for two treatment groups if F is significant, t is significant; if F is not significant, t is not significant.

5.19 MISUSE OF THE t-TEST

The t-test is the most commonly reported statistical procedure in the biological literature. In those research papers in which at least one "p value" is given to announce the significance of the reported data, the t-statistic is usually used. The reasons for the popularity of the t-test are (1) research designs for which the t test is appropriate are used frequently, (2) the software on virtually all calculators and computers includes the t-test, and (3) the t-test is one statistical procedure taught in most elementary statistics courses; consequently, most biologists are familiar with the test.

Unfortunately, in addition to being the most widely used statistical procedure, the t-test is also the most widely abused statistical procedure. This occurs because the t-test is used inappropriately to compare three or more groups two at a time (5.18). The most persistent statistical error in biological research is that independent sample and paired sample t-tests are used to the virtual exclusion of the more appropriate analysis of variance techniques for between-subject, within-subject, and mixed factorial designs (5.18, Chapter 6). *Repeatedly performing t-tests in the same experiment inevitably increases the chance of mistakenly declaring significance* (10.1). For example, in a between-subject design with three groups, a biologist might analyze the data by performing t-tests for each pair of treatment means using as a critical value that for the t-statistic with df's $n_1 + n_2 - 2$ at the $p < .05$ significance level. Three such paired comparisons would be made but the significance level (5.11) would not be at $p < .05$ but at $p < .13$.

If there are not too many comparisons, adding the p values obtained in multiple tests provides a conservative estimate of the true p value for the set of comparisons (Table 10.1). In a three-group between-subject design three t-test comparisons would result in an effective p value of about $3(.05) = .15$. When a four-group between-subject design is used, six possible t-tests could be performed (1 versus 2, 1 versus 3, 1 versus 4, 2 versus 3, 2 versus 4, 3 versus 4). In this case, if the biologist concludes that a significant difference exists between groups 2 and 4 at $p < .05$, the realistic p value is about $6(.05) = .30$ (or about a 30 percent chance of at least one incorrect statement if the biologist concludes that the treatments had an effect, 6.9).

Another common way to misuse the t-test (in a between-subject design with more than three groups) is to examine quickly the means of the groups and calculate only a single t-test on the two groups that have the greatest mean difference. The same strategy also has been used in within-subject designs (4.16) and in mixed factorial designs (4.21); the data are first plotted across time (trials, measurements) and a t-test performed on only the highest and lowest values obtained from each group. Using this strategy, the biologist may assume that because only one or at the most two t-tests were calculated, the real "probability" remains at around .05. Thus, the biologist, in effect, eliminates all apparent nonsignificant comparisons and selects only one or two pairwise comparisons to determine statistical significance. Because a limited number of statistical comparisons are made, the biologist may believe that statistical principles have not been violated. Indeed, after a few moments of reflection these selected comparisons become the only ones of interest to the biologist (planned comparisons, 6.10) and a reasonable scientific "explanation" can be given for these significant (and expected) outcomes! Neither of these post hoc arguments, however, is very convincing. Another disadvantage of multiple t-test comparisons is the limited information extracted from the data collected. When two or more treatment combinations are given within a single experiment (4.21) a more sensitive and appropriate statistical analysis like an analysis of variance (Chapter 6) will permit several hypotheses to be tested within the framework of a single overall analysis.

In summary, the t-test (5.18) may be used correctly to test the hypothesis that two group means are not different, but when the experimental design involves multiple groups or multiple measures, the more appropriate techniques of analysis of variance should be used. The t-test is appropriate for those two groups or condition studies when the dependent (response) variable is continuous and has a normal distribution. The t-test is usually inappropriate for ordinal dependent variables (5.3). If the data have a skewed distribution (not a normal distribution), the robustness of the t-test may still justify its use (5.23). In some cases, the dependent variable may be transformed so that the transformed data have a normal distribution (5.24).

5.20 ONE-TAILED AND TWO-TAILED t-TESTS

The t-test is a special case of the F-test and is used to evaluate two-group studies (5.18). With the F-test, however, the alternative hypothesis (5.5) is *nondirectional* in that differences between two means in either the positive or negative direction are regarded as incompatible with the null hypothesis (5.18). Hence, with $H_0: \mu_1 = \mu_2$ and $H_i: \mu_1 \neq \mu_2$, the null hypothesis would be rejected whenever the F-value falls within the selected critical regions (e.g., $p < .05$) which would occur if $\mu_1 > \mu_2$ or $\mu_1 < \mu_2$. With the t-test the alternative hypothesis may be *directional* (one-tail) or *nondirectional* (two-tail).

An alternative hypothesis that specifies a particular direction of the differences (i.e., $H_i: \mu_1 > \mu_2$ or $H_i: \mu_2 > \mu_1$) may be selected. This type of alternative hypothesis is a *directional hypothesis* and a larger rejection region is permitted. Specifically, a directional test is evaluated at $p = 2(\alpha)$ and if α is normally set at $p < .05$ for a nondirectional test, then $p = 2(.05) = .10$ would be used for the directional test. This doubling of α for the t-distribution is equivalent to locating the entire α level (e.g., .05) in the tail of the t-distribution specified by the directional alternative hypothesis. For this reason, directional and nondirectional hypotheses are commonly known as "one-tailed" and "two-tailed" tests, respectively, with the "tail" referring to the rejection region of the t-distribution (5.8, 5.9). Consequently, a two-tailed test would have rejection regions in both the positive and negative tails whereas a one-tailed test would have a single rejection region, as specified by the directional alternative hypothesis. Because the sampling distribution of F includes differences between means in both directions, a doubling of α adjusts for this difference and increases the region of rejection specified by the directional alternative hypothesis.

Unfortunately one serious disadvantage exists with using one-tailed tests: a true difference in the direction opposite to that specified by the directional alternative hypothesis *must be* statistically ignored. Because in most experiments a researcher would not ignore an effect opposite to the one predicted, the use of one-tailed tests is viewed with scepticism by most reviewers. Of course, a post hoc decision to use a one-tailed test (examine the data and then select a directional test) is not appropriate (5.19). In short, if a directional alternative hypothesis is selected, the rationale for this hypothesis must be very convincing.

5.21 EXPERIMENTAL DESIGN AND STATISTICAL MODELS

Fortunately, an isomorphism exists between many of the theoretical probability sampling models developed by statisticians (5.7) and the designs used by biologists. Hence, for every well-designed experiment an appropriate statistical model usually exists that will properly evaluate the research question(s) being asked. But biologists often select statistical models that do not match their experimental designs (see Chapter 9). In these cases, biologists may either underestimate the statistical significance of their data or artificially inflate their significance levels. Which of these consequences will occur depends on the nature of the experimental design and the statistical model (i.e., sampling distribution) used to evaluate the data.

5.22 STATISTICAL TESTS: PARAMETRIC AND NONPARAMETRIC

All forms of analysis of variance are based on the assumptions that the observations are drawn from a continuous, normally distributed population in which the variances are the same even when the treatments produce changes in the mean values of the groups. The statistical models for analyses of variance require normality and homogeneity of variance for the parameters of the population; consequently, t- and F-tests (5.18) are *parametric* tests (see Chapter 8).

In some situations, experimental data may not be compatible with these parametric assumptions (5.23) or the measurements may be on an ordinal rather than an interval scale (5.3). *Nonparametric* tests make no assumptions about either the variability or the form of the population distribution. These *distribution-free* tests are selected when a particularly high degree of variability is associated with one or more treatment conditions or where the scale of measurement (5.3) makes parametric tests inappropriate. Nonparametric tests can occasionally detect treatment differences not detected by parametric tests when the parametric test is greatly influenced by error variance.

Because of their computational simplicity nonparametric tests are easier to use than analysis of variance, and some researchers prefer nonparametric tests because with their limited assumptions regarding the population more general inferences can be drawn from the sample data (11.1). But, nonparametric tests are (*a*) not as flexible with regard to the types of hypotheses that may be tested as is analysis of variance; (*b*) not as powerful (5.12) and provide less information from the data when the assumptions underlying analysis of variance are met; and (*c*) not available for analysis of mixed factorial designs that are widely used in biological research. Hence, because of their limitations, nonparametric tests are normally used when there are no reasonable alternative parametric tests. Most nonparametric tests are based on some form of combinative analysis like binomial and multinomial distributions (Chapter 11).

5.23 ROBUSTNESS OF A STATISTICAL TEST

Certain assumptions concerning the distribution of scores within the sample groups usually must be met if a given theoretical statistic distribution (e.g., F) is to be used to determine the probability of empirical events (5.7, 5.21). The assumptions of normality, homogeneity of within-treatment variances, and independence underlie the statistical analysis of between-subject designs. However, when a between-subject design with equal sample sizes is used, the sampling distribution of F is very *robust* (insensitive to even flagrant violations of its underlying assumptions). For example, violations of the normality assumption do not constitute a serious problem, except if the violations are especially severe (see 11.1). Likewise, violations of the homogeneity of variance (variances of the different treatment populations are equal) do not appear to distort the F-distribution seriously. The F-test becomes seriously biased (increase in true α level, 5.9) when the largest within-group variance divided by the smallest within-group variable is 9 or higher. Consequently, most biologists do not routinely test the normality and homogeneity of variance assumptions when a between-subject design and about equal sample sizes are used in their experiments (but see Wilcox, 1987a,b).

However, you should become concerned about these assumptions when the observed F-ratio falls close to the critical value of F established for the experiment (5.8, 5.9). Severe violations of the normality assumption might affect the actual α level being used; an α level of .05 may be selected but because of distortions the real α level could be .07 or .08 (5.9). Similarly, relatively extreme heterogeneity (a ratio of the largest to the smallest within-group variance of 9 or higher) may increase the actual α level (Type I error) 2 to 4 percentage points above the assumed significance level.

Violations of the normality and homogeneity of variance assumptions are more serious when unequal sample sizes are present. This is one reason statisticians recommend biologists use equal sample sizes. Violations are also serious when either within-subject (4.16) or mixed factorial (4.21) designs are used. With these latter designs, the practical consequences of such violations have not been determined; consequently, probability corrections should be made (9.6).

5.24 TRANSFORMATION OF DATA

Even though the F-test is a robust statistical test (5.23) the data may still be transformed to a form that most nearly satisfies the basic assumptions underlying the analysis of variance (Chapter 6). The major reasons for using transformations are to obtain homogeneity (equality) of error variance and normality of within-treatment condition distribution. In some analysis of variance models (e.g., those with only one measure in each treatment condition) certain interaction effects are not additive and are completely confounded with experimental error (see Sokal and Rohlf, 1981). Corrections for heteroscedasticity (unequal variance), nonnormality, and nonaddivity are frequently possible by changing (transforming) the data from their original form to a different form.

The most commonly employed transformations are *logarithmic, arcsine,* and *square root* but care must be used to select the appropriate transformation (see Zar, 1974). In general, common logarithm transformation is used when means are positively correlated with variances (greater means have greater variances) or when frequency distributions are skewed to the right, or when effects are multiplicative. When the data are counts (of blood cells, of synaptic active sites, and so forth) transforming the measures to square roots will usually make the variances independent of the means. The arcsine (also known as angular) transformation is especially suited for percentages and proportions. Very often, several departures from the assumption of the analysis of variance are simultaneously corrected by the same transformation to a new scale. Hence, by making the data homoscedastic the data also approach normality and additivity of the treatment effects are ensured. If a transformation of the data does not solve a particular problem, an analogous nonparametric method may have to be selected (Chapter 11). If data must be transformed, a statistician should probably be consulted.

5.25 DERIVED MEASURES (RATIOS AND CEILING OR BOTTOM EFFECTS)

Most biological data are measurements or counts of biological responses or readings of the output of recording instruments (A.7). These observations may be regarded as directly measured dependent variables to distinguish them from derived or computed variables which are based typically on two or more independently measured variables whose relations are expressed in a certain way. Derived or computed measures are ratios, percentages, and rates. Ratios and percentages are basic research quantities in some biological fields, and rates are important in many experimental fields (see Govindarajulu, 1987).

Serious problems may occur when ratios and percentages are used in the statistical analysis and interpretation of biological data. In many cases, for example, ratios are not as accurate as measurements obtained directly, and ratios and percentages may not be approximately normally distributed as required by many statistical tests (5.22). But, the major disadvantage of ratios and percentages (particularly when expressed to an initial baseline measurement) is that information on the two variables whose ratio is being used is not usually reported. In some of these cases, spurious derived data may occur because of either ceiling or bottom effects on one of the variables used in the ratio. Ceiling effects may occur when the value of the dependent variable could not increase greatly for one group because this group's baseline response was at the upper limits of response capability, for example, heart rate at 200–220 beats per minute before treatment conditions were given. Likewise, significant bottom effects may occur when the response output could not decrease for one group as much as it could possibly decrease for any of the other groups. When ratios or percentages are used to determine significant differences among groups *standardized measures may cover up important initial differences* among groups, particularly when classification groups (4.2) are used.

5.26 REGRESSION AND MULTIPLE REGRESSION ANALYSIS

In biological research the identification of associations (relationships) between
and among sets of data is normally done by regression or correlation analysis
(5.27). *Classical regression analysis* deals only with one or more independent
variables and with a dependent variable that is not under the researcher's direct
control. Hence, the independent variable is fixed and only the dependent variable is free to vary (random). In regression analysis one variable (simple) or a
combination of variables (multiple) is used to make predictions about some
other variable. In *simple regression analysis* an independent variable (or predictor variable, X) is used to make predictions about a dependent variable (outcome variable, Y). The *independent variable* is under the control of the
researcher who selects specific values (e.g., drug doses) to be given to different
groups of animals. The use of a single independent variable (X) as the predictor
of a dependent measure (Y) involves simple regression analysis; whereas, when
two or more predictor variables are used, the procedure is known as *multiple
regression analysis* (see Table 5.4).

In simple regression analysis a mathematical procedure is used to fit a straight
line to a set of data points so that for a unit change in X, Y changes by a constant
amount over the range of observations. The line so fitted to the data is a *regression line* and the equation used is called a *regression equation*. Simple regression
which involves the linear relationship between two variables (predictor and
dependent) is also known as *bivariate regression*. In a regression equation, the
dependent (random) variable (Y) is given on the left-hand side of the equation
and the independent (fixed) variable (X) is given on the right-hand side, that is,
the regression of the dependent variable on the independent one. The formula
for simple linear regression is predicted outcome = intercept + slope × (predictor value, X). It should be noted that the regression of a variable Y on a variable X *does not* give the same mathematical relationship as the regression of X
on Y. That is, there is a basic assymmetry in the regression equation, and Y and
X are not interchangeable.

A calculated regression equation is determined on a sample of values so that
the regression coefficient b is a sample estimate of the regression coefficient (β_1)
in the study population (1.3, 4.6). Given certain assumptions (see Table 5.5), the
standard error of the regression coefficient can be computed which gives a confidence interval estimate for the unknown value of β_1. Thus, confidence intervals
and significance tests are available for the regression coefficient (β_1) based on the
standard error of sample values. Tests for the value of the β_0 (the Y intercept) are
also available but these are seldom used.

In some cases in which some kind of curve exists in the set of data points,
transformation of the data (5.24) by taking the logarithm of the variables may
lead to a linear relationship. A linear regression analysis would then be done on
the transformed data. In other cases, a trend analysis of the data may be appropriate to evaluate curvilinear and other relationships (6.16). In a given data set,
a single extreme value (outlier) can have a profound effect on the relation derived
from the regression line. Without remeasurement (of this extreme point) or

using a larger sample, whether the anomalous value is a "fluke" or a representative value of the extreme range of the sampled population cannot be determined. Hence, with very small sample sizes regression analysis may be biased by outlying data points. If regression analysis is used, you should examine the residuals which contain the information in the data *not* explained by the fitted regression line (see Atkinson, 1987; Godfrey, 1986a).

A multiple regression equation can be fitted to observed data by methods similar to those used for simple *bivariate regression*. A multiple regression analysis, however, requires some theoretical model to be postulated that would determine beforehand which variables could be appropriately included (see Sokal and Rohlf, 1981). Multiple regression analysis can be performed by many computer-based programs but questions regarding the optimal number of predictors, the relative importance of various predictors, and the selection of predictors do not have universally accepted answers. For these reasons a statistician should be consulted if a multiple regression analysis is part of the research plan to evaluate biological data. The advantages of multiple linear regression as compared with traditional analysis of variance (Chapter 6) for biological research has been discussed by Slinker and Glantz (1988).

Regression analysis in which the researcher assigns or fixes the level of the independent variable normally allows strong inferences of causality to be drawn. This is not the case when fixed assignment is not used as in *classical correlation analysis* (5.27) in which the subjects "select themselves" for assignment of the predictor variables (see Tables 5.4 and 5.5).

5.27 CORRELATION ANALYSIS

In correlation analysis one variable is used to make predictions about some other variable. But, unlike regression analysis (5.26) neither the predictor variable nor the dependent variable are manipulated by the researcher. Hence, classical cor-

Table 5.4 Similarities and Differences Between Correlation and Regression Analyses (5.26, 5.27)[a]

Correlation	Regression
Purpose: To determine whether two variables are related (data reduction, descriptive function).	*Purpose:* To determine whether one dependent variable (Y) can be predicted from one independent variable (X).
Symbol: r (measure of linear association) ranging from -1.00 thru $+1.00$.	*Symbol:* General equation for straight line, $Y = \beta_0 + \beta_1 (X)$, β_0 is the Y intercept, the value of the Y coordinate where the line crosses the Y axis. β_1 is the slope of the line and measures the amount of change in Y per unit increase in X (measure of linear prediction).
Causality: Correlation does not imply causality.	*Causality:* Statements of causality may be possible.

[a]See this book section.

Table 5.5 Variables and Assumptions of Correlation and Regression Analyses

Correlation (5.27)[a]	Regression (5.26)
Both variables are random (free to vary, i.e., not under the control of the researcher).	Independent variable (X) is fixed (under researcher's control) and dependent variable (Y) is random (free to vary).
Measured on interval or ratio scale.	
Two variables have a bivariate normal distribution.	
Pair of observations independent.	Equal variability about each conditional mean (homoscedasticity).
Measuring the degree of relationship between variables that are linearly related.	For any given value of X, the conditional distribution of Y values is normally distributed.
The square of correlation coefficient, r^2, indicates the proportion of variance in one of the variables accounted for by the variance of scores of the other variable (the coefficient of determination).	Y observations are independent of each other.

[a]See this book section.

relation analysis typically deals with paired variables, both of which are random (i.e., free to vary). Distribution of paired variables (such as height and weight; white cell count and body temperature) are known as bivariate distributions. *Correlation studies* only establish the degree of association (relatedness) between variables and *do not permit causal inference*.

The Pearson correlation coefficient r is a measure of the linear relation between two random variables. The coefficient may vary between -1.00 and $+1.00$ where 0 signifies the absence of a relation and either -1.00 or $+1.00$ indicates a perfect relationship: A *positive correlation* implies a direct relation between the variables, as X increases Y increases, and a *negative correlation* implies an inverse relation, as X increases Y decreases. In summary, the correlation coefficient r is a measure of the strength of the linear association between two variables, X and Y, and the closer r comes to either $+1.00$ or -1.00, the stronger is the relation and the more nearly it approximates a straight line. A scatter diagram (also called a scatterplot or scattergram) allows you to view the relationship between the two variables. The predictor variable traditionally is represented on the abscissa, or X axis, the criterion variable on the ordinate, or Y axis.

One limitation of the correlation coefficient is that it is not a valid measure of the strength of a nonlinear relation. A small correlation between two variables may occur because there is only a weak linear association between the two variables or because large errors in measurement occur. Also, the question of reliability of the correlation when the sample size is fewer than 50 pairs of observations must be considered. *Outliers* (pairs of observations that clearly are out of the range of the other pairs) have a marked effect on the correlation coefficient, often suggest erroneous data, and are likely to give misleading results (Beckman and Cook, 1983). Although these outlier values are substantially remote from the rest of the data they cannot be discarded as being erroneous measurements or miscalculations unless additional independent information is available (e.g., laboratory record indicates the particular tissue sample was dropped). Given these limitations, therefore, correlation analysis has a restricted use in biological research with small sample sizes. But a statistically significant correlation between two variables in the biomedical literature may suggest a hypothesis for subsequent experimental study. Tables 5.4 and 5.5 summarize the important similarities and differences between correlation (5.27) and regression (5.26) analyses.

6

Analysis of Variance (ANOVA)

6.1 ANALYSIS OF VARIANCE: FIXED AND RANDOM FACTOR MODELS

A *fixed factor* structural model is used in most biological research. With a fixed factor structural model, the levels of the independent variables are selected arbitrarily and systematically. Hence, statistical generalizations are limited to the treatment effects observed with the treatment conditions selected by the researcher. A fixed factor model is widely used in biological research because the treatment levels (conditions) included in an experiment usually cover all possible levels of interest to the researcher or the levels selected are thought to be representative of the independent variables.

In contrast, with a *random factor* structural model the levels of an independent variable are selected either randomly or unsystematically from a population of all possible levels (study population, 1.3). This selection procedure produces a random sample from the population of all treatment levels (1.3). The advantage of a random factor model is that statistical generalization (4.6) permits any significant effects observed in the experiment to be extended to the population of all possible levels. A disadvantage of using a *random factor* model is that there is no guarantee that effective levels of the independent variable (e.g., drug dose, stimulation frequency) would be included in the experiment. For this reason biologists systematically select levels of the independent variable, some of which they expect will have significant effects. With a *fixed factor* structural model, fairly simple rules may be specified for the details of the statistical analysis including the selection of appropriate error terms (6.3, 6.4, 6.5, 6.6). Most of the research done by biologists uses independent variables with fixed effects (factors).

In summary, the factors in a study may all be either fixed or all random or some may be associated with fixed effects and others with random effects. The ANOVA statistical models corresponding to these situations are called fixed models, random models, or mixed models, respectively. It is sometimes difficult to decide whether a particular experiment is studying random effects or fixed effects. The criterion which separates random and fixed effects is whether the different levels of the factor selected can be considered a *random sample* of more of such levels or are *fixed treatments* whose differences you wish to contrast (see Sokal and Rohlf, 1981).

6.2. ANALYSIS OF VARIANCE: NESTED FACTORS

Any effects which are restricted to a single level of a factor are said to be nested within that factor. In biological research, nested factors are usually associated with subjects (9.2, 9.3). For example, in a one-factor between-subject design (4.10) the variability due to factor A (the treatment levels a_1, a_2, and so forth) and the pooled variability of subjects treated alike can be isolated. In this case, "subjects" can be considered a factor (S) consisting of s different levels, that is, s different subjects. Because a different collection of s subjects is used in each of the a levels of the independent variable, factor S (subjects) does not cross with the levels (a_1, a_2) of factor A (Table 4.1). The definition of "subjects" as a factor is different at each level of factor A and, hence, factor S qualifies as a nested factor. Thus, the source of variance, S/A, is referred to as the variability of subjects nested within factor A. Whenever the symbol S/A is used *the letter to the left of the diagonal designates the nested factor and the letter to the right of the diagonal designates the factor within which the nesting occurs* (i.e., S within A or S nested in A). Normally, with between-subject experimental designs the factor S is assumed and therefore not described. A two-factor between-subject design (4.13) would be described simply as an A X B factorial design and not as an A X B X S factorial design. The error term (6.6) in this latter design would be S/AB, the variability of subjects nested within factors AB (see Keppel, 1982).

In a one-factor within-subject design (4.16), subjects cross with factor A because each of the s subjects serve in *all* the a treatment levels, an (A $\times$ S) factorial with each subject represented at all levels of factor A. The parentheses in an (A $\times$ S) design mean that factor A is a within-subject manipulation ($\times$ S) and both the independent factor (A) and subjects (factor S) are completely crossed; that is, each subject receives each of the levels (a_1, a_2, and so forth) of treatment A.

6.3 ANALYSIS OF VARIANCE TABLE

The analysis of variance partitions the total variability in an experiment (the total sum of squares) into components (sum of squares) due to between-treatment and within-treatment variability (5.16). These sums of squares are divided by the appropriate degrees of freedom (5.17) to yield mean squares for the various sources of variance. One or more of these mean squares will provide estimates of treatment effects plus experimental error; whereas other sources will provide estimates of experimental error only (within-subject variability). F-ratios of mean squares of treatment-experimental error and mean squares of experimental error (error term) provide a measure of differences among the treatment conditions (5.16).

An analysis of variance (ANOVA) table normally presents the source of variance (6.4), the variance for each source, the degrees of freedom (5.17) for each source, and F-values with their probability of occurrence (5.9). In some tables, the mean squares for each F-value may be given. In most tables, however, the mean squares for the F-values have to be calculated by dividing the variances by their appropriate degrees of freedom (5.17). To determine whether an appropriate statistical model was used to analyze reported data, you must know the sources of variance, the degrees of freedom, and the mean squares for each F-value. If the value of the statistic and its degrees of freedom are presented together in a research paper, you can usually determine whether appropriate comparisons were made. For example, the statement $F(2, 186) = 7.21, p < .001$ indicates that the treatment (condition) mean square has 2 degrees of freedom $F(2, 186)$, its error mean square has 186 degrees of freedom $F(2, 186)$, the magnitude of the F-ratio (7.21) would have occurred by chance only 1 out of 1000 times ($p < .001$). With this information provided for each F-ratio, the analysis of variance model used to assess significance levels can usually be determined (6.4, 6.5, 6.6).

6.4 PARTITIONING OF VARIANCE

A useful system for identifying and labeling the sources of variation in any given experimental design *with all fixed effects* (6.1) is discussed in Lindman (1974, pp. 176–178) and Keppel (1982, pp. 635–643; 1991, pp. 488–498). This system uses capital letters (A, B, and so forth) to represent the factors in an experiment which, alone or with other letters, are used to represent the different sources of variation. From this primary list of factors, df statements (6.5) can be generated and, if required, computational formulas for the sum of squares can also be written from expanded df statements (see Keppel, 1982).

The required rules in this system for a *fixed factor* structural ANOVA model are

Rule 1: List all the factors in the experiment including subjects (Factor S, 6.2) and assume that they all can be multiplied (they all cross).

Rule 2: List all possible main effects (6.7) and tabulate all interactions (6.12) among these factors by multiplying each factor with all other factors.

Rule 3: Substitute nested notation whenever a nested factor appears in the list (6.2).

Rule 4: Delete from the list impossible nested factors which are identified when the same letter (or letters) appears (or appear) on both sides of the diagonal.

In a single-factor design in which factor A is represented by independent groups of subjects (S), the rules of the system would produce the outcomes listed in Table 6.1.

6.5 PARTITIONING OF THE DEGREES OF FREEDOM (df)

For each factor in an experiment (6.3), its degrees of freedom (df, 5.17) will be given by the formula: levels of the factor (a) minus 1, that is, ($a - 1$). In a four-factor experiment (A, B, C, and S), the levels (number) of each factor would be represented by (a), (b), (c), and (s), and the degrees of freedom associated with

Table 6.1 Identifying the Source of Variance, Degrees of Freedom, and Error Term in a Single-Factor Experiment with Two or More Independent Groups: $A \times S^a$

Rule 1	Rule 2	Rule 3	Rule 4 (6.4)[b]
A	A	A	A
S	S	S/A	S/A
	$A \times S$	$A \times S/A$	—

Source of variance (6.4)[b]	df statement (6.5)[b]	Error term (6.6)[b]
A	$(a - 1)$	S/A
S/A	$(s - 1)(a)$	
Total	$(a)(s) - 1$	

[a]Factor S represents subjects and is not normally presented when describing between-subject designs (6.2).
[b]See this book section.

each factor would be $(a - 1)$, $(b - 1)(c - 1)$, and $(s - 1)$. Because the factor S is not used when describing between-subject designs (6.2), this design would be labeled a three-factor experiment (6.14). Also using $(s - 1)$ as the df statement for subjects assumes that an *equal* number of subjects is in each subgroup of the experiment. If not, the following rules will not produce correct df statements when s or $(s - 1)$ are included. Calculation of df for groups with unequal numbers may be found in most biostatistics books (e.g., Rosner, 1990; Sokal and Rohlf, 1981).

Once any source of variance is obtained (6.4), its df statement can be written by the following two additional rules:

Rule 5: If the source contains no nested factors (6.2), multiply the df's associated with the factors listed in the source.

$$df_{A \times B} = (df_A)(df_B) = (a - 1)(b - 1)$$
$$df_{A \times B \times C} = (df_A)(df_B)(df_C) = (a - 1)(b - 1)(c - 1).$$

Rule 6: If the source contains nested factors multiply (1) the product of the df's of the factors given on the left of the diagonal by (2) the product of the *levels* of factors given on the right of the diagonal.

$$df_{S/A} = (df_S)(a) = (s - 1)(a)$$
$$df_{C \times S/B} = (df_C)(df_S)(b) = (c - 1)(s - 1)(b)$$

6.6 SELECTING ERROR TERMS

Once the different sources of variance have been identified (6.4), the appropriate error term for each source of variance can be determined by the following two rules:

Rule 7: If a source contains no repeated factors, the error term is factor S (subjects), that is, S/A, S/AB, S/ABC, and so forth (6.2).

Rule 8: If a source contains a repeated factor or factors, the error term is an interaction of factor S (subjects) with the repeated factor or factors, that is, B X S/A, C X S/AB, and so forth (6.4).

The application of Rules 1 through 8 to identify the sources of variance (6.4), to partition the degrees of freedom (6.5), and to select the appropriate error terms (6.6) for a variety of between-subject, within-subject, and mixed factorial designs are presented in Tables 6.2 to 6.11. These tables may be used as reference sources to reconstruct the ANOVA tables of published reports (6.3).

6.7 ANOVA MAIN EFFECT: TWO TREATMENT CONDITIONS

In a one-factor between-subject design (4.10) with only two groups, a significant F-ratio or t-value (5.18) indicates a significant difference exists between the two treatment conditions (see Table 4.1). Likewise, in a within-subject design (4.16) with only two treatment conditions a significant difference between the means of these two treatment conditions is indicated by a significant F-ratio or t-value.

6.8 ANOVA MAIN EFFECT: THREE OR MORE TREATMENT CONDITIONS

The F-ratio and the theoretical sampling distribution of the F-statistic are used to evaluate the null hypothesis that population treatment means are equal (1.6,

Table 6.2 Identifying the Source of Variance, Degrees of Freedom, and Error Term in a Two-Factor Between-Subject Experiment: A X B X S[a]

Rule 1	Rule 2	Rule 3	Rule 4 (6.4)[b]
A	A	A	A
B	B	B	B
S	S	S/AB	S/AB
	A X B	A X B	A X B
	A X S	A X S/AB	–
	B X S	B X S/AB	–
	A X B X S	A X B X S/AB	–

Source of variance (6.4)[b]	df statement (6.5)[b]	Error term (6.6)[b]
A	$(a-1)$	S/AB
B	$(b-1)$	S/AB
A X B	$(a-1)(b-1)$	S/AB
S/AB	$(s-1)(a)(b)$	
Total	$(a)(b)(s)-1$	

[a]Factor S represents subjects and is normally not presented when describing between-subject designs (6.2).
[b]See this book section.

Table 6.3 Identifying the Source of Variance, Degrees of Freedom, and Error Terms in a Complete Within-Subject Two-Factor Design: (A $\times$ B $\times$ S)

Rule 1	Rule 2	Rule 3	Rule 4 (6.4)[a]
A	A	A	A
B	B	B	B
S	S	S	S
	A $\times$ B	A $\times$ B	A $\times$ B
	A $\times$ S	A $\times$ S	A $\times$ S
	B $\times$ S	B $\times$ S	B $\times$ S
	A $\times$ B $\times$ S	A $\times$ B $\times$ S	A $\times$ B $\times$ S

Source of variance (6.4)[a]	df statement (6.5)[a]	Error term (6.6)[a]
A	$(a-1)$	A $\times$ S
B	$(b-1)$	B $\times$ S
S	$(s-1)$	
A $\times$ B	$(a-1)(b-1)$	A $\times$ B $\times$ S
A $\times$ S	$(a-1)(s-1)$	
B $\times$ S	$(b-1)(s-1)$	
A $\times$ B $\times$ S	$\underline{(a-1)(b-1)(s-1)}$	
Total	$(a)(b)(s)-1$	

[a]See this book section.

Table 6.4 Identifying the Source of Variance, Degrees of Freedom, and Error Terms in a Mixed Factorial Design: A $\times$ (B $\times$ S)

Rule 1	Rule 2	Rule 3	Rule 4 (6.4)[a]
A	A	A	A
B	B	B	B
S	S	S/A	S/A
	A $\times$ B	A $\times$ B	A $\times$ B
	A $\times$ S	A $\times$ S/A	–
	B $\times$ S	B $\times$ S/A	B $\times$ S/A
	A $\times$ B $\times$ S	A $\times$ B $\times$ S/A	–

Source of variance (6.4)[a]	df statement (6.5)[a]	Error term (6.6)[a]
A	$(a-1)$	S/A
B	$(b-1)$	B $\times$ S/A
S/A	$(s-1)(a)$	
A $\times$ B	$(a-1)(b-1)$	B $\times$ S/A
B $\times$ S/A	$\underline{(b-1)(s-1)(a)}$	
Total	$(a)(b)(s)-1$	

[a]See this book section.

Table 6.5 Identifying the Source of Variance, Degrees of Freedom, and Error Term in a Three-Factor Between-Subject Design: A × B × C × S[a]

Rule 1	Rule 2	Rule 3	Rule 4 (6.4)[b]
A	A	A	A
B	B	B	B
C	C	C	C
S	S	S/ABC	S/ABC
	A × B	A × B	A × B
	A × C	A × C	A × C
	A × S	A × S/ABC	–
	B × C	B × C	B × C
	B × S	B × S/ABC	–
	C × S	C × S/ABC	–
	A × B × C	A × B × C	A × B × C
	A × B × S	A × B × S/ABC	–
	A × C × S	A × C × S/ABC	–
	B × C × S	B × C × S/ABC	–
	A × B × C × S	A × B × C × S/ABC	–

Souce of variance (6.4)[b]	df statement (6.5)[b]	Error term (6.6)[b]
A	$(a - 1)$	Ṡ/ABC
B	$(b - 1)$	S/ABC
C	$(c - 1)$	S/ABC
A × B	$(a - 1)(b - 1)$	S/ABC
A × C	$(a - 1)(c - 1)$	S/ABC
B × C	$(b - 1)(c - 1)$	S/ABC
A × B × C	$(a - 1)(b - 1)(c - 1)$	S/ABC
S/ABC	$\underline{(s - 1)(a)(b)(c)}$	
Total	$(a)(b)(c)(s) - 1$	

[a]Factor S represents subjects and is normally not presented when describing between-subject designs (6.2).
[b]See this book section.

Table 6.6 Identifying the Source of Variance in a Mixed Factorial Design: A × B × (C × S)

Rule 1	Rule 2	Rule 3	Rule 4 (6.4)[a]
A	A	A	A
B	B	B	B
C	C	C	C
S	S	S/AB	S/AB
	A × B	A × B	A × B
	A × C	A × C	A × C
	A × S	A × S/AB	–
	B × C	B × C	B × C
	B × S	B × S/AB	–
	C × S	C × S/AB	C × S/AB
	A × B × S	A × B × S/AB	–
	A × C × S	A × C × S/AB	–
	B × C × S	B × C × S/AB	–
	A × B × C	A × B × C	A × B × C
	A × B × C × S	A × B × C × S/AB	–

[a]See this book section.

Table 6.7 Identifying the Degrees of Freedom and Error Terms in a Mixed Factorial Design: A × B × (C × S) (Table 6.6)

Source of variance (6.4)[a]	df statement (6.5)[a]	Error term (6.6)[a]
A	$(a-1)$	S/AB
B	$(b-1)$	S/AB
C	$(c-1)$	C × S/AB
S/AB	$(s-1)(a)(b)$	
A × B	$(a-1)(b-1)$	S/AB
A × C	$(a-1)(c-1)$	C × S/AB
B × C	$(b-1)(c-1)$	C × S/AB
A × B × C	$(a-1)(b-1)(c-1)$	C × S/AB
C × S/AB	$(c-1)(s-1)(a)(b)$	
Total	$(a(b)(c)(s)-1$	

[a]See this book section.

Table 6.8 Identifying the Source of Variance in a Mixed Factorial Design: A × (B × C × S)

Rule 1	Rule 2	Rule 3	Rule 4 (6.4)[a]
A	A	A	A
B	B	B	B
C	C	C	C
S	S	S/A	S/A
	A × B	A × B	A × B
	A × C	A × C	A × C
	A × S	A × S/A	–
	B × C	B × C	B × C
	B × S	B × S/A	B × S/A
	C × S	C × S/A	C × S/A
	A × B × S	A × B × S/A	–
	A × C × S	A × C × S/A	–
	B × C × S	B × C × S/A	B × C × S/A
	A × B × C	A × B × C	A × B × C
	A × B × C × S	A × B × C × S/A	–

[a]See this book section.

Table 6.9 Identifying the Degrees of Freedom and Error Terms in a Mixed Factorial Design: A × (B × C × S) (Table 6.8)

Source of variance (6.4)[a]	df statement (6.5)[a]	Error term (6.6)[a]
A	$(a-1)$	S/A
B	$(b-1)$	B × S/A
C	$(c-1)$	C × S/A
S/A	$(s-1)(a)$	
A × B	$(a-1)(b-1)$	B × S/A
A × C	$(a-1)(c-1)$	C × S/A
B × C	$(b-1)(c-1)$	B × C × S/A
B × S/A	$(b-1)(s-1)(a)$	
C × S/A	$(c-1)(s-1)(a)$	
B × C × S/A	$(b-1)(c-1)(s-1)(a)$	
A × B × C	$(a-1)(b-1)(c-1)$	B × C × S/A
Total	$(a)(b)(c)(s)-1$	

[a]See this book section.

Table 6.10　Identifying the Source of Variance in a Complete Within-Subject Three-Factor Design: (A $\times$ B $\times$ C $\times$ S)

Rule 1	Rule 2	Rule 3	Rule 4 (6.4)[a]
A	A	A	A
B	B	B	B
C	C	C	C
S	S	S	S
	A $\times$ B	A $\times$ B	A $\times$ B
	A $\times$ C	A $\times$ C	A $\times$ C
	A $\times$ S	A $\times$ S	A $\times$ S
	B $\times$ C	B $\times$ C	B $\times$ C
	B $\times$ S	B $\times$ S	B $\times$ S
	C $\times$ S	C $\times$ S	C $\times$ S
	A $\times$ B $\times$ C	A $\times$ B $\times$ C	A $\times$ B $\times$ C
	A $\times$ B $\times$ S	A $\times$ B $\times$ S	A $\times$ B $\times$ S
	A $\times$ C $\times$ S	A $\times$ C $\times$ S	A $\times$ C $\times$ S
	B $\times$ C $\times$ S	B $\times$ C $\times$ S	B $\times$ C $\times$ S
	A $\times$ B $\times$ C $\times$ S	A $\times$ B $\times$ C $\times$ S	A $\times$ B $\times$ C $\times$ S

[a]See this book section.

5.5). In a single-factor between-subject design (4.10) one mean square (MS_A) in addition to estimating experimental error also reflects the presence of any treatment effect in the population. This mean square is divided by a mean square ($MS_{S/A}$) which estimates only experimental error (5.16). Hence, the F-ratio formed ($MS_A/MS_{S/A}$) to evaluate the null hypothesis is often called the *overall*, or *omnibus*, F-test.

Table 6.11　Identifying the Degrees of Freedom and Error Terms in a Complete Within-Subject Three-Factor Design: (A $\times$ B $\times$ C $\times$ S) (Table 6.10)

Source of variance (6.4)[a]	df statement (6.5)[a]	Error term (6.6)[a]
A	$(a-1)$	A $\times$ S
B	$(b-1)$	B $\times$ S
C	$(c-1)$	C $\times$ S
S	$(s-1)$	
A $\times$ B	$(a-1)(b-1)$	A $\times$ B $\times$ S
A $\times$ C	$(a-1)(c-1)$	A $\times$ C $\times$ S
A $\times$ S	$(a-1)(s-1)$	
B $\times$ C	$(b-1)(c-1)$	B $\times$ C $\times$ S
B $\times$ S	$(b-1)(s-1)$	
C $\times$ S	$(c-1)(s-1)$	
A $\times$ B $\times$ C	$(a-1)(b-1)(c-1)$	A $\times$ B $\times$ C $\times$ S
A $\times$ B $\times$ S	$(a-1)(b-1)(s-1)$	
A $\times$ C $\times$ S	$(a-1)(c-1)(s-1)$	
B $\times$ C $\times$ S	$(b-1)(c-1)(s-1)$	
A $\times$ B $\times$ C $\times$ S	$(a-1)(b-1)(c-1)(s-1)$	
Total	$(a)(b)(c)(s)-1$	

[a]See this book section.

In a two-treatment experiment (6.7), this omnibus F-ratio tests directly whether a significant difference exists between the two treatments given to the same subjects (within-group design, 4.16) or between experimental and control subjects (between-group design, 4.10). If four groups of subjects are used in a between-subject design with only one factor or four treatments are given to the same group of subjects in a within-subject design, the F-ratio would be based, in each case, on the deviation of four means (see Table 4.3). In these cases, a significant overall F-test indicates *at least* two of the treatment means are significantly different but does not indicate which means are significantly different from each other or even if more than one pair of comparisons is significant.

In these experiments, the null and alternative hypotheses (1.6, 5.5), formally stated, are

$$H_0: \mu_i = \mu_2 = \mu_3 = \mu_4 \quad \text{and} \quad H_i: \text{ not } H_0.$$

The omnibus F-test, which is the proper analysis to test these hypotheses, is the most conservative test that could be used. This overall F-test requires a very large difference between means to attain significance and reject H_0. The reason for this conservatism is that there are 25 possible combinations of mean comparisons (pairs and combinations) when there are four treatment means (6.9). The F-test evaluates all these 25 comparisons and maintains the overall level of significance at some previously specified level (e.g., .05 or .01). If the F-test is significant, H_0 is rejected, and the alternative hypothesis (H_i: not H_0) is asserted. But, the alternative hypothesis, H_i, is very vague, indicating only that at least 1 of the 25 pair comparisons of means is significantly different from zero. Determining which of the pair comparisons of means are significantly different from zero requires further analyses using *unplanned* (post hoc) multiple comparison tests (6.9, Chapter 10).

6.9 POST HOC MULTIPLE COMPARISON TESTS

Multiple treatment comparisons may be classified into two types: *planned* and *unplanned* comparisons. If a detailed analysis plan (including individual pairwise comparisons) is formulated *before* the data are collected these individual (analytical) comparisons are called planned comparisons (6.10). In contrast, unplanned comparisons (post hoc multiple comparisons) are comparisons that are suggested after the data are evaluated by an overall analysis (6.8), that is, they are not specifically predicted (not expected) before the start of an experiment. A significant overall F-ratio (6.8) in which three or more treatment means are compared would indicate that subsequent post hoc multiple comparisons are necessary to determine which treatments differ significantly from each other (6.8). In this situation, therefore, you would use a significant overall F-ratio to guide subsequent analysis of differences among treatment means.

The major problem in performing a series of post hoc comparisons is that as the number of comparisons increases so does the likelihood of making Type I errors (5.10). Type I errors accumulate in a predictable manner with each statistical test performed in a series of such comparisons. If several comparisons are made in an experiment, each at $\alpha = .05$, the probability of making a Type I error would be .05 for each of the comparisons. But, the probability of making one or more Type I errors *in the total set of comparisons* would be greater than .05. This increased Type I error rate has been called the *familywise (FW) error rate* to distinguish it from the *Type I error per comparison (pc)*.

The relationship between these two Type I error rates is given by the formula:

$$\alpha(FW) = 1 - [1 - \alpha(pc)]^c$$

where c represents the number of orthogonal (independent) comparisons that are conducted. With the pc error set at $\alpha = .05$ and with *three comparisons*, the FW type error rate is

$$\alpha(FW) = 1 - (1 - .05)^3 = 1 - (.95)^3 = 1 - .857 = .143.$$

As may be seen, the FW type error increases directly with the number of comparisons made. With $c = 6$, for example, the FW type error rate is

$$\alpha(FW) = 1 - (1 - .05)^6 = 1 - (.95)^6 = 1 - .735 = .265.$$

The familywise error rate may be approximated by the formula FW = $c[\alpha(pc)]$, that is, for three comparisons and $\alpha(pc)$ set at .05, the resulting value would be 3(.05) = .15; whereas, the correct probability would be .143. Likewise, for six comparisons and $\alpha(pc)$ set at .05, the approximation value would be 6(.05) = .30 whereas the correct probability would be .265. The importance of familywise error rate is obvious when the total number of possible differences between pairs of mean comparisons in an experiment is considered. For example, in a single-factor between-group experiment with three groups ($a = 3$), there are three such comparisons; for $a = 4$ there are six and for a = 5 there are 10 (see Table 10.1). If you consider all possible comparisons (both pairs of treatment means and complex combinations, 6.10), then the potential number of post hoc tests increases dramatically. If $a = 3$ the total number of pairwise *and* complex comparisons is six. If $a = 4$ the total number of pairwise *and* complex comparisons is 25. If $a = 5$ the total number of pairwise *and* complex comparisons is 90. Fortunately, most biologists are concerned only with evaluating the differences between pairs of treatment means (Chapter 10).

Many statistical procedures are available to deal with the increased FW error rate associated with post hoc comparisons (Chapter 10). Unfortunately, statisticians do not agree as to how best to correct for the increase in FW error rate. All suggested approaches, however, use the same basic strategy to cope with this problem, namely to reduce the size of the critical region—that is, to lower progressively the significance level as the number of means to be compared increases (5.8, 5.9). If the size of the rejection region is reduced, fewer Type I errors will be committed and consequently the FW error rate will be lowered. The various test statistics proposed differ in the ways in which the reduction in pc rate is made. Decreasing the size of the critical region, however, makes it more difficult to reject the null hypothesis; consequently, Type II error would increase (5.10). Increasing Type II error decreases the power of the multiple test procedure (5.12), and *each post hoc multiple comparison procedure must cope with the relation between the two types of errors of statistical inference* (5.10). Many multiple comparison procedures are available for selection, and they range from "liberal" (those that will detect many differences, and make more Type I errors) to "conservative" (those that will detect few differences, and make more Type II errors). The most widely used multiple comparison tests, in order of decreasing power (5.12), are the Duncan multiple range test, the Student-Newman-Keuls test, the Tukey test, and the Scheffe' test (Chapter 10, Table 10.2).

6.10 PLANNED COMPARISONS: ORTHOGONAL CONTRASTS

The primary requirement for analytical *planned* comparisons is that the analysis plan be formulated *before the data are collected* (6.9). Two additional restrictions in using planned comparison are (1) the number of comparisons should not exceed the number of degrees of freedom, df (6.5), for treatment conditions, and (2) the comparisons should be orthogonal (i.e., independent of each other).

An experiment using planned comparisons produces the greatest statistical power (i.e., the highest likelihood of finding a significant difference if the null hypothesis is false, 5.12) because, given their restriction, planned comparisons require the least difference between means to obtain significance (5.8, 5.9). With planned comparisons, a significant overall F value (6.8) is not required before making these specific comparisons. If the plan of your experiment lists specific a priori comparisons, you are justified in making these comparisons.

The simple rule to follow is: specify the experimental hypotheses and make exact tests of their statistical alternatives. If the statistical hypothesis requires an overall F-test then this comparison should be made. As more experiments are done in a particular research area, it may become possible to design an experiment to explicitly test a set of particular hypotheses. In a single experiment, several explicit hypotheses can be tested. These hypotheses may contrast two means (pairwise comparison) or two sets of means (complex comparison). In a four-group between-subject design, for example, you may only be interested in three specific comparisons. The three null hypotheses and their alternatives may be

Null hypothesis I	H_0:	$\mu_1 = \mu_2$
Alternative hypothesis I	H_i:	$\mu_1 \neq \mu_2$
Null hypothesis II	H_0:	$\mu_3 = \mu_4$
Alternative hypothesis II	H_i:	$\mu_3 \neq \mu_4$
Null hypothesis III	H_0:	$(\mu_1 + \mu_2) = (\mu_3 + \mu_4)$
Alternative hypothesis III	H_i:	$(\mu_1 + \mu_2) \neq (\mu_3 + \mu_4)$

In this example, you would not make an overall F-test because this test would not evaluate any of the specified comparisons. Note, that the three null hypotheses are orthogonal to each other (i.e., they are independent comparisons). Also, because the planned comparisons of pairs of means and combinations of means are orthogonal three specific tests can be made given the number of df's available (5.17, 6.5). In a between-subject design with four groups, there would be three df's ($a - 1 = 3$) available for planned comparisons. The difference between means required for significance is less for these three planned comparisons than required for an overall F-test in a between-subject design with four groups. The reason is that only 3 of the 25 possible comparisons (pairs and combinations) are being evaluated (6.9). Hence, the likelihood of obtaining a significant difference by chance alone is much less when only three comparisons are planned, and the value of the test statistic necessary to achieve statistical significance is consequently reduced. For planned comparisons the method of orthogonal contrasts using sets of orthogonal coefficients is described in many applied statistics books (e.g., see Keppel, 1982, pp. 103–124; Keppel and Zedeck, 1989, pp. 150–159; Howell, 1987, pp. 337–339; Sokal and Rohlf, 1981, pp. 232–242).

Unfortunately, planned comparisons in biological research are rare events; therefore, a strong rationale for each planned comparison should be given. Reviewers and editors must be convinced that these comparisons were the only ones of interest, and were not selected after the data were examined by the researcher, that is, post hoc (6.9). In some cases, various treatment conditions may be compared with the same control condition. In this situation, the comparisons are not independent of each other (not orthogonal) as the same control group is used in all of the comparisons. A Dunnett test, however, may be used to make these types of comparisons (Chapter 10, 10.6).

6.11 THE SEARCH FOR SIGNIFICANCE

The conceptual distinction between planned (6.10) and unplanned (6.9) analytical comparisons cannot be overemphasized. Unfortunately, some biologists become concerned primarily with obtaining significance in the statistical analysis of their data. A significant difference among the treatment conditions (i.e., a positive experimental result) is more likely to lead to a publication then when only negative results (no significant differences among groups) are found. After the data have been examined, it is relatively easy to convince oneself that the comparisons of interest are only those that show the largest differences among the treatment means. Hence, these comparisons may evolve into planned comparisons which makes it easier to reject the null hypothesis and to publish the experimental results.

Even if the distinction between planned and unplanned comparisons is maintained, the post hoc multiple-test procedure (Chapter 10) selected may be the one which produces a significant difference between the most "interesting" treatment means. Most statisticians are familiar with the researcher who complains that "I know there is a significant difference between these two conditions but the statistical test I used was not significant. What should I do? Is there any test that will confirm a significant difference does exist between the two conditions?" In these cases, the multiple comparison test is not selected by a careful consideration of the possible errors of statistical inference, but rather on whether a significant difference among the groups of interest can be obtained.

6.12 INTERACTION: DEFINITIONS

An interaction assesses the joint effects of two factors (or the simultaneous effects of three or more factors) on a given biological response. An interaction can be defined in various ways; each definition emphasizing different aspects of the same concept. Two such definitions for an A X B interaction would be

Table 6.12 Partitioning of the Total Sum of Squares in a Two-Way Analysis of Variance: A × B

Total variability	
Between-group variability	Within-group variability
Effects of factor A (main effects of A) Effects of factor B (main effects of B) Joint effects of factors A and B (A × B interaction)	Estimate of the variability of subjects treated alike (S/AB): Effects of uncontrolled or "chance" factors (estimate of experimental error)

1. An interaction is present when the effects of one independent variable (A) on a biological response *change* at different levels of the second independent variable (B).
2. An interaction is present when the simple main effects of one independent variable (A) *are not* the same at different levels of the second independent variable (B).

In summary, the dependence of the effect of one factor (A) on the level of another factor (B) is called an interaction. A significant interaction is present when the effects of two treatment conditions (A, B) applied together cannot be predicted from the averaged response of the separate factors, A and B. These averaged responses of A and B are called main effects. The presence of a significant interaction requires researchers to qualify their statements regarding main effects because, in most instances, an overall statement for each separate treatment condition would have little meaning. The relation among main effects and the A × B interaction (6.13) in a two-way analysis of variance is illustrated in Tables 6.12 and 6.13.

Table 6.13 Analysis of an A × B Interaction for a 2 × 2 Factorial Design (6.12, 6.13)[a]

	Levels of factor A		
Levels of factor B	A_1	A_2	Row means
			(Main effects of factor B)
B_1	Ma_1b_1	Ma_2b_1	$\bar{M}B_1$
B_2	Ma_1b_2	Ma_2b_2	$\bar{M}B_2$
Column means	$\bar{M}A_1$	$\bar{M}A_2$	
	(Main effects of factor A)		

M is the mean (average) of an individual treatment condition (e.g., Ma_1b_1, Ma_2b_1, and so forth). $\bar{M}$ is the general (overall) mean of either a column (i.e., $\bar{M}A_1$ and $\bar{M}A_2$) or a row ($\bar{M}B_1$ and $\bar{M}B_2$). A comparison between the two column means ($\bar{M}A_1$ and $\bar{M}A_2$) determines whether a significant main effect exists for factor A. Similarly, a comparison between the two row means ($\bar{M}B_1$ and $\bar{M}B_2$) determines whether a significant main effect exists for factor B. A comparison among the four cell means (Ma_1b_1, Ma_2b_1, Ma_1b_2, Ma_2b_2) determines whether a significant interaction exists; that is, whether significant variance *remains* after the variances due to the column and row effects are subtracted from the total variance among the cell means.

[a]See this book section.

Two general procedures are used to analyze significant interactions. Both procedures decompose the original factorial design into smaller components. The first method divides the factorial design into a set of single-factor experiments (4.10, 6.13). This approach examines the effect of one factor at *each* of the levels of the other factor. Hence, the *analysis of the simple effects of factor A* at level 1 (b_1) and level 2 (b_2) of factor B would be done (6.13). The second general method of analyzing a significant interaction is to transform the original factorial design into a set of smaller factorials (6.14). This second approach has been called the *analysis of interaction comparisons* (see Keppel, 1982, 1991). The types of smaller factorial designs analyzed will depend on the research hypothesis to be evaluated.

6.13 TWO-WAY INTERACTION (A × B)

The significance of an interaction is tested by an interaction mean square. With a two-way (A × B) design an interaction is defined formally as the deviation remaining when the deviations due to the rows (B_1, B_2) and columns (A_1, A_2) are subtracted from the deviations among subgroups (Table 6.13). The interaction mean square (A × B) provides an estimate of this remaining variance (after main effects variances have been removed). This estimate is then divided by an appropriate estimate of experimental error to provide an F-value (5.18). Hence, when the effects of two treatments (factors) applied together cannot be predicted from the averaged responses of the separate factors (main effects) a significant interaction is probably present.

From the definitions of an interaction (6.12) what does it mean to infer that the A × B interaction mean square is not significant? If this interaction mean square is not significant the difference between the means a_1 and a_2 for the first level of B (b_1) *is not* significantly different from the difference between the means of a_1 and a_2 for the second level of B (b_2). If the A × B interaction sum of squares is exactly zero, the difference between the means of a_1 and a_2 for b_1 would be exactly equal to the difference between the means of a_1 and a_2 for b_2. With a non-

Table 6.14   Relative Magnitudes of Mean (M) Values for Evaluating an A × B Interaction

Levels of factor B	Levels of factor A			Examples		
	A_1		A_2	A_1		A_2
B_1	Ma_1b_1	<	Ma_2b_1	100	<	200
B_2	Ma_1b_2	>	Ma_2b_2	75	>	25
	A_1		A_2	A_1		A_2
B_1	Ma_1b_1	>	Ma_2b_1	100	>	50
B_2	Ma_1b_2	>	Ma_2b_2	100	>	50

> = greater than; < = less than.

significant $A \times B$ interaction, the A effect, the difference between a_1 and a_2, is independent of B; that is, there is approximately the same difference between a_1 and a_2, regardless of the levels of B.

The null hypothesis (5.5) for this $A \times B$ interaction would be

$$H_0: \quad a_1 - a_2 \text{ at } b_1 = a_1 - a_2 \text{ at } b_2.$$

The alternative hypothesis (5.5) for this $A \times B$ interaction would be

$$H_i: \quad a_1 - a_2 \text{ at } b_1 \neq a_1 - a_2 \text{ at } b_2.$$

A quick method for revealing a significant $A \times B$ interaction is to examine the means of the original data table. Data showing an interaction would yield *the pattern* of relative magnitudes illustrated in the top half of Table 6.14.

When the pattern of signs expressing relative magnitudes is *not uniform* an interaction is indicated. When the pattern of signs expressing relative magnitudes is uniform, as shown in the bottom half of Table 6.15, an interaction *may* or *may not* be present. Often an interaction is present without a change in the direction of the differences. In these cases, the *relative magnitudes* are affected.

For the two data sets of means given in Table 6.14 the main effects of factor A (column means) and of factor B (row means) are presented in Table 6.15. Using the data in the top half of this table the differences between A_1 and A_2 at B_1 is -100 ($100 - 200 = -100$) and at B_2 this difference is 50 ($75 - 25 = 50$). For the data in the bottom half of the table, the difference between A_1 and A_2 at B_1 and B_2 is the same ($100 - 50 = 50$). In summary, for the data in the top half of the table, the effects of factor A change at the two different levels of factor B and an interaction is present (6.12). For the data in the bottom half of the table, the effects of factor A are the same at both levels of factor B and, therefore, an interaction is not present.

Another definition of an $A \times B$ interaction is that an interaction is present when the simple main effects of factor A *are not* the same at different levels of factor B (6.12). If they are the same, then an interaction is absent. For the data in the bottom half of Table 6.15, the difference between the marginal (column)

Table 6.15 Mean (M) Values for Evaluating an $A \times B$ Interaction

Levels of factor B	Levels of factor A			Row means
	A_1		A_2	
B_1	100	<	200	150
B_2	75	>	25	50
Column means	87.5		112.5	
	A_1		A_2	
B_1	100	>	50	75.0
B_2	100	>	50	75.0
Column means	100		50	

> = greater than; < = less than

means for A_1 and A_2 $(100 - 50 = 50)$ is identical to the differences found between A_1 and A_2 for B_1 $(100 - 50 = 50)$ and B_2 $(100 - 50 = 50)$. The same outcome is found if we consider factor B, the difference between marginal (row) means $(75 - 75 = 0)$ is identical to the differences found between B_1 and B_2 for A_1 $(100 - 100 = 0)$ and A_2 $(50 - 50 = 0)$. For the data in the top half of Table 6.15, the marginal means do not reflect accurately the actual experimental means and, therefore, an interaction is present.

To evaluate interactions, the means of the four subgroups are normally plotted across the two factors which provides a graphic representation of the data. Examples of nonsignificant A $\times$ B interactions from four experimental outcomes are shown in Figure 6.1. As may be seen, if the two individual curves in each experiment were displaced vertically, they would fall on top of one another. Thus, the pair of curves in each experiment (1, 2, 3, and 4) are parallel to each other. In these examples the simple main effects show the same pattern of results; consequently, no interaction is present because the simple main effects of factor A do not change as a function of variations in factor B.

From the pattern of the four group means (Ma_1b_1, Ma_1b_2, Ma_2b_1, Ma_2b_2) for each of the four experimental outcomes (Figure 6.1) the following results and interpretations would be most likely. In Experiment 1, both main effects (A, B)

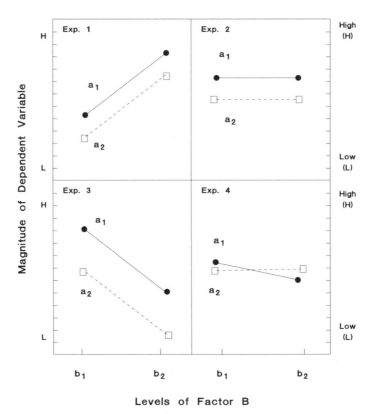

Figure 6.1 Examples of nonsignificant A $\times$ B interaction mean squares where both factors have only two levels (6.12, 6.13).

would be significant as higher values of the dependent variable are observed for a_1 at both levels of B (b_1 and b_2) compared with a_2, and higher values of the dependent variable are observed for b_2 at both levels of A (a_1 and a_2) compared with b_1 (see Table 6.13). In Experiment 2, the main effect of A would be significant but the main effect of B would not be significant. In Experiment 3, both main effects (A, B) would be significant; whereas, in Experiment 4, neither the main effect of A nor of B would be significant (Figure 6.1).

If the simple main effects show a different pattern of results, a significant interaction is present (6.12). Examples of significant A × B interactions are shown in Figure 6.2. As may be seen, if the individual curves in each experiment were displaced vertically, they would *not* fall on top of one another; that is, the pair of curves in each section are not parallel to each other. Hence, in these experimental outcomes the simple main effects show different patterns indicating an interactive effect.

From the pattern of the four group means (Ma_1b_1, Ma_1b_2, Ma_2b_1, Ma_2b_2) for each of the four experimental outcomes (Figure 6.2) the following results and interpretations would be most likely: In Experiment 1, the A × B interaction and both main effects (A and B) would be significant. In Experiment 2, the A × B interaction and the main effect of A would be significant, but the main effect

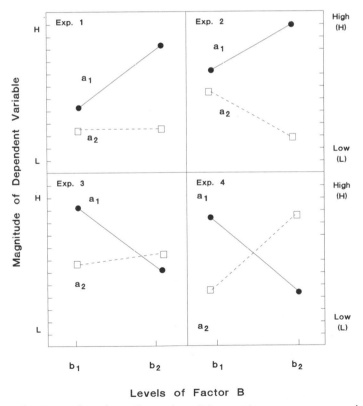

Figure 6.2 Examples of significant A × B interaction mean squares where both factors have only two levels (6.12, 6.13).

of B would not be significant. In Experiment 3, both the A × B interaction and the main effect of B would be significant but the main effect of A would not be significant. In Experiment 4, the A × B interaction would be significant but neither the main effect of A nor of B would be significant (Figure 6.2).

These examples are from a 2 × 2 factorial design, but the same principles apply to two-way interactions from other A × B factorial designs with different levels of the two factors, for example, a 2 × 3, a 3 × 3, and so forth. Illustrative experimental outcomes for a 3 × 3 factorial design are given in Figure 6.3. An interaction is absent when the functions depicting the simple main effect are parallel (Figure 6.3, Panel B); an interaction is present when the functions are not parallel (Figure 6.3, Panel A).

Because chance factors operate in every experiment, significant interactions *cannot* be determined by *simply inspecting* a graphic representation of the data.

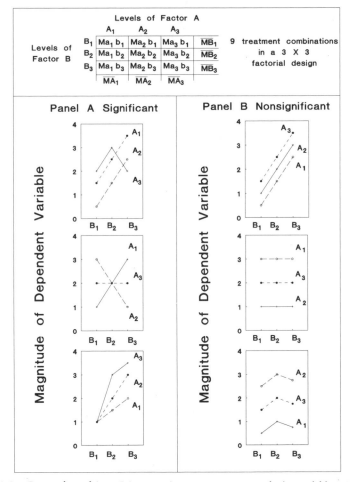

Figure 6.3   Examples of A × B interaction mean squares that would be significant (Panel A) and not significant (Panel B) for a factorial design having three levels of each factor (6.12, 6.13).

Unfortunately this interpretative procedure is so common in biological research that it is referred to as the "eye-ball" analysis. Appropriate statistical analysis must be done before a probability statement about an interaction can be made. In most cases, an overall F-test of the A $\times$ B interaction mean squares is used to determine whether a significant interaction is present and, if so, post hoc statistical tests are performed to determine significant differences among treatment conditions (6.9, Chapter 10). In mixed factorial designs [e.g., an A $\times$ (B $\times$ S) design] a significant A $\times$ B interaction may also be evaluated by trend analysis (6.16).

A very useful procedure for analyzing data which contain a significant interaction is the testing of simple effects. A *simple effect* is defined as the effect of one factor *at one level of the other factor*. In a two-factor ANOVA an examination of the cell means in the individual rows refers to the simple effects of the column factor (Table 6.13). For instance, in Table 6.16 the column factor is factor A and a_1, a_2, and a_3 examined first at b_1, then at b_2, and finally at b_3, would be an evaluation of the simple effects of factor A. Likewise, an examination of the cell means in the individual columns refers to the simple effects of the row factor which in Table 6.16 would be the simple effects of factor B. Hence, the A by B matrix is split into separate single-factor experiments and the simple effects are the detailed or specific effects of an independent variable. In short, the simple effects of a factor are revealed by examining the treatment means within the body of the A by B matrix either row by row or column by column.

The simple effects of a factor should not be confused with the main effects of a factor. Main effects are the general or averaged effects of an independent variable; these averaged effects are given by the marginal means, that is, the row and column means (Table 6.13, Figure 6.3). Tests of simple effects can be used to clarify both significant main effects and interactions. Simple effects, however, are seldom examined and tested unless a significant interaction exists in the data. The construction of appropriate error terms for testing simple effects is usually a weighted average for the revelant main effect and interaction (see Howell, 1987; Keppel, 1982; Winer, 1971). One potential limitation of an analysis of simple effects is that the analysis is sensitive to both interaction effects and to

Table 6.16 Analysis of the Simple Effects of Factor A in a 3 $\times$ 3 Factorial Design[a]

	Examination of the simple effects of factor A (all three levels, a_1, a_2, and a_3) at each level of factor B[b]
b_1	Single-factor design (the effects of factor A at only b_1, 4.13[c])
b_2	Single-factor design (the effects of factor A at only b_2)
b_3	Single-factor design (the effects of factor A at only b_3)

[a]Three levels of factor A (a_1, a_2, and a_3) and three levels of factor B (b_1, b_2, and b_3) are in a 3 $\times$ 3 factorial design.
[b]Depending upon the research question asked and the experimental design used the simple effects of factor B could be examined instead of factor A.
[c]See this book section.

main effects. Consequently, when large main effects are present, analyses of simple effects may not help you interpret significant interactions (see Keppel and Zedeck, 1989, pp. 213–237).

If a significant A × B interaction is not present, the simple effects of either independent variable are assumed to be the same at all levels of the other independent variable. Consequently, you would then interpret the significant main effects of the variables. The term *additive* is often used to describe the joint influence of two simple main effects when an interaction is not present; that is, the effect of one variable (A) simply adds to the effect of the second variable (B). When an interaction is present, the combination is *nonadditive*. What this indicates is that an additional effect, the interaction, must be used to specify the joint effects of the two main effects. Hence, *the A × B interaction serves a critical role in the analysis of a two-factor design indicating whether to analyze in detail the interaction or to focus instead on the two main effects* (Figure 6.3).

In some statistics books flowcharts are used to guide you to the appropriate statistical test (see 12.1) or through an analysis of higher-order interactions. Unfortunately, for some biologists these flowcharts become obligatory statistical blueprints for the statistical analysis of their data. But statistical tests should be chosen to evaluate those comparisons relevant to the given research question (1.1). With this caution in mind, Table 6.17 provides a summary of a common order of hypothesis testing in an A × B factorial design.

6.14 THREE-WAY INTERACTION (A × B × C)

Significant higher-order (three-way) interactions are more difficult to interpret than are significant two-way interactions (6.13). *The A × B × C interaction serves a critical role in the analysis of a three-factor design and refers to the joint effect of all three factors.* A three-way interaction is present when the interaction of two of the independent variables is not the same at all levels of the third variable (i.e., a three variable interaction exists when the interaction of two of the

Table 6.17   Order of Hypothesis Testing in an A × B Factorial Design (Table 6.2), a Complete Within-Subject Two-Factorial Design (Table 6.3), and an A × (B × S) Mixed Factorial Design (Table 6.4)

A × B interaction (6.13)[a] is	
Not significant	Significant
Analysis of main effects[b] (Table 6.13)	Analysis of the simple effects of one of the factors (Table 6.16)
	or
	Analysis of interaction comparisons (6.12)[c]

[a]See this book section.
[b]If significant and more than two levels of either factor A or B use post hoc multiple comparison tests (Chapter 10). If not significant calculate power of statistical test (5.15).
[c]If A × B interaction is significant the analysis and interpretation of main effects could still be important depending upon the research question asked and the experimental design used.

variables *changes* at different levels of the third variable). In a three-factor design, there are three main effects, three 2-way interactions (6.13), and one 3-way interaction (Tables 6.5 and 6.7).

If a significant A × B × C interaction is not present, the results of the three-way experiment can be described in terms of two-way designs—an A × B design (collapsing over factor C), an A × C design (collapsing over factor B), or a B × C design (collapsing over factor A). Thus, the three-way design is collapsed into less complex two-way designs for analysis and interpretative purposes (6.13). Which variable (factor) is collapsed across will depend upon the experimental plan.

A significant A × B × C interaction can be analyzed systematically into a set of increasingly focused statistical tests. Figure 6.4 illustrates schematically an analysis of a significant A × B × C interaction. A 2 × 2 × 2 factorial design is

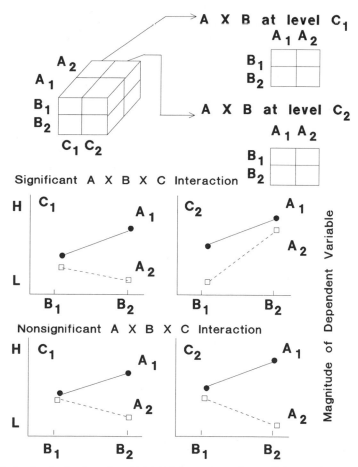

Figure 6.4 Analysis of an A × B × C interaction where all factors have only two levels (6.12, 6.14). In this 2 × 2 × 2 factorial design the A × B interaction mean squares is evaluated at each level of factor C (see Figures 6.1 and 6.2).

used for illustrative purposes. One way to consider an A × B × C interaction is to regard the A × B interaction (6.13) itself interacting with factor C. Note that the A × B interaction for C_1 is different from the A × B interaction at C_2. Hence, the A × B interaction depends upon the level of factor C which produces a significant A × B × C interaction. The same analytical procedure can be used with the A × C interaction at different levels of B, or the B × C interaction at different levels of A. A second general method of analyzing interactions is to transform the factorial design into a set of smaller factorials. Keppel (1982) gives a detailed description of the use of miniature factorial designs in the analysis of significant A × B and A × B × C interactions.

6.15 FOUR-WAY INTERACTION (A × B × C × D)

In biological research, significant three-way interaction can sometimes be interpreted (6.14) but four-way interactions (A × B × C × D) are normally impossible to interpret. Consequently, in most cases four-factor experimental designs should not be used; rather, sequential two-factor experiments should be planned (4.24).

In biological research, additional factors are usually added as different control procedures are considered for the experimental treatment condition. Hence, in thesis research the overall design recommended by the candidate's committee may include several groups to control for suspected nuisance factors (4.24). Unfortunately, a balanced design using various control groups can evolve quickly into a four-factor design. If a four-way interaction is necessary to answer the proposed research question, a statistician should be consulted *before* data are collected.

6.16 TREND ANALYSIS

When a quantitative independent variable is manipulated, you may be interested in the shape or the form of the function relating the independent and dependent variables. Essentially, with a quantitative independent variable, the treatment levels represent different amounts of a single common variable. This independent variable may be different dosages of a particular drug (0, 2 mg/kg, 4 mg/kg, 8 mg/kg, and so forth) or different stimulation frequencies (0, 10, 20, and 40 spikes per second, sps). Rather than determine whether differences exist among contiguous means (i.e., Is there a significant difference between 4 mg/kg and 8 mg/kg?), a more revealing question may be What is the general relation between the independent and dependent variables? Does the outcome of the experiment represent a *linear* function (a steady rise or fall in the treatment means as the independent variable is increased) or a *nonlinear* function?

In biological research, trend analysis would commonly be used to determine the simplest function that would describe the data adequately. For example, the data presented in Figure 6.5 represent the effects of stimulation of L_7 (a motoneuron in the invertebrate *Aplysia*) on gill muscle contraction in two groups of animals. In this experiment a 2 × (7 × 8) design (4.21) was used and a com-

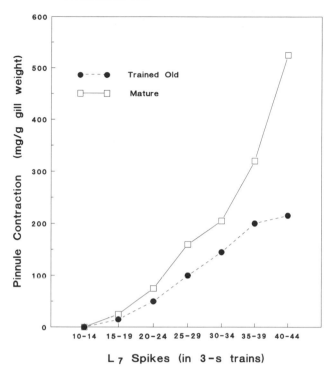

Figure 6.5   Mean gill contraction is related to L_7 spike rate for normal adult animals and for old animals given siphon/gill withdrawal training. *(Adapted from Zolman and Peretz, 1987.)*

parison between pinnule (gill) contraction elicited by L_7 stimulation in old trained animals and mature animals revealed no significant group effect, $F(1, 14) = 2.97$, a significant spike frequency effect, $F(6, 84) = 28.8$, $p < .001$ and a significant Group $\times$ Spike Frequency interaction, $F(6, 84) = 4.76$, $p < .05$. Rather than using post hoc multiple comparison tests (6.8, Chapter 10) to evaluate differences among the 14 means contributing to the significant two-way interaction (6.13), a trend analysis was used to describe the relation between spike train frequency and gill contraction in the two groups.

For comparison, representative curves of pure (ideal) cases of a different component of trend in an experiment containing seven equally spaced intervals on some quantitative independent variable (like spike train frequency) are given in Figure 6.6. The first curve reflects a *linear* component in which the curve rises (or may drop) at the same rate along the extent of the independent variable. The second curve reflects a *quadratic* component as the curve shows *concavity*, a single bend upward (or in other cases downward). The other two curves are more complex with the third reflecting a *cubic* trend component and the fourth a *quartic* trend component. These curves of greater complexity are distinguished by the number of times the function reverses direction. A linear function has no reversals, a quadratic function has one reversal, a cubic function has two reversals, and a quartic function has three reversals (Figure 6.6). In actual experiments, the observed curves are not generally pure cases as chance factors normally distort

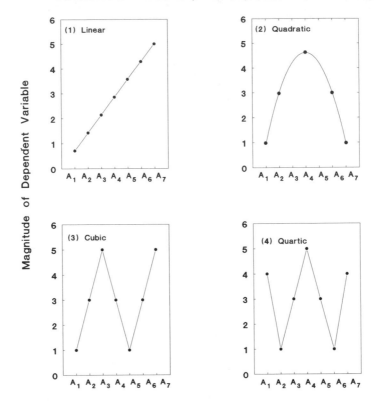

Levels of Independent Variable (factor A)

Figure 6.6 Ideal examples of linear, quadratic, cubic, and quartic trend components (6.16).

the experimental curve and more than one of the trend components may be represented in the functional relation. Trend analysis provides an objective method for assessing the separate contributions of each of the pure components by using a technique called the *analysis of orthogonal polynomials.*

Essentially, a polynomial equation is used to determine the functional relation between the quantitatively manipulated variable and the dependent variable (biological response). The general form of the equation is

$$Y = \alpha + \beta_1 X^1 + \beta_2 X^2 + \beta_3 X^3 + \beta_4 X^4 + \cdots$$

In this equation β_1, β_2, β_3, β_4, and so forth represent the population regression coefficients for the first degree, second degree, third degree, fourth degree, and so forth—terms which correspond to the linear, quadratic, cubic, quartic, and higher-order components, respectively.

With 6 df for the significant Group $\times$ Spike Frequency interaction (Figure 6.5), six regression components can be extracted from the data, each with 1 df (see 5.17). The formal statistical statements (5.5) are

| Statistical hypothesis I | H_0: | $\beta_i = 0$ |
| Alternative hypothesis I | H_1: | $\beta_i \neq 0$ |

| Statistical hypothesis II | H_0: | $\beta_2 = 0$ |
| Alternative hypothesis II | H_1: | $\beta_2 \neq 0$ |

.   .

.   .

.   .

| Statistical hypothesis VI | H_0: | $\beta_6 = 0$ |
| Alternative hypothesis VI | H_1: | $\beta_6 \neq 0$ |

If the proper procedures have been followed, each of the statistical hypotheses presented is independent of the five other hypotheses. Thus, it is possible for one, two, or all six components to be significant. As might be expected for significant higher-order trends, the difficulty of interpretation increases considerably. Hence, in most biological experiments only the first two or three regression components (if significant) may be interpretable. For example, a trend analysis of the significant Group × Spike Frequency interaction shown in Figure 6.5 revealed significant linear, $F(1, 14) = 4.73, p < .05$, quadratic, $F(1, 14) = 9.98, p < .01$, and cubic, $F(1, 14) = 6.32, p < .05$, component differences between the two groups. The significant linear trend difference between the two groups indicates that the pinnule contraction increase produced by increased spike rate in old animals was not as great as that shown by the mature animals. The two higher-order trend component differences (i.e., quadratic and cubic) probably reflect the lower and apparent asymptotic level of contraction found in the old animals as compared with the mature animals (see Figure 6.5).

In a trend analysis, values of the manipulated variable are normally selected at equally spaced intervals as in Figure 6.5. The assumption of equal spacing is required to use simple computational procedures to obtain the regression data. Also, if the function is not known before the experiment is run it is better to use equal intervals to make it more likely that important changes in the biological dependent measure will be covered. There are, however, procedures to extract the same information if the independent variable is unequally spaced. In this latter situation, a statistician should be consulted before the data are collected.

One limitation of trend analysis is that the knowledge concerning the under-lying function for the population is based on the limited number of points selected for the experiment. If spacings between the values are very large, it may not be accurate to draw a continuous function between the data points in the sample (experiment). Note, in the experimental data shown in Figure 6.5, this problem did not occur as a progressively increasing frequency range was used. Normally, if the data points are not too far apart, the regression predictions are reasonably accurate. A related but more serious problem concerns the extrapolation of the function outside the two extreme values on the independent variable included in the experiment. For example, in Figure 6.5 if the stimulation frequency had been restricted to the range of 10 to 34 sps, only a significant linear component difference between the two groups would have been observed. Obviously, if only a significant linear difference between the two groups had been extrapolated to higher frequencies, this conclusion would have been wrong. What about extrapolation of the trend analysis results beyond the 40–44 sps used in the experiment? By increasing spike frequencies the curves would be expected to change. At higher spike frequencies even the mature animals should reach an asymptotic level of contraction and then show a decline because of physiological fatigue. The reason higher spike frequencies were not used in the representative experiment shown in Figure 6.5 was because higher spike frequencies were well beyond the range of normal neuronal function in this species. Note the old animals had apparently reached their asymptotic level of responding but because higher frequencies were not used a definite statement could not be made. Across the range of normal physiological values the shape of the two curves in Figure 6.5 represent an accurate functional relation. However, if the normal physiological range of the manipulated variable is unknown, subsequent extrapolations of the experimental data must be viewed with caution.

6.17 MULTIVARIATE ANALYSIS OF VARIANCE (MANOVA)

The simultaneous analysis of several dependent variables is called *multivariate analysis*. When an analysis focuses on *one* single dependent variable it is called a *univariate analysis*. All the methods described in Section II have been *univariate* methods as the effects of treatment conditions are determined separately for each dependent variable (Chapter 6 and 12). Suppose, for instance, that the purpose of a study is to compare the effects of treatment conditions on diastolic blood pressure, heart rate, and serum cholesterol. If three separate ANOVA's are used with each one analyzing treatment effects on one of the three different dependent variables then each of these analyses would be *univariate*. A *single simultaneous analysis* of the effects of treatment conditions on the three dependent variables is a *multivariate analysis*.

For most univariate methods, an analogous multivariate method is available. As examples, the multivariate analogue of the t-test or single-factor ANOVA (5.18) for comparing the means of two groups is the Hotelling's T^2-test and, likewise, multivariate regression analysis, multivariate analysis of variance, and multivariate analysis of covariance procedures are available.

The two main advantages for using a multivariate analysis rather than doing a set of univariate analyses are (1) a multivariate analysis controls for the increase in familywise error rates (6.9, 10.1) when the number of statistical tests is increased. As the number of statistical tests performed at a given significance level increases so does the probability of finding a significant difference (10.1), and (2) a multivariate analysis is more sensitive in detecting group differences that depend on certain relationships among the dependent variables (see Elston and Johnson, 1987, pp. 234–235).

Some of the disadvantages of using multivariate analysis are (1) the mathematical assumptions are more stringent than those for univariate analysis; (2) the statistical analysis is more difficult to understand; (3) few multivariate analyses have been used in biological research; (4) the abuse of multivariate analysis in educational, psychological, and social sciences has hindered their acceptance by biological scientists; and (5) many biologists, including editors and reviewers, do not fully understand univariate analyses; consequently, a research paper containing multivariate analysis probably would have difficulty being accepted for publication.

Multivariate problems are common in medical research and substantial development in statistical techniques and applications of multivariate analysis have occurred in recent years. Discriminant analysis is one example of multivariate techniques that have been applied to medical problems (see Bourke, Daly, and McGilvray, 1985). Although multivariate techniques will come into greater use, they are conceptually more difficult to understand than univariate techniques and are easily misapplied. Hence, they are rarely used in biological research. The interested reader is referred to Kachigan (1986), Stevens (1986), and Glantz and Slinker (1990) for general introductions to multivariate methods.

6.18 ANALYSIS OF COVARIANCE (ANCOVA)

A reduction in the magnitude of error variance (5.16, 6.4) may be achieved either directly through experimental design or indirectly by statistical procedures. With direct control, important sources of error (nuisance) variance are identified, included in the experimental design, and their influence directly removed in the partitioning of the total sum of squares (6.4, 9.4). For example, a single-factor within-subject design reduces error variance by using the same subjects in all the treatment conditions (4.16). The variability due to subjects is then removed from the error estimate (see Table 4.5). Reducing nuisance variability could also be done when age is known to have an effect on the dependent variable. If subjects of different ages were used in the experiment this age variance would become part of the error variance. However, before the experiment, subjects could be matched for age (block), and the matched subjects within each block randomly assigned to the different treatment conditions (4.8). Variations associated with blocks (the main effect and interaction) are isolated in the randomized block statistical analysis (see Table 9.3). Without blocking, these age sources of variance would contribute to the error variance in a completely randomized design (4.10).

A reduction in error variance may also be achieved by a statistical procedure which adjusts the results of an experiment for particular differences existing in subjects before the start of the experiment. *Analysis of covariance* (ANCOVA) is a statistical analysis which consists of the combined application of linear regression (5.26) and analysis of variance (Chapter 6) techniques. ANCOVA is used when experimental treatments are compared in the presence of concomitant (associated) variables which can be neither eliminated or experimentally controlled. In experiments ANCOVA would be used to correct for chance differences between groups that occur when animals are assigned randomly to the treatment groups. ANCOVA procedures adjust the group means for these preexisting differences and reduce the size of the error term used in subsequent statistical analysis. Both these adjustments are made from prior information about the animals that may be correlated with the dependent (response) measure. As might be expected the mathematical assumptions of ANCOVA include those of the appropriate analysis of variance as well as of linear regression analysis. If some of these assumptions are violated, the interpretation of an ANCOVA becomes difficult. ANCOVA encompasses a large body of statistical methodology too extensive to be covered briefly. Useful discussions of the ANCOVA along with additional references may be found in Howell (1987), Keppel (1982), and Sokal and Rohlf (1981). The different types of control of factors which may influence treatment-induced experimental outcomes are summarized in Figure 6.7.

6.19 MISSING DATA: UNEQUAL SAMPLE SIZES AND ESTIMATION PROCEDURES

In most cases, unequal sample sizes are not planned but occur because animals are lost during the experiment. In these situations, the loss of animals may be

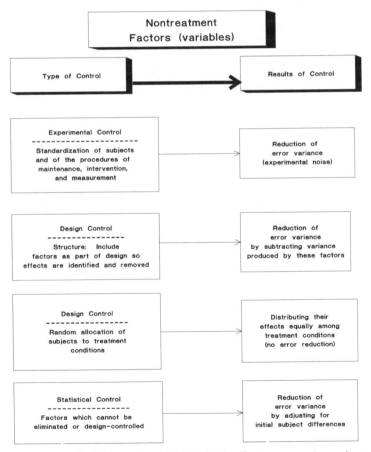

Figure 6.7 Control of factors (variables) which affect error variance in statistical tests. The significance of treatment-induced experimental outcomes is dependent upon the amount of experimental error (5.16).

related to treatment conditions (4.12). If treatment- related loss occurs the randomness of assignment of animals to the treatment conditions is destroyed. This loss may add a systematic bias to the differences among the experimental means which cannot be disentangled from any significant treatment effects. But, if animal loss is not related to treatment effects statistical procedures are available for analysis of the unequal n data. When equal sample sizes have been planned but animal loss has produced unequal sample sizes, the *analysis of unweighted means* is an appropriate method to use (see Keppel, 1982, pp. 346–356). An alternative procedure is the *method of least squares*. This latter method is replacing the analysis of unweighted means because of the widespread availability of computer programs designed to apply this method to experiments with unequal sample sizes (A.5).

In within-subject or mixed factorial designs in which numerous repeated measurements are taken, a few measures of a given animal in a particular group may be lost (equipment failure, loss of a tissue sample, and so forth). In these cases two alternatives are available to the biologist, either all the data from this animal could be eliminated from the study (unequal *n* analysis) or *the few missing data points could be estimated* (see Sokal and Rohlf, 1981). In general for each missing data point which is replaced by an estimated value 1 degree of freedom is lost in the subsequent statistical analysis (5.17, 6.5).

6.20 THE INTERPRETATION OF NONSIGNIFICANCE

A safe rule of thumb is to *not interpret nonsignificant findings* particularly if the power of your statistical test is low (5.12, 5.13). A corollary rule is to be certain that your rationale for doing the study does not rely upon proving the null hypothesis (5.5). Many biologists often report no statistically significant difference among treatment conditions, and proceed to discuss their results as if they had *proved* that the treatments had no effects. What was done, of course, was that the biologists failed to demonstrate that their selected treatments had any effects (1.6, 1.7, 5.4, 5.5, 5.10). A nonsignificant result means that if the treatment conditions were given to a large number of subjects there is no certainty that the actual sample results would be observed in the larger sample. Nonsignificant results may be due to inadequacies of the measures used, low statistical power because of small sample size, large experimental error, or no significant relationship between the measured variables. Hence, if a biologist wishes to obtain nonsignificant results for certain comparisons the likelihood of this outcome may be increased by using small sample sizes and increasing experimental error (be sloppy). For these reasons, nonsignificant results are usually uninterpretable and typically are obtained by decreasing the power of the statistical test (5.13) even when true treatment effects exist.

One of the most common problems in thesis research is the small sample sizes used for many of the "required" control groups (6.15). Usually, a member of the thesis committee suggests that a "few" preparations be done to control for some particular variable. Everyone agrees that this control would be important, another member recommends another control and it is accepted, and so forth. The candidate may protest that only a certain number of animals are available or that each preparation is time-consuming or that a post doctoral position only will be held for another six months. Rarely does the candidate inform the committee members that such comparisons with low power which fail to detect a statistically significant effect are meaningless (5.12, 5.14). Even if this rationale was advanced by the candidate, some committee members probably still would insist that a few preparations are better than none and even eye-ball comparisons are important (see 4.24).

6.21 BIOLOGICAL AND STATISTICAL SIGNIFICANCE

Biologists must distinguish between a biologically important result and a statistically significant result. Biological importance relates to the magnitude of the observed effect whereas statistical significance refers to whether or not the observed result is because of chance and sampling error (spurious). A significant difference between two treatment conditions may not be biologically important if a large sample was necessary to reject the null hypothesis (1.6, 1.7, 5.9, 5.15). If sample size is enormous, trivial biological differences in populations may be statistically significant. Furthermore, a statistically significant finding even with a small sample does not eliminate the possibility that the observed effect may be confounded by subject-, time-, or environment-related extraneous variables (4.11, 4.12, 4.15, 4.19, 4.23, 4.26). A confounded treatment condition may be statistically significant but not biologically important because of the confounding variable.

Even a significant and nonconfounded treatment effect found with a small sample size is no guarantee of its biological importance. The result may have limited generalization given the animal model (4.27) or the experimental conditions used (4.28). For example, in vitro preparations are widely used to study biological mechanisms. But a major problem with in vitro preparations is determining how normal the preparation remains when placed in an abnormal laboratory environment (4.28, Table 4.15). Hence, a statistically significant treatment effect may be biologically unimportant because of its small magnitude, its confounding with other variables, the inappropriateness of the animal model, the abnormality of the experimental preparation, and so forth.

7

Post Hoc Analysis

7.1 GENERATION OF HYPOTHESES

Experienced biologists go far beyond their original plans for analyzing a set of data. This unplanned data analysis is post hoc (6.9) and is *not* guided by significant overall F-ratios (6.8). Rather, this post hoc analysis is exploratory and is a search for trends and outcomes not expected by the biologist. This process has been called "data dredging" and is a common procedure used in thesis research. In most situations, the experienced researcher is well aware that interesting, unexpected outcomes may only be caused by chance factors; consequently, this *exploratory data analysis usually is not included in the results section of an experimental report* (Chapter 2). In thesis research, the candidate should be candid about the nature and amount of "data dredging" that has occurred.

The analysis of data in depth is both necessary and laudable. Some methods are available to protect this post hoc exploratory analysis from extreme values (outliers) and to ensure that the distributional assumptions are modest (see Chambers, Cleveland, Kleiner, and Tukey, 1983; Everitt and Dunn, 1983; Hoaglin, Mosteller, and Tukey, 1982; Tukey, 1977; Velleman and Hoaglin, 1981, for reviews). These types of data analyses, however, should not be confused with hypothesis-testing analyses (5.5, 5.16). *These data explorations are hypothesis-generating efforts,* that is, this post hoc exploratory analysis may provide information for the formulation of subsequent research questions (1.1). In some cases, nonsignificant outcomes in a particular direction may appear consistently in a number of experiments and statistical procedures are available to determine whether a significant *pattern of results* exists across a number of experiments (7.2).

7.2 TRENDS ACROSS EXPERIMENTS

In a series of experiments, a particular treatment condition may not produce a significant effect (no basis to reject the null hypothesis). Yet in every experiment the treatment condition may have always produced a greater amplitude of the biological response compared with a control condition. The nonsignificant F tests in each experiment (5.18) cannot measure the consistency of the data obtained in independent experiments.

Several statistical procedures can be used to evaluate the consistency of data across a series of replication studies (7.3, 7.5). A useful summary and illustration of some of these statistical methods is given in Rosenthal (1984). All these methods use the difference between two means, which is a problem for studies in which there are more than two conditions. In this latter situation, the experimental design may be treated as a factorial with the treatments as one factor and the independent replication as another (see Winer, 1971, pp. 391–394; Keppel, 1982, pp. 76–77).

In some situations, an unexpected outcome found in post hoc exploratory data analysis (7.1) may also be apparent upon closer examination in other similar experiments. In this case the researcher by determining the significance of the consistency of the pattern of results may design an experiment to test a research question based upon extrapolations from this consistency.

7.3 THE TRUE TEST: INDEPENDENT REPLICATION

A distinction between *replication* and *extension* studies can be made (see Cooper and Rosenthal, 1980). A replication study provides *an additional test* of an already tested research hypothesis. An extension study evaluates a research question *based upon* a previously tested research hypothesis. Subsequent studies vary in the closeness with which they duplicate the original experimental procedures. In *exact*, or strict, replications all assumed critical features between the two studies are duplicated (a replication study). In *partial* replication usually one critical feature is purposely changed in the new study (an extension study). An exact replication adds little new information, but provocative new findings are usually quickly replicated to determine whether the original finding was a Type I error (5.10). Partial replications produce useful new information because a successful replication indicates that the phenomenon extends beyond the boundary conditions of the original study (1.8,4.25).

An unsuccessful replication, however, provides ambiguous information about the original phenomenon. Three possible explanations for a failure to replicate are generally accepted: (*a*) inadequate statistical power (5.12), (*b*) unsatisfactorily reproduced experimental conditions, and (*c*) spurious or artifactual results of the original experiment, a Type I error (5.10). Hence, an unsuccessful replication raises many questions. Was the first experiment a Type I error or was the second experiment a Type II error? Were the experimental conditions duplicated exactly or was some critical variable left out of the replication study?

The failure to replicate often is not resolved by a second experiment and many unsuccessful replications usually are required before incorrect published data become suspect. Indeed, extensive research is often necessary before the spurious or artifactual results of original experiments can be identified and corrected (see Dworken and Miller, 1986). For this reason, the erroneous search for significance (6.11) by a scientist may result in a considerable waste of the time and effort of other biologists who may use spurious published data to design extension studies which are not successful.

7.4 SYSTEMATIC RESEARCH AND REPLICATION

In a systematic research program, the different types of replication can be incorporated into a single experiment. In such an experiment, one set of treatments may be an exact replication of one part of a previous experiment and another set of treatments may be a partial replication (an extension) of the previous experiment (7.3). This *systematic replication* approach combines the value of different kinds of replication. By including an exact replication of certain treatment conditions you can, besides evaluating the reliability of the original findings, provide a baseline to compare the effects of another treatment condition. Systematic replications of this sort are factorial designs and can be analyzed by standard statistical procedures (4.13, 4.21). The self-correcting nature of science is based primarily upon the repeating and extending of prior research.

7.5 META-ANALYSIS

A statistical procedure for combining and evaluating data from separate but similar studies is *meta-analysis*, and scientists from all fields are now using meta-analysis when they review a body of scientific literature. Meta-analysis is a quantitative synthesis that uses formal statistical procedures to retrieve, select, and combine results from previous separate studies (see Wachter, 1988). Meta-analysis is a controversial statistical method which supposedly provides a quantitative synthesis of all available data. Proponents believe that meta-analysis will replace traditional scientific reviews of research fields written by experts (see Mann, 1990). Aspiring meta-analysts may purchase computer software systems which perform a full complement of meta-analytic statistical functions (e.g., Johnson, 1989; Mullen, 1989). Hence, doing a meta-analysis of a research area is becoming easier but doing a valid meta-analysis is still difficult. Meta-analysis is essentially an observation study (the observations are the studies done by other investigators) and all the pitfalls of observational studies must be carefully considered (4.1, 4.3). To do a meta-analysis you must examine the data included in the article and cannot just read the abstract of the article. The interested reader is referred to Cooper and Rosenthal (1980), Gerbarge and Horwitz (1988), Hedges and Olkin (1985), Light and Pillemer (1984), Oakes (1986), Rosenthal (1984), and Wolf (1986) for reviews of meta-analysis.

III
STATISTICAL TESTS

8
Parametric Tests

8.1 ASSUMPTIONS AND POWER

Sections I and II focused on a particular form of statistical analysis and inference, namely hypothesis testing using analysis of variance (ANOVA) techniques (Chapter 6). In these sections emphasis was given to experimental design (Section I) and to the rationales, interpretations, and applications of the most commonly used ANOVA procedures for between-subject, within-subject, and mixed factorial designs (Section II).

One of the most compelling reasons for using these ANOVA tests when their underlying theoretical assumptions are met is that, for any given sample size, these parametric tests are more powerful than their nonparametric counterparts (5.22). In general, a statistical test with a large number of restrictions (e.g., a parametric test) will be more powerful than a test with few restrictions (e.g., a nonparametric test). But, if the normality and equal variance assumptions of parametric tests are grossly violated a nonparametric test can be as powerful as, or even more powerful than, the parametric test it replaces (Chapter 11).

Many statistical software packages have incorporated methods for checking the assumptions of statistical models and the data to which they are fitted. These methods are used to identify potential problems in the regression analysis of a given set of data. Graphic methods are also used to compare sample distributions and to detect outliers. Outliers are values that are clearly out of the range of all other values (5.27). Two useful data-plotting methods developed by Tukey (1977) are the stem-and-leaf display (8.2) and the box-and-whisker-plot (8.3). These two procedures are valuable for preliminary data exploration and require minimal assumptions.

8.2 STEM-AND-LEAF PLOTS

The graphical presentation of data is used for data reduction (5.1), for exploratory data analysis (7.1), and for diagnostic regression analysis (8.1).

A stem-and-leaf plot is a simple display of the original data, is easily constructed, retains information about each data point, and makes the distribution of the data apparent. Stem-and-leaf displays provide information about the central tendency, variability and shape of the sample distribution, and also identify outliers (5.1, 5.27). Table 8.1 presents a stem-and-leaf display of 46 measurements of current flow (pA) in hippocampus neurons. The particular program

Table 8.1 Computer Printout of Stem-and-Leaf Plot

Stem and Leaf Plot of Variable: Current, N = 46

Minimum is: 29
Lower Hinge is: 74
Median is: 129
Upper Hinge is: 158
Maximum is: 446

```
0    23
0    4455555
0H   6677
0    999
1    001
1M   222233
1H   4444444455
1    677
1
2    01
2    2
2    4
     ***OUTSIDE VALUES***
3    047
4    4
```

used to display this information, as well as the subsequent box-and-whisker plot (8.3), was the GRAPH module of SYSTAT, but similar results can be obtained from other statistical packages. The left side of a stem-and-leaf plot shows stems (the vertical axes of the pattern) which are the most significant digits (sometimes called the leading digits). The right side (the horizontal numbers) shows leaves which are the next digits after each stem. These digits are the least significant (or trailing) digits. In the data represented there are one 2, one 3, two 4s, five 5s, two 6s and · · · one 30, one 34, one 37, and one 44. These values would have to be multiplied by 10 to approximate the real numeric data, that is, 44 actually represents 446, the maximum value.

In this plot, the minimum and maximum are the lowest and highest scores and the median is the value of the score at the 50th percentile of the distribution (see 5.1). The lower and upper hinges (H_L and H_U) are related to the 25th and 75th percentiles and the distance between them is a measure of spread. This distance, called the H-spread, is used to identify outliers in the sample (see Myers and Well, 1991). In the plot four outliers (outside values) are identified. Outliers could be legitimate values that happen to be extreme and may reflect skewed or heavy-tailed distributions (see 11.1). Outliers could also be produced by the misreading of recorded values, errors in data calculation or errors in data entry.

8.3 BOX-AND-WHISKER PLOTS

Box-and-whisker plots (or box plots) provide a simple graphical display of the distribution of a single dependent variable. The same data for hippocampus neurons given in Table 8.1 are also displayed in a box plot in Figure 8.1. As may be

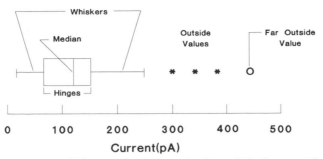

Figure 8.1   Diagram of a box-and-whisker plot (box plot) of current flow data.

seen, the median is marked by a central vertical line. The edges of the box are
the lower and upper hinges of the distribution and enclose about 50 percent of
the data (see stem-and-leaf plot, 8.3). Box plots are very useful for visualizing
dispersion of data, for screening for errors, and for identifying potential problems. As examples, the central portion of the distribution in Figure 8.1 is not
symmetrical because the median is not in the center but lies toward the right of
box. The distribution is positively skewed—the whisker on the right is longer
than the one on the left. The relative position of the four outliers are highlighted.
Box plots are useful tools for describing the responses of single units (e.g., the
characteristics of a single ionic channel).

In both stem-and-leaf and box plots the skewness of data and the occurrence
of heavy tails indicate the data sampled may not be from a normally distributed
population. This assumption of normality can be examined by using more formal graphic diagnostic regression methods (8.1). More information on such
plots may be found in Atkinson (1987); Hoaglin, Mosteller, and Tukey (1982);
Tukey (1977); or Velleman and Hoaglin (1981).

Special ANOVA Designs and Analyses

9.1 SPECIAL ANOVA DESIGNS

It is a unique research question that cannot be successfully answered with one or another of the ANOVA designs (Chapter 6) introduced in Tables 6.1 thru 6.11. Nevertheless, other designs exist which may improve the power and efficiency of a particular experiment. Each of these special designs has its own analysis of variance model (6.1) with an accompanying set of statistical assumptions (5.7). In each case, however, the basic principle of the analysis of variance is the same: Data are collected in such a way that the total variation can be separated into its component sources, including an estimate of the treatment effects and an estimate of the relevant error variance. With these estimates an appropriate F-ratio may be formed to test for treatment effects (Chapter 6). There are designs, for example, that permit a study of many variables at once (drug type, drug dosage, intake regimen, and so forth) without having to use every possible combination of the levels of the various variables, a requirement which is often impractical or uneconomical. These designs, however, require stringent assumptions about the absence of interaction effects (6.12). Details of these designs can be found in advanced statistics books under the headings of *fractional factorial designs, nested designs, latin square designs, graeco-latin square designs* and *orthogonal array designs*, to name the most common ones (Mead, 1988). If a research project requires the use of a specialized design, a statistician should be consulted or included as a member of the research team.

9.2 CORRELATED OBSERVATIONS: INTRODUCTION

In within-subject designs (4.16, 4.17), repeated measures of the same variable from the same subject are taken and these observations on the same subject are correlated rather than independent (4.9). Biologists who inadvertently use experimental designs with correlated observations risk making several types of errors. Depending on the nature of the error, the biologist may end up with a test of significance that yields negatively or positively biased F-ratios (Table 4.5).

The statistical principle to remember is that *the variance among correlated observations is less than the variance among independent observations sampled from the same population.* Identical twins, repeated measures on the same subject (4.16, 4.17), and littermates are examples of correlated observations (4.9,

5.27). In biology, littermates are often used in developmental research; consequently, littermates will be used to illustrate the potential problems with correlated measures (9.3, 9.4, 9.5, 9.6).

In Table 9.1 the design of an experiment is given in which four animals from each of eight litters are measured on a given biological response (each litter is designated by a different letter, A, B, . . ., H, and each animal in the litter by a numerical subscript). The analysis of variance in Table 9.1 shows two sources of variation: $MS_{between}$ and MS_{within}. The between variation compares independent observations because no basis exists for assuming a significant correlation among the randomly selected eight litters. The within source represents variation among littermates. If no correlation existed among littermates in this sample, litter variability (within) would be about the same as $MS_{between}$ (in the population the variances would be identical, 1.6, 1.7). But, if a positive correlation (5.27) exists among the littermates, the MS_{within} variation will be less than the $MS_{between}$ variation and *the F-ratio will become greater than 1.00 without any treatment effect* (5.16).

The value of the average correlation (5.27) among animals (designated r_i) can also be obtained from the MS values shown in Table 9.1 where n is the number of animals in each litter.

$$r_i = \frac{MS_{between} - MS_{within}}{MS_{between} + (n - 1)MS_{within}}.$$

Table 9.1 Experimental Design with Four Animals per Litter and the ANOVA Table

Litter[a]	A_1	A_2	A_3	A_4	
	B_1	B_2	B_3	B_4	
	C_1	C_2	C_3	C_4	
	D_1	D_2	D_3	D_4	Estimate of MS_{within}–variance
	E_1	E_2	E_3	E_4	
	F_1	F_2	F_3	F_4	
	G_1	G_2	G_3	G_4	
	H_1	H_2	H_3	H_4	

Estimate of $MS_{between}$–variance

Analysis of variance (ANOVA) table (6.3)[b]

Source (6.4)	df (6.5)	MS (5.18)
Litters	7	$MS_{between}$
Subjects within litters	24	MS_{within}
Total	31	
Null hypothesis: No correlation among littermates (5.27)		Alternative hypothesis: Positive correlation among littermates (5.27)
$MS_{between}/MS_{within} = 1.00$		$MS_{between}/MS_{within} > 1.00$

[a]Each litter is designated by a different letter (i.e., A, B, . . ., H) and each animal within a given litter by a subscript (e.g., C_3 indicates the third animal in litter C).
[b]See this book section.

If the F-test, $MS_{between}/MS_{within}$ is significant, the litters differ among themselves on the biological measure. Equivalently, a significant F indicates a significant correlation among the littermates, that is, the F-test to evaluate $MS_{between}$ is also the proper test of significance to evaluate r_i (see Denenberg, 1979, 1984).

9.3 NESTED DESIGNS

Correlated subjects (e.g., littermates, 9.2) can be assigned to either within-treatment conditions or across-treatment conditions. An experiment in which littermates are assigned to the same treatment is called a *nested design;* whereas, the situation in which littermates are assigned to different treatments is called a *randomized-blocks design* (9.4).

As an example of a nested design, in a prenatal drug experiment pregnant rats would be assigned to one of four chronic drug treatment groups: vehicle-control and low, medium and high doses of the drug. In this hypothetical experiment two females are randomly assigned to each of the four drug conditions. At birth four male pups are randomly selected from each litter and have several brain neurochemicals measured. The design of the experiment and the analysis of variance (ANOVA) table are shown in Table 9.2. Note the two sources of error

Table 9.2 Design of a Nested Experiment and the ANOVA Table

	\multicolumn{4}{c}{Dose of drug}			
	None	Low	Medium	High
Litter[a]	A_1	C_1	E_1	G_1
	A_2	C_2	E_2	G_2
	A_3	C_3	E_3	G_3
	A_4	C_4	E_4	G_4
	B_1	D_1	F_1	H_1
	B_2	D_2	F_2	H_2
	B_3	D_3	F_3	H_3
	B_4	D_4	F_4	H_4

Analysis of variance (ANOVA) table (6.3)[b]

Source (6.4)	df (6.5)	MS (5.18)
Drug (treatments)	3	MS_{drug}
Litters within treatments	4	$MS_{litters}$
Subjects within litters within treatments	24	$MS_{subjects}$
Total	31	

[a]Each litter is designated by a different letter (i.e., A, B, . . ., H) and each animal within a given litter by a numerical subscript (e.g., B_2 indicates the second animal in litter B).

[b]See this book section.

variance in this design: litters and rat pups are both random variables (6.1). A nested design exists because litters are nested within treatments and the rat pups are doubly nested within litters and treatments (6.2). Because the aim of the experiment is to make generalizations to a population of rats, $MS_{litters}$ is the proper denominator for the F-test evaluating the drug variable (5.16, 5.18). However, $MS_{litters}$ has only 4 df and thus has very low statistical power (5.12, 5.13, 5.15, 5.17). Although eight litters are used in the experiment, two each are assigned to each treatment condition; consequently, the value of only one litter per treatment can vary; hence, 4 df are available. In contrast, $MS_{subjects}$ has 24 df. If this error estimate could be pooled with $MS_{litters}$ a combined error term with 28 df and with much greater statistical power would be available. To determine whether the two MS values can be combined, a preliminary F-test ($MS_{litters}/MS_{subjects}$) is normally performed. Winer (1971) recommends that the level for rejecting the null hypothesis of this preliminary test be set relatively high (between .20 and .30) to avoid a Type II error (i.e., accepting the hypothesis of a zero litter effect when it should be rejected, 5.10, 5.12).

If a significant correlation exists among littermates, $MS_{litters}$ will be significantly greater than $MS_{subjects}$ and these two sources of variance should not be pooled into one common error term (9.2). The common mistake made when using a littermate-nested design is to ignore the litter classification and assume that all the observations are independent (4.9). Because littermates are probably correlated, ignoring the litter classification produces an error term which underestimates error variance (9.2) and thereby results in an inflated F-ratio (5.16).

If litters are to be used (e.g., Table 9.2), the experiment should be designed on the assumption that each litter will probably yield only one independent observation, and sufficient litters should be used to ensure a statistical test with adequate power. To conserve animal resources other important biological measures should be taken from the other littermates (4.9). In summary, a researcher should never ignore a litter variable and assume before the fact that a littermate correlation does not exist. In short, strong and compelling evidence is required before pooling animals across litters is justified.

9.4 RANDOMIZED-BLOCKS DESIGNS

Using related subjects within a treatment condition is usually not helpful (9.3). In contrast, having correlated subjects present across treatment conditions is very helpful. Suppose a developmental biologist wanted to determine the effects of a drug treatment given immediately after birth on the young rat's behavior. Four female littermates from each of eight litters may be selected and the four females of each litter randomly assigned to the four drug doses. With this assignment each litter becomes a randomized block. The experimental design and the analysis of variance are presented in Table 9.3.

Because the variable of interest, drug dose, is within a litter, the proper error term to evaluate this is $MS_{interaction}$ which is also a within-litter term. If a positive correlation exists among littermates, the $MS_{interaction}$ will be smaller than $MS_{litters}$

Table 9.3　Design of a Randomized-Blocks Experiment and the ANOVA Table

	Dose of drug			
	None	Low	Medium	High
	A_1	A_2	A_3	A_4
	B_1	B_2	B_3	B_4
	C_1	C_2	C_3	C_4
Litter[a]	D_1	D_2	D_3	D_4
	E_1	E_2	E_3	E_4
	F_1	F_2	F_3	F_4
	G_1	G_2	G_3	G_4
	H_1	H_2	H_3	H_4

Analysis of variance (ANOVA) table (6.3)[b]		
Source (6.4)	df (6.5)	MS (5.18)
Between litters	7	$MS_{litters}$
Within drug	3	MS_{drug}
Interaction	<u>21</u>	$MS_{interaction}$
Total	31	

[a]Each litter is designated by a different letter (i.e., A, B, . . ., H) and each animal within a given litter by a subscript (e.g., B_4 indicates the fourth animal in litter B).

[b]See this book section.

by an amount determined by the correlation. The value of the average correlation among animals, r_i, can be obtained by the equation:

$$r_i = \frac{MS_{litters} - MS_{interaction}}{MS_{litters} + (n - 1)MS_{interaction}}$$

where n is the number of animals in each litter. Because MS_{drug} will remain about the same whether subjects are assigned to within- or between-treatment conditions, the use of $MS_{interaction}$ to evaluate MS_{drug} is more likely to yield a significant finding. The common mistake made when using this type of randomized-blocks design is to ignore the litter classification and treat the data as though all the observations are independent. In other words, the sum of squares (5.17) values for litter and interaction are pooled and divided by 28 (summation of df for the two sources of variation). Because the pooled value will be larger than $MS_{interaction}$, when a positive correlation exists among littermates, the outcome of this error summation procedure is to produce an F-ratio smaller than it should be. Hence, the biologist by ignoring the litter classification would underestimate the level of significance (5.16).

9.5　CORRELATED OBSERVATIONS: CONCLUSIONS

The failure to deal properly with correlated observations is a major problem in biological research. A common error in biological research is the assumption that littermates or tissue samples from the same animal are independent observations (4.9). The consequence of making this erroneous assumption of independency depends on the experimental design used. If a nested design (9.3) has been used, the error will produce falsely inflated F-ratios. If a randomized-blocks design has been used (9.4) the error will produce an underestimation of the F-ratios for all the "within" conditions.

If designed properly the use of related animals is a simple yet powerful way to increase the efficiency of an experiment. *The general rule is to assign related animals to the different treatment conditions*, thus using a randomized-blocks design (9.4). When related animals are assigned to the same treatment condition, a nested design is obtained which presents special problems (9.3). Indeed, nested designs in biology are usually inefficient and arranging the experiment so that there are independent observations is a better alternative. Within the context of littermates, only one animal per litter would be selected for each specific treatment condition and the other animals in the litter would be used for other experiments or assays (9.4). In a few cases, a nested design may be an efficient method to answer a given research question. If a research project requires the use of a specialized nested design, a statistician should be consulted before data are collected.

9.6 PROBABILITY CORRECTIONS FOR WITHIN-SUBJECT DESIGNS

Analyses of variance of within-subject designs (4.16, 4.17, 4.18) are not very robust (5.23) and violations of the underlying mathematical assumptions of normality, homogeneity of within-treatment variances, and independence may cause significant problems in statistical inference. Another assumption which is unique for within-subject designs is that the correlations between all possible pairs of treatments are equal. With three treatments, the correlations between levels a_1 and a_2, between levels a_1 and a_3, and between levels a_2 and a_3 are assumed to be equal (homogeneity of covariances). Even when minor violations are present the actual theoretical sampling distribution shifts to the right of the normal (null) F-distribution. Hence, the critical F-ratio values in the tabled (normal) values of the F-distribution are too small. The F-ratio values from the correct sampling distribution (shifted) would be larger than those listed in the normal F-tables (Figure 1.11). With three or more levels of a within-subject variable the normal F-test is biased in a positive direction; consequently, a more lenient significance level is actually being used.

Several ways to correct this bias have been proposed. A sphericity test is normally done to test the assumption of compound symmetry (homogeneity of covariances) in repeated-measures designs with three or more levels of the within-subject factor. In the outputs of some computer programs three significance levels may be provided: the normal (classical) two-tailed F-levels, Greenhouse-Geisser adjusted levels, and Hulyh-Feldt adjusted levels. The Greenhouse-Geisser adjustment reduces the numerator and denominator degrees of freedom (5.17) to adjust for the fact that the classical two-tailed F tends to be too liberal. The Greenhouse-Geisser adjustment, however, tends to overcorrect and this produces a reduction in the number of null hypotheses falsely rejected as expected by theory. The adjusted F-ratios are biased in a negative direction. The Hulyh-Feldt correction adjusts the numerator and denominator degrees of freedom by a factor that reflects the degree of heterogeneity *actually present* in the experimental data. Hence, the Hulyh-Feldt correction is the method of choice if the complicated calculations are done by a computer program.

9.7. NESTED INDEPENDENT VARIABLES

A factorial design (4.13) is normally used when more than one independent variable is manipulated in an experiment. In some multifactor designs, however, an independent variable may be nested within the levels of another independent variable. A nested analysis of variance is where a subordinate classification is nested within the higher level of classification. This type of design is also called a *hierarchical analysis of variance* and the groups representing a subordinate level of classification must be randomly selected. Both simple and rather complicated forms of nested designs are found in the biological and biomedical literature. The two general uses of nested ANOVA are (1) to specify the magnitude of error at various stages of an experiment and (2) to determine the magnitude of the variance attributable to different levels of variation in such fields as quantitative genetics (see Sokal and Rohlf, 1981, pp. 271–308).

10

Popular Post Hoc
Multiple Comparison Tests

10.1 NEED FOR POST HOC TESTING

With three or more treatment conditions and an overall significant F (rejection of the null hypothesis), at least one of the population means can be concluded to be different from the others (6.9). But, an infinite number of other possible deviations from the $\mu_1 = \mu_2 = \cdots \mu_i$ situation exist. Should every possible pair or combination of measures be tested (6.10)? If so, how should the significance level be determined for so many possible comparisons? No simple answers exist for these questions and many different statistical procedures have been proposed as solutions for this multiple comparison problem (see Hochberg and Tamhane, 1987, Jaccard, Becker, and Woods, 1984; Miller, 1985; Wilcox, 1987a,b for reviews).

Suggested solutions to this problem are named after pioneer workers in the field, including Fisher, Scheffe', Tukey, Duncan, Newman, Keuls, and Dunnett. These individuals have developed procedures to deal with the increased familywise (FW) error rate associated with post hoc comparisons (6.9). The same basic strategy is used by all statistical methods, namely to lower the significance level to control for the FW error rate associated with an increase in the number of individual comparisons. The various test statistics proposed differ in the ways in which a balance is achieved between the two types of errors (Type I and Type II) of statistical inference (5.10). Each of the tests is an "a posteriori" (post hoc) contrast test, which is a systematic procedure for comparing all possible pairs of group means. Typically, these post hoc tests are used after the data have been examined and differences noted previously, usually by a significant overall F-test (5.18). The number of pairwise comparisons among pairs of treatment means is given by the formula: $a(a - 1)/2$, in which a = the number (levels) of the treatment condition. The primary function of the post hoc test procedures is to protect against reporting too many Type I errors. If there are c comparisons each at the α level of significance (5.9), the total risk of making a Type I error is

$$\alpha_T = 1 - (1 - \alpha)^c$$

This total risk has also been called the FW error rate (6.9). In the case of 18 comparisons with an $\alpha = .05$, the total chance of obtaining $p < .05$ at least once by chance is $\alpha_T = 1 - (1 - .05)^{18} = .60$. Hence, an *important general rule for all experimental designs is design the experiment to minimize the total number of tests of hypotheses that need to be done in the statistical analysis.* Planned (a priori) comparisons are preferred because they have greater power than post hoc comparisons for any given level of α (6.10). With planned comparisons some of the possible comparisons in the experiment are not made (must be ignored). If you want to make all possible comparisons the results will be the same whether this decision is made a priori or post hoc (see Table 10.1).

10.2 LSD TEST AND DUNCAN'S TEST

The *least significant difference (LSD)* test is essentially a student's t-test between group means except that this test uses the error term from the overall analysis of variance thus pooling the within-treatment variances and degrees of freedom (Chapter 6). The LSD test holds the per-comparison error rate to alpha (5.9) but is normally not used because as the number of groups increases, so does the familywise (FW) error rate (6.9, 10.1). For example, with six samples from the same population the probability of some pair showing a significant difference at the .05 alpha level is 39 percent (Table 10.1).

The *Duncan multiple range test* (DMR) attempts to avoid the increase in FW error associated with the LSD test by using a different range value for subsets of different means. In this test the larger the potential subset, the larger the difference in means required to be declared significant. The Duncan procedure uses a special protection level rather than a significance level, that is, the probability of finding a significant difference, given that the two groups are in fact equal, is less than or equal to the specified protection level. The Duncan MR test does not maintain its claimed protection level even with equal sample sizes, is only approximate with unequal sample sizes, and, therefore, is not recommended (see 10.8).

Table 10.1 Probability of Having at Least One Significant Comparision ($p < .05$) When All Possible Pairs of Means Are Tested

Number of means and (tests)	Approximate value[a]	Tests are independent[b]	Tests are nonindependent[c]
2 (1)	.05	.05	.05
3 (3)	.15	.14	.11
4 (6)	.30	.26	.21
5 (10)	.50	.40	.30
6 (15)	.75	.50	.39
7 (21)	1.05	.64	.47

[a]Approximation formula is $n(\alpha)$ when n = number of tests and α = probability level selected for single test.
[b]Test's independent formula is $1 - (1 - \alpha)^n$ where n = number of tests and α = probability level selected for single test and the assumption is that the tests are statistically independent. This assumption of independence is not correct for normal multiple comparison situations; hence this formula is conservative and overestimates the probability of a Type I error (Table 5.1).
[c]Probabilities for nonindependent situations (see Godfrey, 1986b).

10.3 STUDENT-NEWMAN-KEULS TEST

The Student-Newman-Keuls (SNK) test is very similar to Duncan's MR test (10.2) as different range values are used for different subsets of treatment means. SNK test holds the familywise (FW) error rate to alpha for each stage of the testing procedure (6.9, 10.1). Hence, alpha is neither familywise nor per-comparison. SNK test is only approximate if the group sizes are unequal. In many statistics books, the SNK test is listed as the Newman-Keuls test and is a commonly used multiple comparison procedure (Howell, 1987; Winer, 1971). But, the SNK test has been found to be inadequate in its control of Type I errors in certain situations (see Holland and Copenhaver, 1988; Jaccard, Becker, and Woods, 1984). The DMR (10.2) and the SNK tests are known as sequential tests because significance testing follows a series of sequential tests, each with a different critical value to establish the significance between pairs of means (see 10.8).

10.4 TUKEY HSD TEST AND TUKEY-KRAMER TEST

The Tukey HSD (Honestly Significant Difference) test maintains the familywise (FW) error rate (6.9) at the chosen value of α_{FW} for the entire set of pairwise comparisons. It uses the same value as the largest used in the SNK procedure (10.3); hence, with the Tukey test a single range value is used for all comparisons, regardless of how many means are to be in a subset. Of the three most commonly used multiple comparison tests, the Duncan (10.2), the Student-Newman-Keuls (10.3) and the Tukey, the latter test is usually recommended because of its favorable power characteristics relative to the two sequential procedures (10.8). The Tukey test, like the other two, is only approximate for unequal group size but gives reasonably accurate results if sample sizes are nearly equal. The Tukey test is recommended for between-subject designs (4.10) in which all pairwise comparisons are of interest. The Tukey-Kramer test is recommended for unequal sample sizes (see 10.8).

10.5 THE SCHEFFÉ TEST

The Scheffé test uses a single range value for all comparisons, which is appropriate for examining all possible linear combinations of group means, not just pairwise comparisons. Hence, the Scheffé test is stricter than the other multiple comparison tests (10.2, 10.3, 10.4) because the familywise (FW) error rate (6.9) is held at a particular value regardless of the number of comparisons actually conducted. The Scheffé test is exact, even with unequal group sizes, and requires no special tables because it is based on the values of the F-statistic appearing in standard F-tables. The *Scheffé test is used primarily to evaluate arbitrary combinations of groups against each other*, for example, the mean of groups 1 and 3 versus the mean of groups 2, 4, and 5 (see 10.8). The Scheffé test should not be used when all pairwise comparisons are to be made (see Howell, 1987).

10.6 THE DUNNETT TEST

The Dunnett test is a specialized correction technique for familywise (FW) error rate (6.9) that compensates for the increased number of Type I errors. The Dunnett test is not as "corrective" as are other post hoc tests because it takes into consideration only a limited number of comparisons, the control-experimental contrasts. Hence, this test is applicable when there is a control group (or a standard treatment group) and your *only* interest is in comparing each of the other groups with the single control or standard treatment group. Unfortunately, the Dunnett test has a great potential for abuse as researchers may quickly examine their data, conclude that the control and experimental group comparisons are the only ones of interest (because the experimental group means are similar), use this planned comparison test (6.10), achieve significance (6.11), and publish their papers (see 10.8).

10.7 THE BONFERRONI t-TEST

The Bonferroni procedure (also called Dunn's test) has been gaining popularity because it is easy to apply, has the widest range of applications, and, if the number of planned comparisons can be limited, provides critical values that are lower than those of other procedures. Even if many comparisons are made the Bonferroni t-test critical values are only slightly larger than those of other procedures. The Bonferroni statistic is a modified t-statistic which corrects for the number of comparisons being made in between-subject designs, and a paired-samples form is used for repeated-measure designs (see Godfrey, 1986b; Holland and Copenhaver, 1988; Jaccard, Becker, and Wood, 1984).

The determination as to which comparisons are to be tested must be made before the data are inspected. Hence, the planned-unplanned comparison problem (6.10) may be associated with this test statistic. Usually, only a few comparisons are planned because as more comparisons are done, the critical values of the Bonferroni t become larger. With an increase in the number of comparisons the Bonferroni procedure overestimates the true probability of making a Type I error (and increases the probability of making a Type II error); hence, this procedure becomes too conservative (less power) when many pairwise comparisons are made in a fixed effects, between-subject (4.10) design (see 10.8).

10.8 SUMMARY OF MULTIPLE COMPARISON POST HOC TESTS

Several multiple comparison procedures are available to test which pairs of means are significantly different (10.2, 10.3, 10.4, 10.5, 10.6, 10.7). The simplest (Fisher's least significance difference test, 10.2) is to perform t-tests on all the pairwise comparisons. Normally, a significant overall F-test would be required before using the least significance difference test. The t-tests are done using the pooled estimate (s^2) of the population variance given by the error term in the analysis of variance (Chapter 6). The Bonferroni t-test (10.7) also uses multiple t-tests but each of these tests must reach significance at the α/c level where c is the total number of comparisons made, to ensure an overall significance level of α (5.9).

Several multiple comparison procedures (Duncan, 10.2; Newman-Keuls, 10.3; Tukey, 10.4) begin by comparing the largest mean with the smallest, and continue with the next largest difference, and so on, until either a nonsignificant comparison is encountered (Duncan, Newman-Keuls) or until all pairwise comparisons have been made. With these range tests the difference between means is compared at each step to an appropriate null distribution. The Scheffé test (10.5) allows for testing more complex contrasts as well as all pairwise comparisons of means. The Dunnett test (10.6) identifies group means that are significantly different from the mean of a particular group (normally the control group).

The multiple comparison literature is enormous, and arbitrariness and ambiguity confront the interested researcher. Multiple comparison tests are used in three distinct situations which are (*a*) planned comparisons (6.10), (*b*) post hoc comparisons 6.9, and (*c*) post hoc comparisons that are guided by a significant overall F-ratio (10.1). Biologists normally apply these tests only after a significant F-ratio (5.16) has been obtained. But many multiple comparison tests (e.g., Bonferroni t-test, Dunnett, Scheffé, Tukey, Tukey-Kramer) will control adequately the Type I error probability (5.10) regardless of whether the F-ratio is significant or not (see Wilcox, 1987a,b). Given that the experimentalwise error rate should be maintained at the indicated level (e.g., $p < .05$) the choice of multiple comparison procedure will depend primarily upon power considerations (5.12) and the robustness of the test (5.23). The power and robustness of a multiple comparison test depends upon the type of design used (e.g., between-subject, within-subject) and the consequences of violating the statistical assumptions of equal sample size, homogeneous population variances, and normality (see Jaccard, Becker, and Woods, 1984; Sokal and Rohlf, 1981, table 9.3, p. 261). Table 10.2 summarizes the recommendations of Jaccard, Becker, and Woods (1984).

Table 10.2 Recommendations for Multiple Comparison Test Based Upon Experimental Design and Statistical Assumptions

Type of design[a]	Assumptions of: Equal sample n, homogeneous population variances, and normality (optimal conditions)	Violation of assumptions (suboptimal conditions)
Between-subject (4.10)	Tukey HSD test (10.4)	[b]Unequal n: Tukey-Kramer test (10.4) [b]Unequal variance: Games and Howell test
Within-subject (4.16)[d]	Tukey HSD test (10.4)	[c]Bonferroni paired t-test (10.7)

[a]Mixed factorial designs (4.21) would use between- and within-subject design recommendations.
[b]Calculation procedures are given in Games, Keselman, and Rogan (1981).
[c]Calculation procedures are given in Shott (1990).
[d]See this book section.

Table 10.3 Summary of Multiple Comparison Test Procedures

Test	Error rate[a]	Comparison[b]	Type of test[c]
Planned (a priori)			
1. Individual t-tests	PC	Pairwise	t
2. Orthogonal contrasts	PC	Orthogonal	F
Unplanned (post hoc)			
1. Bonferroni t (Dunn's test)	PE or EW	Any contrasts	t
2. Newman-Keuls	EW	Pairwise	Range
3. Tukey (HSD)	EW	Pairwise	Range
4. Tukey (WSD)	EW	Pairwise	Range
5. Scheffé	EW	Any contrasts	F
6. Other tests (e.g., T-method, GT2-method, Welsch step-up procedure, SS-STP (see Sokal and Rohlf, 1981, table 9.3, p. 261)			
Planned (control compared with all experimental groups)			
1. Dunnett's test (see Howell, 1987; or Rosner, 1990)			

[a]PC = per comparison, PE = per experiment, EW = experimentwise
[b]Some tests use means in calculations, others use totals.
[c]Calculation examples may be found in Howell (1987) or Rosner (1990).

Other recommendations have been made in popular textbooks. As examples, Howell (1987) and Glantz (1987) recommend the Newman-Keuls test when post hoc comparisons are guided by a significant F-ratio. But, Keppel (1991) indicates that the Tukey test is preferred over the Newman-Keuls test, and Sokal and Rohlf (1981) recommend a variety of methods but not the Newman-Keuls test. Wilcox (1987a) recommends that ". . . multiple comparison procedures based on the assumption of equal variance never be used, and that procedures for unequal variances always be used, instead" (p. 185). Relatively few studies have evaluated multiple comparison procedures in repeated-measures designs when statistical assumptions are violated. And, these are the most popular designs in biological research.

In essence, the relative merits of the various multiple comparison procedures depends on how you regard the importance of the two types of error (Type I and Type II) of statistical inference (5.10) for your study. The recommendations given in Table 10.2 for the various experimental designs are reasonable compromises. If multiple comparison testing is to be guided by a significant overall F-ratio, then the Tukey tests would be reasonable choices for *both* between- and within-subject comparisons. Common sense should be used in making decisions based upon the outcomes of any multiple comparison procedure. If a pairwise comparison difference just reaches or just misses significance (5.9, 6.11) all the qualifications of the particular test should be considered carefully. And, if this comparison is biologically important then a replication (7.3, 7.4) using planned comparisons (6.10) should be done. Table 10.3 summarizes the features of some of the most common multiple comparison procedures and refers to those textbooks in which calculation procedures are given.

11

Nonparametric Tests

11.1 ADVANTAGES AND DISADVANTAGES OF NONPARAMETRIC TESTS

Distribution-free nonparametric methods do not have restrictive assumptions as to the normality of observations (5.22), are appropriate for ordinal measurements (5.3), and are easy to calculate. The general disadvantages of these methods, compared with parametric tests, are that they are less powerful (5.12), the hypotheses tested are less specific, and they do not take advantage of all the known information about the sample distribution. Hence, nonparametric techniques should be regarded as complementary statistical methods rather than attractive alternatives to parametric methods (5.22).

An inherent characteristic of nonparametric statistics is that they deal with ranks rather than values of the observations (see Conover, 1980). The observations are normally arranged in an array and ranks are assigned from 1 to n. Numerous nonparametric methods exist, but only a few have direct applicability for experimental data in the biological sciences. In complete within-subject designs and mixed factorial designs in which *more than two observations* are obtained from each animal, no nonparametric tests are available to analyze all the data. Indeed, nonparametric tests are typically limited to relatively simple experimental designs because no error terms are available to assess complex interactions among variables (6.12, 6.13, 6.14).

In some cases a nonparametric test may be more powerful than a corresponding parametric test. An extreme score in a data sample (an outlier, 5.27) may make a parametric test less powerful because it inflates the error term (5.16). For example, the parametric t-test is more powerful than its nonparametric alternative, the Mann-Whitney U test (11.5), when two treatment conditions are being compared and the population is normally distributed. However, when the population of values is not normally distributed, some nonparametric tests may be more powerful. Tests based on ranks can be more powerful than parametric tests when the sample data are drawn from populations that are skewed or have more values in their tails (heavy-tailed distributions) than is true of the normal distribution (see Myers and Well, 1991). These outcomes are known because computer simulations with populations which are heavy-tailed or severely skewed have been used to make comparisons between parametric and nonparametric tests. Therefore, you should plot your data to try and identify flagrant violations of normality. Many statistical packages include stem-and-leaf plots and box-and-whisker plots of sample data (see Chapter 8).

11.2 CHI-SQUARE (χ^2) TEST

One of the most commonly used nonparametric methods (11.1) is the application of the χ^2 test of independence to row (r) $\times$ column (c) contingency tables in which expected frequencies are obtained from the set of data itself. The χ^2 statistic is used to determine if the observed frequencies of occurrence of a categorical value of a qualitative variable differ significantly from expected or theoretical frequencies of occurrence (5.3). The expected frequency, for example, may be what would be expected by chance, that is, for 100 occurrences and two categories the expected frequency for each of the two cells would be 50. This expected frequency would be used to evaluate the results obtained (the observed frequencies). Statistically, whether the observed data fit the model specified by the null hypothesis (5.16) is determined. If the observed data do not conform at a specified probability level, the null hypothesis is rejected and the alternative hypothesis is asserted. A test of this sort is known as a *goodness-of-fit* test because it ascertains the fit between an empirical observation and a theoretical model (5.5).

Just as the t- and F-test statistics (5.18) are associated with degrees of freedom (5.17) and have their accompanying sampling distributions, so does the χ^2 statistic. Although the χ^2 statistic is discrete in the values that it can assume, it approximates very closely a continuous distribution also known as the χ^2 distribution. The χ^2 distribution differs in shape depending upon its degrees of freedom. The approximation of the test statistic, χ^2, with the χ^2 distribution is very good provided that all expected cell frequencies are 5 or greater. *To use the χ^2 test, frequencies and not percentages must be the data, the frequencies in the various cells must be independent of one another, and the cells must be mutually exclusive and exhaustive.*

In biological and biomedical research, both the independent and dependent variables are often discrete variables. Usually in this research the independent variable is one type of treatment compared with either a placebo condition or another form of treatment. The dependent variable is commonly a mutually exclusive and exhaustive two-category variable, such as the survival status of the individual (live or dead). In such studies the important question is whether the proportion of survivors is significantly greater in one treatment condition than in another. With a small sample size *Fisher's exact probability* test would be used to answer this research question. With intermediate sample size, the χ^2 test of the independence of categorical variables would be the appropriate test of significance if n is sufficiently large (expected frequencies of 5 or more in at least 80 percent of all cells in the $r \times c$ contingency table).

11.3 WILCOXON TESTS: GENERAL CONSIDERATIONS

The *Wilcoxon* tests convert the scores or values of a variable to ranks, require calculation of a sum of the ranks, and provide critical values for the sum necessary to test the null hypothesis at a given significance level (11.1). The Wilcoxon tests are randomization tests for ranked data and the statistic is easy to calculate. But, the quantitative information inherent in the scores is lost when they are converted to ranks, that is, two adjacent scores, 100 and 80, assume a difference of only 1 in the rankings. Hence, the loss of statistical power must be considered when any nonparametric test is used (11.1). Calculation procedures for the various Wilcoxon tests may be found in Howell (1987), Rosner (1990), or Runyon (1985).

11.4 WILCOXON SIGNED RANK TEST: ONE SAMPLE CASE AND PAIRED MEASURES

The Wilcoxon signed rank test is a nonparametric test (11.1) for ordinally scaled variables (5.3). The procedures for calculating the test statistic in the one-sample case and paired measures are about the same. In the one-sample case, the mean that is hypothesized under H_0 is subtracted prior to ranking the differences (5.5). For paired measures (either before-after or matched-pairs measures), the second score is subtracted from the first for each pair before ranking the differences. Hence, the Wilcoxon signed rank test is the nonparametric analogue to the paired t-test (11.3).

11.5 MANN-WHITNEY U TEST (WILCOXON RANK SUM TEST): TWO INDEPENDENT MEANS

The *Wilcoxon rank sum test* is used to test the null hypothesis that there is no difference in the distributions of two populations (5.5). Based on the ranks from two independent samples, this nonparametric test corresponds to the t-test, except that no assumptions are necessary as to normality or equality of variances (11.3). The scores in both groups are ranked together from low to high, the sum of the ranks of each group is obtained, and given the null hypothesis (the average of the ranks is approximately equal for both groups), the test statistic W_i (the sum of the ranks of the first sample) should not differ significantly from W_e (the expected sum of the ranks).

The Mann-Whitney U test and the Wilcoxon rank sum test are equivalent in that exactly the same *p* value is obtained by applying either test to the same data. Therefore, in this situation choosing what test to use is a matter of convenience but the Mann-Whitney test is the best known nonparametric test for two independent means.

11.6 KRUSKAL-WALLIS TEST (WILCOXON ONE-WAY ANALYSIS BY RANKS)

A nonparametric alternative to a one-way ANOVA (single factor, 6.7, 6.8) may be required to compare means among more than two samples where the underlying distributions are far from being normal (5.22) or where ordinal data are only available (5.3). The logic of the Wilcoxon rank sum test (11.5) is generalized to compare more than two samples. The observations in all treatment groups are pooled and ranks are assigned to each observation in the combined sample. The average ranks for the individual treatment groups are then compared. If the average ranks are far apart, the null hypothesis (H_0) is rejected and the alternative statistical hypothesis (H_i) is asserted (some of the treatments are different). If the average ranks are close to each other, there is no basis for rejecting H_0.

The test procedure for comparing the average ranks among three or more groups is known as the *Kruskal-Wallis* test and it tests the hypothesis that all samples were drawn from an identical population. If the overall test is significant, procedures are available to determine which pair of treatment means are significantly different (see Rosner, 1990, pp. 470–472). The Wilcoxon one-way analysis by ranks does not provide an overall test of significance as does the Kruskal-Wallis test. Rather, the Wilcoxon one-way analysis by ranks provides a test of pairwise comparisons among the treatment conditions (see Runyon, 1985, pp. 248-250). The Kruskal-Wallis test may only be used with equal sample sizes.

11.7 FRIEDMAN TWO-WAY ANALYSIS BY RANKS

The Friedman two-way analysis by ranks is the nonparametric analogue to the randomized-blocks design (9.4). The column variables represent the various treatment conditions and the rows represent the matched groups or repeated measures on the same individuals. The null hypothesis is that the treatment groups are drawn from the same population (5.5). The calculation procedures involve rank-ordering the values of the variable in each row from low to high, summing the resulting ranks in each column, calculating the test statistic $\chi^2 r$, and determining the probability of the observed $\chi^2 r$ given the appropriate degrees of freedom (see Runyon, 1985, pp. 250–252). The Friedman test provides an overall test of significance. If $\chi^2 r$ is significant, the Wilcoxon signed rank test may be used to test for significant differences between pairs of means (11.4).

11.8 RANK CORRELATION COEFFICIENT

The product moment correlation coefficient r is used to measure the degree of linear relationship between the paired values of two continuous random variables (5.27). If the population distributions of the two variables required for interpretation of r are questionable, the raw scores on each variable may be converted into ordinal values (ranks) and these two rank orders correlated. The n values of one variable are ranked 1 through n, and the n values of the other variables are also ranked 1 through n. It makes no difference whether rank 1 refers to the lowest or highest score in the distribution as long as *the same ranking method is used for both variables*. The outcome is n pairs of ranks and it is these ranks which are correlated resulting in the rank correlation coefficient.

The rank correlation coefficient is free of the assumptions of a joint bivariate normal population distribution as is required for the product moment correlation coefficient (5.27). But, the two coefficients are similar in that neither implies a causal relationship between the correlated variables (4.1). Measures of correlation are available for most types of relationships not within the domain of the product moment correlation coefficient or the rank correlation coefficient for two ordinally scaled variables (5.3). As examples, there are the *biserial correlation coefficient*, for relating a continuous normally distributed variable with a dichotomized variable which has an underlying normal distribution; the *point biserial correlation coefficient*, for relating a continuous normally distributed variable with a truly dichotomized variable; the *tetrachoric correlation coefficient*; the *four fold point correlation*, the *contingency coefficient*; and the *correlation ratio* or *eta coefficient*. The details of the assumptions, definitions, and mathematical properties of these coefficients may be found in advanced reference books on correlation methods.

12

Selection of Statistical Tests

12.1 ADVANTAGES AND DISADVANTAGES OF STATISTICAL FLOW CHARTS

Flowcharts of appropriate methods of statistical inference are presented in many biostatistics books. In the best case, these flowcharts provide a quick reference to the statistical methods covered in the particular biostatistics book. In the worst case, these flowcharts become a simple cookbook for the selection of the "appropriate" statistical method for any given set of data. Sometimes these flowcharts are presented in a decision tree format in which at each branch (choice-point) a yes-no response is required to select the correct path to the appropriate statistical method. Unfortunately, for some readers these flowcharts become an obligatory blueprint for the statistical analysis of their research data. A similar menu-driven selection of methods is also becoming routine in "user-friendly" statistical computer packages. A more recent trend is the development of *statistical expert systems*. Biologists who are not statistically qualified may use these systems to protect themselves from errors in their data analysis (see Brent, 1989; Gale, 1985; Hand, 1984, 1985). Unfortunately, expert statistical systems still cannot eliminate all the serious blunders that novices may make (see Murry, 1990, pp. 1066–1067).

Despite their potential for misuse, flowcharts can be valuable *reference aids* in the selection of appropriate statistical procedures and Figures 12.1–12.11 summarize tests discussed previously. The guiding rule in the selection of any statistical method is to know the research hypotheses and plan exact tests of their statistical alternatives (6.10). Before this rule can be applied some knowledge of experimental design and statistical inference (12.2) and the logic of hypothesis testing (12.3) must be obtained. For this reason, each reference figure (Figure 12.1–12.11) provides a listing of the statistical methods available and identifies the chapter section in which a brief description of the method is given.

12.2 REVIEW OF EXPERIMENTAL DESIGN AND STATISTICAL INFERENCE

Section I focused on the interdependence among experimental design, statistical inference, and the validity of research conclusions. The core of this material may be reviewed quickly by reading the following: 1.5, 4.4, 4.5, 4.10, 4.16, 4.21, 4.22, 4.23 and 5.21.

12.3 REVIEW OF STATISTICAL HYPOTHESIS TESTING

Section II focused on the logic of hypothesis testing, statistical inference, and parametric and nonparametric statistical procedures. The core of this material may be reviewed quickly by reading the following: 1.6, 1.7, 5.5, 5.10, 5.16, 5.22, 9.5, 10.1, and 11.1.

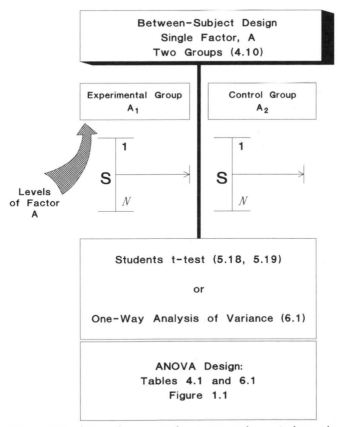

Figure 12.1   Statistical tests between the means of two independent groups (12.4).

12.4 STATISTICAL TESTS BETWEEN THE MEANS OF TWO INDEPENDENT GROUPS

The essential features of these statistical tests are that different subjects are used in each of the two treatment groups (4.10) and one and only one measure for each subject is analyzed (4.9). In Figure 12.1 the chapter sections in which these tests, their assumptions, and ANOVA tables are given are enclosed in parentheses.

12.5 STATISTICAL TESTS BETWEEN THE MEANS OF TWO DEPENDENT SAMPLES

The essential feature of these statistical tests is that the same subjects are used in both treatment conditions (4.16). These tests are called repeated measures or

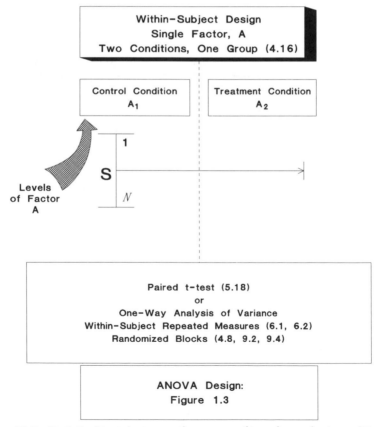

Figure 12.2 Statistical tests between the means of two dependent conditions for one independent group (12.5).

within-subject tests because two correlated measures from each subject are analyzed. In Figure 12.2 the chapter sections in which these tests, their assumptions and ANOVA tables are given are enclosed in parentheses.

12.6 STATISTICAL TESTS AMONG THE MEANS OF THREE OR MORE INDEPENDENT GROUPS (SINGLE FACTOR)

The essential features of these statistical tests are that different subjects are used in each of the three or more treatment groups, only the levels of one factor are

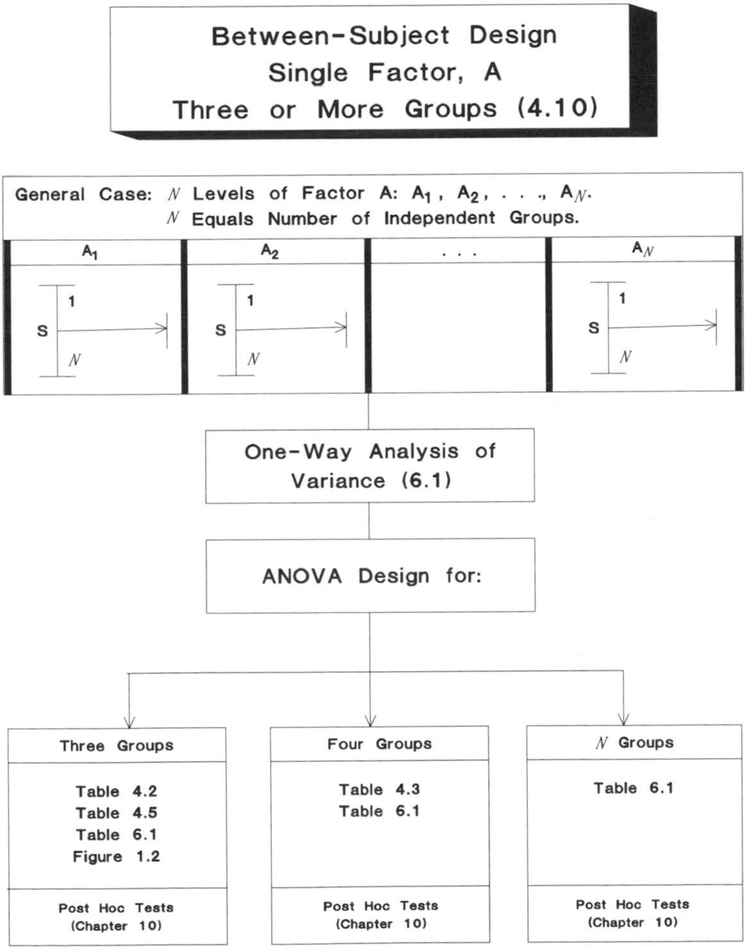

Figure 12.3 Statistical tests among the means of three or more independent groups in a single-factor design (12.6).

manipulated, and one and only one measure for each subject is analyzed. In Figure 12.3 the chapter sections in which these tests, their assumptions, and ANOVA tables are given are enclosed in parentheses. Post hoc multiple comparison tests *are* also necessary to determine which of the groups are different from each other (Chapter 10).

12.7 STATISTICAL TESTS AMONG THE MEANS OF THREE OR MORE DEPENDENT TREATMENT SAMPLES (SINGLE FACTOR)

The essential features of these statistical tests are that the same subjects are used in all the treatment conditions and only the levels of one factor are manipulated. These tests are also called repeated-measures or within-subject tests because

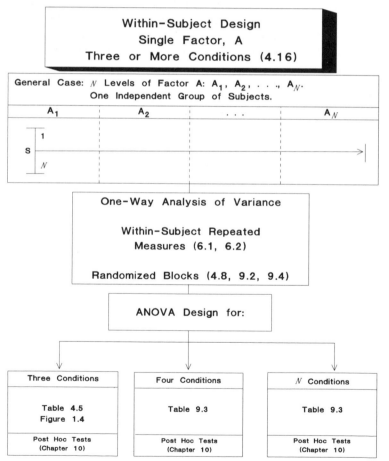

Figure 12.4 Statistical tests among the means of three or more dependent conditions for one independent group in a single-factor design (12.7).

three or more correlated measures of the same dependent variable from each subject are analyzed. In Figure 12.4 the chapter sections in which these tests, their assumptions, and ANOVA tables are given are enclosed in parentheses. Post hoc multiple comparison tests *are* also necessary to determine which of the correlated measures are different from each other (Chapter 10).

12.8 STATISTICAL TESTS FOR BETWEEN-SUBJECT FACTORIAL DESIGNS

The essential features of these statistical tests are that the levels of two or more factors (A, B, and so forth) are manipulated together and a different group of

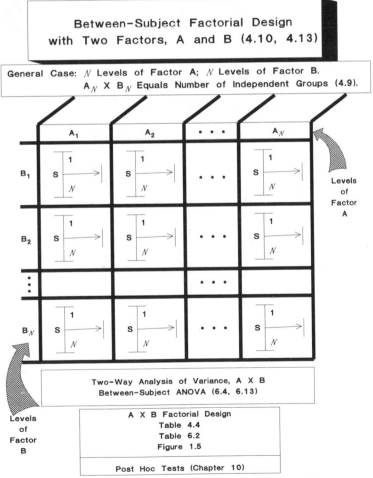

Figure 12.5 Statistical tests for between-subject A × B factorial designs (12.8).

subjects is used for each of the different treatment combinations (A_1B_1, A_2B_2, A_1B_2, and so forth). In Figure 12.5 (two factors) and Figure 12.6 (three factors) the chapter sections in which these between-subject factorial tests, their assumptions, and ANOVA tables are given are enclosed in parentheses. Post hoc multiple comparison tests (Chapter 10) *are* also necessary to evaluate significant main effects with more than two comparison means (6.8) and to interpret two-way and higher-order interactions (6.13, 6.14) in these factorial statistical tests.

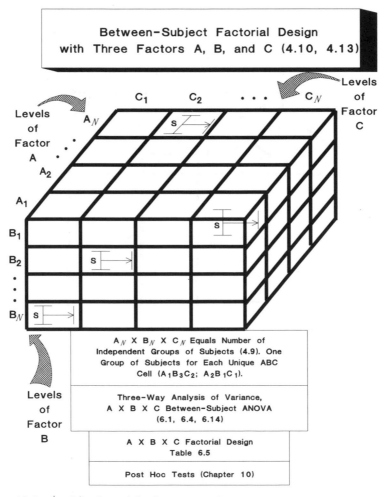

Figure 12.6 Statistical tests for between-subject $A \times B \times C$ factorial designs (12.8).

12.9 STATISTICAL TESTS FOR WITHIN-SUBJECT FACTORIAL DESIGNS

The essential features of these statistical tests are that the same subjects are used in all treatment combinations and the levels of two or more factors (A, B, and so forth) are manipulated together. Hence, the *same* group of subjects is given each different treatment combination (A_1B_1, A_2B_2, A_1B_2, and so forth). These tests are also called repeated measures as correlated measures of the same depen-

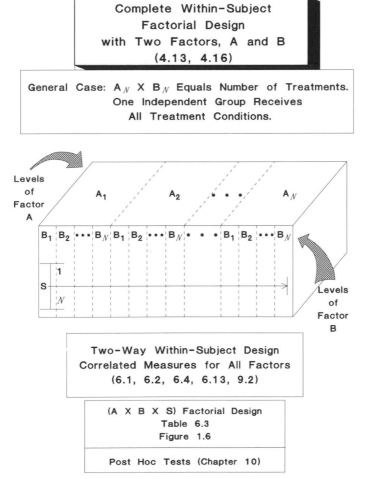

Figure 12.7 Statistical tests for within-subject A × B factorial designs (12.9). Within-subject factors are enclosed in parentheses with subjects (A × B × S) to identify correlated measurements (9.2, 9.5).

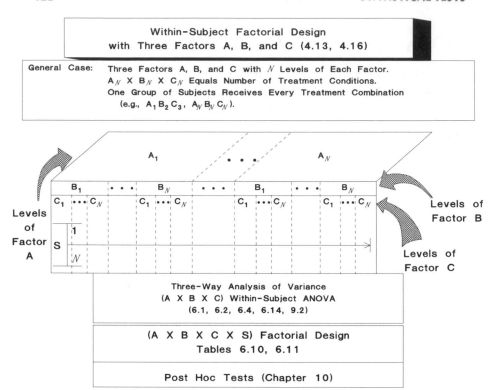

Within–Subject Factorial Design
with Three Factors A, B, and C (4.13, 4.16)

General Case: Three Factors A, B, and C with N Levels of Each Factor.
A_N X B_N X C_N Equals Number of Treatment Conditions.
One Group of Subjects Receives Every Treatment Combination
(e.g., $A_1 B_2 C_3$, $A_N B_N C_N$).

Three–Way Analysis of Variance
(A X B X C) Within–Subject ANOVA
(6.1, 6.2, 6.4, 6.14, 9.2)

(A X B X C X S) Factorial Design
Tables 6.10, 6.11

Post Hoc Tests (Chapter 10)

Figure 12.8 Statistical tests for within-subject A × B × C factorial designs (12.9). Within-subject factors are enclosed in parentheses with subjects (A × B × C × S) to identify correlated measurements (9.2, 9.5).

dent variable from each subject are analyzed. In Figures 12.7 (two repeated factors) and Figure 12.8 (three repeated factors) the chapter sections in which these complete within-subject factorial tests, their assumptions, and ANOVA tables are given are enclosed in parentheses. Post hoc multiple comparison tests (Chapter 10) *are* also necessary to evaluate significant main effects with more than two comparison means (6.8) and to interpret two-way and higher-order interactions (6.13, 6.14) in these factorial statistical tests.

12.10 STATISTICAL TESTS FOR MIXED FACTORIAL DESIGNS

The essential features of these statistical tests are that both between-subject (12.4, 12.6) and within-subject (12.5, 12.7) components are included in the design and in the subsequent analysis of the data. Two different groups of sub-

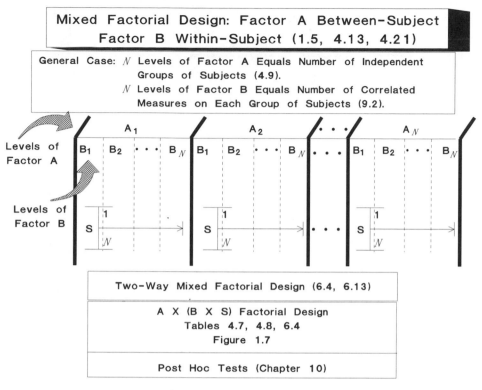

Figure 12.9 Statistical tests for mixed A × (B × S) factorial designs (12.10). The within-subject factor is enclosed in parentheses with subjects to identify correlated measurements (9.2, 9.5).

jects (between-subject component) with two repeated (correlated) measures (e.g., heart rates) for each subject would be a 2 × (2 × S) mixed factorial design, an A × (B × S) design. Hence, in a mixed two-factor experiment (A, B) independent groups are the levels of one factor (factor A) and repeated measures are the levels of the other factor (factor B) (see Figure 12.9). In a mixed factorial design the within-subject components are identified by their association in parentheses with subjects (B × S). In an A × (B × C × S) mixed factorial design (see Figure 12.10) factor A would be the between-subject component and repeated measures would be associated with the last two factors, B and C (4.21, 4.22, 4.23). Likewise, in an A × B × (C × S) mixed design factors A and B would be the between-subject components and repeated (dependent, correlated) measures would be the last factor, C (see Figure 12.11).

In Figures 12.9–12.11 the chapter sections in the text where these various mixed factorial designs, their statistical assumptions, and ANOVA tables are

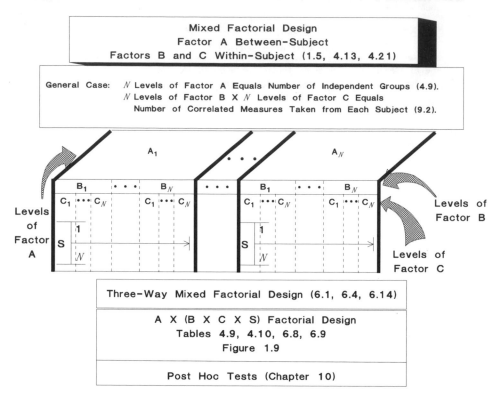

Figure 12.10 Statistical tests for mixed A × (B × C × S) factorial designs (12.10). The within-subject factors are enclosed in parentheses with subjects to identify correlated measurements (9.2, 9.5).

given are enclosed in parentheses. Post hoc multiple comparison tests (Chapter 10) *are* also necessary to evaluate significant F-ratios for main effects with more than two comparison means (6.8) and to interpret two-way and higher order interactions in these mixed factorial statistical tests.

12.11 STATISTICAL TESTS OF ASSOCIATION AND OF PREDICTION OF FUNCTIONAL RELATIONSHIPS

In biological research, the identification of relationships between and among sets of data is normally done by correlation or regression analysis. The essential similarities and differences between statistical tests of association and of prediction of functional relationships (regression) are summarized in Table 5.4. The chapter sections in which these statistical tests are discussed briefly are correlation (5.27), linear regression (5.26), analysis of covariance (6.18), and multiple regression (5.26).

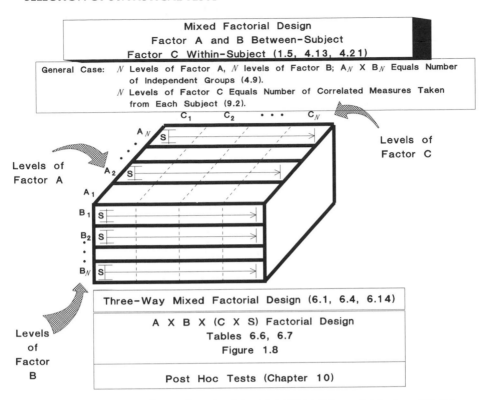

Figure 12.11 Statistical tests for mixed A × B × (C × S) factorial designs (12.10). The within-subject factor is enclosed in parentheses with subjects to identify correlated measurements (9.2, 9.5).

IV
RESEARCH DESIGN PROBLEMS AND THEIR CRITIQUES

13

Introduction to Design Problems

13.1 PURPOSE OF DESIGN PROBLEMS

In "Chapter 14," the essentials of experimental design and statistical inference (Sections I thru III) are reviewed by illustrating their applications and misapplications in 100 research design problems. In a number of disciplines, design and statistical principles are now being taught by showing their misapplications (see Friedman and Friedman, 1980; Hooke, 1980, 1983; Jaffe and Spirer, 1987). A few flawed research studies in medicine (Riegelman and Hirsch, 1989) and physiology (Scott and Waterhouse, 1986) have also been reviewed.

The 100 problems in "Chapter 14" are briefs of biological studies. For each brief you should decide whether the author's conclusion should be accepted or rejected. In many of the experimental designs, the treatment conditions may be confounded by subject-, environment-, or time-related extraneous variables, proper control groups may be absent; and so forth. In other studies, both the statistical treatment of the data and the author's conclusion may be incorrect or the statistical treatment may be correct but the conclusion of the author may be wrong. In some studies, the statistical treatment of the data may be inappropriate but the author's conclusion may be correct. If you do not accept the author's conclusions, try to identify the reason or reasons why these conclusions should be rejected. For each brief you may want to identify the factors and their levels by reconstructing the experimental design and, when appropriate, the ANOVA table used for the statistical comparisons. After you have made your decision, review the subsequent critique to identify any problems which may exist. Each critique includes a restatement of the research hypothesis, the ANOVA table (if appropriate), and whether the inferences of the researchers are appropriate. If serious design or statistical errors do exist in the research brief, citations are provided to the relevant topics in Sections I thru III.

Although emphasis is given to design and inference errors, a critical, not a cynical, perceptive should be cultivated in your evaluations. To be critical is not to demolish or to deride but to make exact and discriminating judgments. Errors may occur in biological studies but every flaw is not fatal. In your evaluations assume that all omitted portions of the experiment were performed properly; that is, make your decisions from the relevant facts presented in each brief.

In the following briefs, many common abbreviations and statistical symbols are used. For convenience, these abbreviations and symbols, their meaning, and the chapter section in which some are discussed in more detail are listed (e.g., Factorial designs 4.13):

Symbol	Meanings and definitions
$=$	Equal to
$<$	Less than
NS	Not significant
F	The F-statistic (5.18)
$>$	Greater than
F (df numerator, df denominator)	The designation of the numerator and denominator associated with a particular F. In a given brief, numbers would replace df numerator and df denominator; that is, $F(1,68) =$ value of F (5.18)
p	Probability: the proportion of times out of 100 that a particular value of a statistic (F, t, etc.) will occur by chance (5.6)
$p < .05$	Probability of obtaining the given value is less than 5 out of 100
SD	Standard deviation of scores (5.2)
SE or SEM	Standard error of the mean (5.2)
t	The t-statistic (5.18)
t (df denominator)	The designation of the denominator degrees of freedom associated with a particular t. In a given brief, a number would replace the df denominator, that is, $t(18) =$ the value of t.
r	The product-moment correlation (5.27)
s or n	Sample size, number of animals per treatment condition, number of pairs of scores in linear regression/correlation (4.9)
χ^2 (chi–square)	The chi-square statistic (11.2)
ANOVA	Analysis of variance statistical method (6.1, 6.3)
A $\times$ B design	A two-factor between-subject design, also called an A $\times$ B factorial design or a completely randomized factorial design. A 2×2 factorial design indicates there are two levels of both factor A and factor B. A 2×3 factorial design indicates there are two levels of factor A and three levels of factor B, and so forth (4.10, 4.13)
A $\times$ B $\times$ C design	A three-factor between-subject design, that is, a $4 \times 4 \times 3$, a $2 \times 2 \times 4$, and so forth (4.10, 4.13)
(A $\times$ S) design	A single-factor within-subject design. Also called a repeated-measures design. The within-subject (or repeated) factor is enclosed in parentheses (4.16) to identify dependent (correlated) measurements (9.2, 9.5).
(A $\times$ B $\times$ S) design	A two-factor complete within-subject design (4.16). The within-subject factors are enclosed in parentheses to identify dependent (correlated) measurements (9.2, 9.5).

Symbol	Meanings and definitions
(A × B × C × S) design	A three-factor complete within-subject design (4.16). The within-subject factors are enclosed in parentheses to identify dependent (correlated) measurements (9.2, 9.5).
A × (B × S) design, A × (B × C × S), A × B × (C × S), and so forth	Mixed factorial designs. Also called split-plot designs (4.21). Within-subject factors are enclosed in parentheses [(B × S), (B × C × S)] to identify dependent (correlated) measurements (9.2, 9.5).

13.2 RESEARCH DESIGN PROBLEM: EXAMPLE

A biologist wanted to determine whether functional auditory receptors were located on the legs of a cockroach. To test this hypothesis an aversive conditioning paradigm was used to train a group of cockroaches ($n = 100$) to respond to a vocal signal ("Jump") and, after this training, when the biologist said "Jump" all the cockroaches jumped (to avoid a brief shock to their feet). Under anesthesia, the legs of these trained cockroaches were then amputated using sterile operative procedures approved by the Animal Research Committee of the university. Following adequate recovery from surgery when the biologist said "Jump" not a single cockroach did. From these results the biologist concluded that the cockroaches could not hear the conditioned vocal signal because their auditory receptors had been removed.

Critique

The research hypothesis is whether functional auditory receptors are located on the legs of a cockroach. A complete within-subject design (4.16) was used. Because the scale of measurement (5.3) was ordinal (a jump or a no-jump response) a nonparametric test (5.22, Chapter 11) would be appropriate to evaluate the numerical data. Unfortunately, the biologist did not control for any differential carry-over effects (4.19) that may occur when a within-subject design (4.16) is used. The removal of the cockroach's legs following training would have affected significantly the cockroach's ability to make the required response. If the biologist had counterbalanced the treatment conditions (4.20); that is, removed the legs of one-half of the cockroaches before training, the biologist would probably have realized (when this group of cockroaches did not learn) that a conceptual problem existed in the design of the experiment (1.1, 1.2).

The Outcome of This Experiment

Being unaware of the serious design problem, the biologist submitted the frequency data of his experimental study for publication in a prestigious biology journal. The submitted manuscript was returned immediately by the editor because no statistical analysis was included. The biologist did a paired t-test (5.18) on his data (significant at a $p < .0001$ level), and resubmitted the revised paper along with a blistering letter condemning the editorial policy of the journal for emphasizing statistical analyses rather than scientific understanding.

After this revised manuscript received favorable peer reviews, the journal editor forwarded the manuscript to the journal's statistical consultant (see A.6). This statistician recommended further revision of the manuscript because the paired t-test was not the correct statistical method to use with ordinal data. The statistician indicated a Wilcoxon signed rank test (11.4) should be done; a recommendation forwarded promptly by the editor to the biologist. On principle, the biologist refused to do another statistical test on such clear-cut data and sent the manuscript with the paired t-test analysis to another respected biology journal which accepted the manuscript without major revisions.

In a subsequent electrophysiological study some pressure receptors on the cockroaches' legs were found to respond (produced action potentials) to auditory stimuli. In their article's discussion, the neurophysiologists concluded that these auditory receptors apparently had functional significance for the cockroach as a previous study by an eminent biologist showed striking behavioral changes when these receptors were removed. Subsequently, one of the favorite questions of the eminent biologist to Ph.D. candidates was—"Can you describe one important biological discovery that could be attributed to the statistical analysis of a given set of data?" *None of the successful* Ph.D. candidates could!!

13.3 TOPIC INDEX OF RESEARCH DESIGN PROBLEMS

The research design problems in "Chapter 14" focus on *general* design and statistical errors with an emphasis on studies in the neurosciences. Most biologists should be able to evaluate all the problems as specialized terms have been defined and jargon has been avoided. If you wish to concentrate on a specific discipline the following index provides a guide to various biological areas:

Field	Problems
Biomedical	1, 2, 3, 12, 14, 17, 18, 21, 25, 30, 39, 45, 64, 76, 77, 95
Cardiovascular physiology	8, 14, 15, 17, 23, 28, 29, 38, 42, 54, 57, 64, 78, 84, 96
Endocrinology and renal physiology	4, 9, 24, 27, 30, 36, 37, 38, 44, 48, 51, 57, 72, 73, 78, 79, 99
Exercise physiology	13, 37, 41, 65, 74, 92, 96
Neurophysiology	5, 6, 10, 11, 16, 22, 42, 47, 49, 61, 63, 68, 70, 71, 72, 75, 83, 85, 88, 89, 93, 97
Pharmacology and toxicology	33, 34, 35, 41, 44, 46, 50, 52, 53, 55, 60, 61, 62, 65, 66, 80, 81, 86, 91, 94
Psychology (behavioral neuroscience)	16, 19, 31, 32, 40, 48, 49, 52, 53, 58, 61, 63, 72, 75, 79, 81, 85, 86, 87, 89, 90, 100
Respiratory physiology	7, 10, 20, 26, 53, 62, 67, 69, 98
Zoology	33, 35, 41, 44, 46, 53, 55, 60, 61, 65, 94

14

Research Design Problems and Critiques

RESEARCH DESIGN PROBLEM 1

Herpes infects about 1 out of 500 adults and thus is a major health problem in the United States. A cell biologist developed a drug that effectively destroyed monkey herpes virus in a cell culture preparation. In a double-blind clinical research trial, 400 sexually active normal males and females (between 21 and 35 years old) in New York City were randomly assigned equally to two treatment groups, a drug and a placebo group. The treatment conditions were given for 1 year and all subjects were interviewed monthly, sample cultures were taken, and the appropriate injections were given. At the end of the year a between-subject ANOVA was used to determine whether there were significant differences in herpes infections among the four groups. The following results were obtained: drug effect $F(1, 296) = 1.02$, NS, sex effect $F(1, 296) = -0.89$, NS, Drug $\times$ Sex interaction, $F(1, 296) = 1.35$, NS. Because there were no significant differences in herpes infections among the groups, the physicians concluded that the monkey herpes virus drug was not effective in preventing herpes in sexually active males or females in New York City.

Critique

The research hypothesis is not stated explicitly but apparently is whether monthly injections of a particular drug prevents herpes infections in sexually active males and females. Differences in infected individuals at the end of the study were evaluated by a 2 (male vs. female) $\times$ 2 (drug vs. placebo) between-subject ANOVA (4.10). The general ANOVA table for this experiment is given in Table 6.2. The specific ANOVA table for this study would be

Source	df	Error term
Drug (D)	1	S/Drug $\times$ Sex
Sex (S)	1	S/Drug $\times$ Sex
D $\times$ S	1	S/Drug $\times$ Sex
S/Drug $\times$ Sex	396	
Total	399	

Many serious problems exist in this experimental report. First, the power of any statistical test (5.12, 5.13), given the sample sizes used, would be extremely low. By chance, less than one herpes-infected case would be expected in the control group. Another major problem is that a parametric, rather than a nonparametric, test was used (5.22). In this study, the number of individuals infected by the virus was the dependent variable; consequently, nonparametric statistical methods would have to be used because of the ordinal scale of measurement (5.3). Most of the individual data would be zero values (no infection) and some groups would be expected to have no variance! In the parametric F-test that was used, the degrees of freedom for the error term, S/AB, are not correct (6.5, 6.6). The correct degrees of freedom for the S/AB error term would be $(s - 1)/(a)(b)$ or $(100 - 1)(2)(2) = 99 \times 2 \times 2 = 396$. (If there was a 25 percent loss of subjects, from 400 to 300 then the df used would have been correct.) Even though multiple measurements were taken on each subject (monthly sample cultures), only the number of infected cases in each group at the end of the 1-year treatment (i.e., a between-subject ANOVA) was used.

RESEARCH DESIGN PROBLEM 2

When labor has to be induced the mother's cervix can fail to soften and enlarge thereby prolonging labor. To investigate whether the cervix can be softened and dilated by treating it with a gel containing prostaglandin E_2, physicians applied such a gel to the cervixes of 60 women who were having labor induced and a placebo gel that contained no active ingredients to 30 other women who were also having labor induced. The two groups of women were of similar ages, heights, weeks of gestation, and initial extent of cervical dilation before gel application. The labor of women treated with prostaglandin E_2 averaged 8.5 hours and the labor of control women was 13.9 hours (h). The standard errors of the mean for these two groups were .22 and .43 h, respectively. An ANOVA with unequal n indicated a significant group effect, $F(1,88) = 154.48, (p < .001)$ and the investigators concluded that prostaglandin E_2 applied to the cervix of labor-induced women facilitates their labor.

Critique

The research hypothesis is whether a woman's cervix during labor can be softened and dilated by applying prostaglandin E_2. The difference in the length in labor of an experimental and a control group of women (groups matched on a number of relevant variables) was determined. The general ANOVA for this study is presented in Table 6.1. The specific ANOVA table for this study is

Source	df	Error term
Group	1	S/Group
S/Group	88	
Total	89	

If you thought that an ANOVA test was inappropriate for a two-group between-subject design see 5.18. Although a balanced design would require the women to be equally and randomly assigned to the treatment conditions (4.7), no reason exists for rejecting the author's conclusions given the methods used and the results obtained. There may be a question regarding the extra 30 women in the experimental group but because the standard deviations (5.2) of the groups were about the same no basis exists for assuming that the experimental group had a "bimodal" distribution. A description of any blind control procedures used (4.26) would have been helpful. In this case, we must assume that neither the physicians nor the women knew which treatment condition was being applied. If the physicians knew which gel they were applying they may change unconsciously their method of gel application. Similarly, women who knew they were receiving a helpful therapy would be expected to be less stressed compared with women who knew they were just being used as controls. Hence, a more thorough description of experimental procedures would have helped in the review of this report, but the conclusion of the authors is appropriate.

RESEARCH DESIGN PROBLEM 3

In a nutritional study of southern adolescent females, the effect of diet on tooth decay was analyzed. Eighty-three girls (11.5 to 16.5 years old at the beginning of the study) were examined by a dentist in the spring of 1988 and again in the spring of 1990 (2 years later). Nutritionists conducted two 24-h dietary recalls for each girl during each of the testing years. The calculated nutrient intakes were averaged for the 2 days. Other data collected at the same time included fluoride treatments, presence of braces, and fluoride content of drinking water.

The mean number of decayed, missing, and filled teeth (DMFT) was $3.4 \pm .3$ (SD) in 1988 and $5.2 \pm .3$ (SD) in 1990 indicating a period of active tooth decay during the 2-year study. Using a multiple regression analysis (including the following factors: water fluoride, dietary fat, protein, sucrose and calcium:phosphate ratio), the DMFT in 1988 and the change in DMFT over 2 years were significantly related to dietary fat, protein, and calcium:phosphate ratio. The authors concluded that alterations in diet must be made to reduce tooth decay in southern adolescent females.

Critique

The research hypothesis is whether the diet of southern adolescent females is correlated with tooth decay. A multiple regression analysis (5.26) was used and both the independent variables and the dependent variables were random (free to vary). Hence, the study is based upon correlational data (Table 5.4). But, cause-and-effect conclusions cannot be made from the correlational data (5.27) presented in the study. The proposed aim of the reported study was to determine . . . "the effect of diet on tooth decay. . . ." If the term *effect* had not been used perhaps the authors would not have made the inappropriate cause-and-effect statement in their conclusion.

RESEARCH DESIGN PROBLEM 4

A renal physiologist was interested in defining the mechanisms involved in the relationship between antidiuretic hormone (vasopressin) and prostaglandins in the kidney. This relationship was to be examined specifically in collecting tubules microdissected from the papillary collecting duct in the rat kidney. Freshly microdissected collecting tubules from 10 rats were aspirated into individual wells of cell culture plates suspended in about 1 μL of microdissection solution. Each sample comprised 4–6 mm total tubule length. As a first step in the experimental program, the effect of osmolality on the prostaglandin synthesis in the papillary collecting duct was determined. Prostaglandin synthesis was measured with a radioimmunoassay method. Forty tissue sample cultures were randomized equally into four osmolalities; that is, the osmolality of the standard 300-mOsm KRB was increased to 800, 1400, and 2000 mOsm by appropriate procedures. A completely randomized single-factor ANOVA indicated a significant osmolality effect, $F(3, 36) = 5.36$, $p < .001$, and Tukey's HSD test showed that every group was significantly different from every other group ($p < .05$). Because significant increases in prostaglandin synthesis occurred as osmolality increased, the renal physiologist concluded that prostaglandin synthesis in the papillary collecting tubules of the rat kidney increases significantly with increases in local osmolality conditions.

Critique

The research hypothesis is not stated explicitly but apparently is whether prostaglandin synthesis in the papillary collecting tubule is increased by local osmolality conditions. The general ANOVA (6.3) for this experiment is presented in Table 6.1. The specific ANOVA used to evaluate the data was

Source	df	Error term
Group (G)	3	S/Group
S/Group	36	
Total	39	

However, in this experiment, only 10 animals were used and 40 measurements were obtained. In a completely randomized single-factor ANOVA the number of animals is equal to the number of independent observations (4.9, 4.10). The renal physiologist treated each tubule as an independent observation even though more than one tubule was taken from each animal. Because the tubules from each animal were not identified some of these correlated observations (9.2) were nested with osmolality (9.3), and this type of nested design usually produces inflated F-ratios (9.3, 9.4).

A slight change in the design of the study would have produced meaningful data. A randomized-blocks design (9.4) could have been used by treating all the tubules from each rat as a single block. The experimental design and general analysis of variance table for a randomized-blocks design are presented in Table 9.3.

In the suggested experimental design, four tubules from each of the 10 rats would be selected and randomly assigned to the four osmolality conditions. The specific ANOVA table for this experiment would be

Source	df	Error term
Between subject (rats)	9	
Within Osmolality	3	Osmolality × Subject
Osmolality × Subject	27	
Total	39	

RESEARCH DESIGN PROBLEM 5

A prenatal regimen of glucocorticoid hormones (synthetic) given to mothers decreases the incidence of infant respiratory distress syndrome. Presumably this beneficial effect occurs by hastening alveolar maturation which increases the production of alveolar surfactants necessary for efficient lung function (i.e, gas exchange). Hormones can also exert a profound organizing influence on the developing central nervous system by altering the developmental fate of post-natally differentiating cell populations. Therefore, a physiologist was interested in whether hormone administration in the young rat would affect subsequent neurophysiological activity in the hippocampus. Pregnant Sprague-Dawley rats were obtained from a commercial supplier. Following the day of birth each litter was culled to 8 pups and the pups randomly assigned to one of three treatment conditions: control (0.1 mL of physiological saline, $n = 16$ pups), low dose (1 mg/kg dexamethasone in 0.1 mL saline, $n = 16$), and high dose (10 mg/kg dexamethasone in 0.1 mL saline, $n = 24$). All pups were injected on the fourth day after birth. Two rat pups in the control and low-dose groups died and 10 pups died in the high-dose group, but 14 pups in each group were available for the neurophysiological experiments.

In these experiments single-barrel micropipettes were used for recording extracellular field potentials in the dentate gyrus. Recordings were begun when the rats were around 70 days old, all rats were treated exactly alike (coordinates, anesthesia), and rats from the three groups were counterbalanced for day of recording. Once prepared, stimuli from a constant voltage source were delivered to the area using a stainless steel concentric bipolar electrode. Depth profiles of dentate granule cell responses evoked by entorhinal stimulation were obtained. At the conclusion of the recording, anodal dc voltage was passed through the recording micropipette and stimulating electrode to aid in histological verification of electrode placement. All rats were then sacrificed and their brains removed, stored, and sectioned for histological analysis.

Depth profile data were a determination of the level of transmembrane current sink (sink) and current source (source). A completely randomized ANOVA indicated that there was a significant group effect, $F(2, 39) = 8.32, p < .001$, for sink data and a Tukey's HSD test indicated that both drug groups were significantly different from the control ($p < .05$), but the two drug groups did not differ one from the other. A separate ANOVA on source data found the same significant results observed for the sink data. The physiologist concluded that dexamethasone could change depth profile but an increase in the hormone (beyond 1 mg/kg) did not produce a greater effect because hormone receptors in the hippocampus at the critical period were probably already saturated at the lower dose.

Critique

The research hypothesis is whether dexamethasone, a synthetic glucocorticoid hormone, given shortly after birth would affect subsequent neurophysiological activity in the hippocampus of the 70-day-old rat. The general ANOVA for the reported experiment is presented in Table 6.1. The specific ANOVA table for this study would be

Source	df	Error term
Group	2	S/Group
S/Group	39	
Total	41	

The selective subject loss (4.12) in the high-dose group was probably responsible for this group not being different from the low-dose group. About 42 percent of the animals in the high-dose group died before neural recordings were taken whereas only 13 percent of the animals in the control and the low-dose groups died. Consequently, the animals in the high-dose group were probably not representative of those in the other two groups. The random assignment of animals to treatment conditions controls for subject-related confounding of the treatment conditions (4.11), but if the loss of animals produces a loss of this randomness then the experiment becomes flawed. Only the "best" animals may have survived the acute injection of the high dose of the hormone, and, therefore, these selected animals may not have shown a greater effect than the wider range of animals given the low dose of the hormone.

Another design problem exists for the reported experiment as eight littermates were randomly assigned to three treatment conditions, hence some correlated observations (9.2) would be nested within treatments (9.3) and this type of nested design usually produces inflated F-ratios (9.3, 9.5). A randomized-blocks design (9.4, Table 9.3) would have been more appropriate but only three animals per litter could be used. If sex had been added as a classification variable (4.2) then six pups (three males, three females) could have been used. But, a randomized-blocks design would not solve the problem of selective loss of subjects in the high-dose treatment.

Table 14.1 Mean (M) Percentage of Initial Amplitude
Response ($\pm$ SEM) for the Three Age Groups Across Trials

| Age | Sequential blocks of five trials | | | |
	1^a	2	3	4
Old	99(1)	98(2)	98(3)	97(2)
Mature	80(3)	60(2)	40(1)	30(2)
Young	79(2)	61(3)	42(2)	31(3)

[a]First block is the average of only four trials (trials 2 to 5). All other blocks are
the average of five trials.

RESEARCH DESIGN PROBLEM 6

A physiologist wanted to determine whether significant age-dependent differences in gill-withdrawal habituation occur in the invertebrate *Aplysia*. Sixty *Aplysia* from three distinct populations (20 days old, 100 days old, and 400 days old) were used in the experiment. The animals in each age group ($n = 20$) were individually tested by stimulating their siphons every 30 sec with a jet of water (30 g) for 20 trials. When the siphon of the adult *Aplysia* is stimulated, the siphon, mantle shelf, and gill all contract vigorously and withdraw into the mantle cavity. Data from all animals were analyzed as percentage (%) of amplitude withdraw of their initial withdrawal force which was set at 100%. Gill-withdrawal responses were measured by a thread connected to the gill and attached to a sensitive pressure (force) transducer.

A mixed factorial ANOVA was used to determine whether differences existed among the three age groups. The following results were obtained: age $F(2, 57)$ = 5.20, $p < .01$; trials $F(18, 1026) = 3.10$, $p < .01$; Age $\times$ Trial, $F(36, 1026)$ = 2.01, $p < .01$ (see Table 14.1). Newman-Keuls post hoc multiple comparisons indicated that the old *Aplysia* did not change significantly across trials whereas the other two groups showed a significant decrease across trials ($p < .05$). The physiologist's major conclusion from these results was that the old *Aplysia* was probably deficient in the neural mechanisms underlying habituation.

Critique

The research hypothesis is whether significant age-dependent differences in gill-withdrawal habituation occur in *Aplysia*. The general ANOVA for the mixed factorial design used is presented in Table 6.4. The specific ANOVA table for this experiment is

Source	df	Error term
Age (A)	2	S/Age
Trials (T)	18	Trials $\times$ S/Age
S/A	57	
Age $\times$ Trials	36	Trials $\times$ S/Age
Trials $\times$ S/A	1026	
Total	1139	

The selected statistical test is appropriate for the 19 measurements (excluding the first) used from each animal. However, the use of percentage of amplitude withdraw of initial response as the dependent variable makes it impossible to determine whether the author's conclusion is reasonable (5.25). The normal (initial) amplitude of the *old Aplysia's* gill-withdrawal response may be so low that further reductions would be unlikely to be recorded reliably. If the author had presented the mean amplitudes of the initial gill-withdrawal responses for the three groups, any "bottom" effect which might have affected the response outcomes could have been determined. The use of derived measures (5.25) and classification variables (4.2) in the same experiment makes it likely that the groups may differ initially. Consequently, initial response data *must* be presented.

RESEARCH DESIGN PROBLEM 7

It is well known that smoking is positively correlated with increased lung cancer, cardiovascular problems, and other diseases. An investigator wanted to determine whether smokers who could be induced to stop smoking would have lower incidences of these problems than smokers who continued to smoke. From a voluntary population of 200 smokers who smoked two or more packs a day, the researcher administered a "drug-support" therapy treatment for one month to all these smokers. At the end of the treatment period most of the smokers did reduce significantly their number of cigarettes and 50 of the subjects stopped smoking completely. These 50 nonsmoking subjects were then matched with 50 smoking subjects from the original population (matched on length of smoking, number of packs, age, sex, etc.) and these two groups were given extensive annual physical examinations for the next 10 years. Using appropriate nonparametric statistical tests, the investigator found a significant decrease (90%) in the number of cases of lung cancer and cardiovascular problems in the nonsmoking group. The investigator concluded from this data that if all smokers could be trained to stop smoking, about a 90 percent decrease in these smoking-related diseases would be expected in the total smoking population.

Critique

The research hypothesis is whether smokers who could be induced to stop smoking would have lower incidences of "smoking-related problems" than smokers who continued to smoke. The 50 smokers who stopped smoking *were not* representative of the total population of smokers. Indeed, these individuals represented only one-fourth of the general smoking population, that is, they were the 50 out of the 200 smokers who could stop completely when given a one-month drug support program. These nonsmokers were an example of subject self-selection (4.2) and, hence, their results cannot be extrapolated (generalized) to the total smoking population. If the investigator had remembered the research question the answer to the question was given by the data obtained; that is, smokers who could stop smoking do have lower incidences of "smoking-related problems" than smokers who could not stop smoking.

RESEARCH DESIGN PROBLEM 8

Elevated levels of plasma high-density lipoprotein (HDL) cholesterol may be associated with a *lowered* risk of coronary heart disease. Several previous studies had suggested that vigorous exercise may result in increased levels of HDL. To determine whether running is associated with an increase in HDL concentration, plasma HDL concentrations in middle-age (35–45 years old) marathon runners, joggers, and inactive men were determined.

Mean Plasma HDL Concentrations and Standard Deviations (SD)

Inactive men (n = 30)	48.3 mg/dL ± 10.2 SD
Joggers (n = 30)	50.3 mg/dL ± 19.6 SD
Marathon Runners (n = 30)	64.8 mg/dL ± 11.9 SD

A between-subject ANOVA was done and there was a significant group effect $F(2, 87) = 5.63$, $p < .01$ and a Scheffé multiple comparison test indicated that the runners were significantly different from the inactive men ($p < .05$) but did not differ from the joggers, and the joggers and inactive men did not differ significantly. From these results, the researchers concluded that only very strenuous exercise will significantly increase HDL concentration, that is, jogging had no significant effect on HDL concentration.

Critique

The research hypothesis is whether HDL concentrations differ in middle-age men who either run, jog, or are inactive. The general ANOVA for this study is presented in Table 6.1. The specific ANOVA table for this study is

Source	df	Error term
Group	2	S/Group
S/Group	87	
Total	89	

This study, however, was not an experiment and does not permit causal inferences to be made. Classification variables are the independent variables in this study and classification variables are always subject-confounded (4.2). Inactive men, joggers, and marathon runners probably differ in their diets, their response to stress, their self-esteem, their body weight, and so forth. Because these subject-related confounded variables cannot be controlled by the researcher, cause-and-effect conclusions are impossible when only classification variables are used. The data presented also makes the author's conclusions suspect. Inactive men and marathon runners are classes of individuals that are relatively easy to define. Inactive men do not walk, jog, or run. Marathon runners run in marathons (26 miles). But joggers may jog very slowly once a week or rather briskly four to seven times a week. Notice that the SD for the joggers is about twice that of the other two groups (5.2). Consequently, this group would appear to have individuals who vary greatly in their HDL levels and probably also in the amount of their weekly exercise. Individuals who jog briskly for 40 minutes at least 3 times a week may have the same HDL concentrations as marathon runners. High HDL concentrations may, therefore, be *associated* with both moderate and strenuous exercise. But the author's conclusion that only very strenuous exercise will significantly increase HDL concentration is not justified because classification variables were used.

RESEARCH DESIGN PROBLEM 9

A renal physiologist wanted to determine whether a newly developed clinical drug (S-130) affected prostaglandins in the kidney. This effect was examined specifically in collecting tubules microdissected from the papillary collecting duct in the rat kidney. Freshly microdissected collecting tubules from 90-day-old rats ($n = 12$) were aspirated into individual wells of cell culture plates suspended in about 1 μL of microdissection solution. Each sample comprised 4–6 mm total tubule length. One hundred and twenty tissue sample cultures were randomized equally into four treatment conditions, 0.00 mg (vehicle control), 0.25 mg, 0.50 mg, and 0.75 mg of drug S-130. All samples were exposed to their treatment condition for the same amount of time and prostaglandin synthesis was measured with a very sensitive radioimmunoassay (RIA) method using coded samples (blind procedure).

A completely randomized single-factor ANOVA was used but there was no significant treatment effect, $F(3, 116) = 1.01$. Therefore, the renal physiologist concluded that under his experimental conditions prostaglandin synthesis in the papillary collecting tubules of the rat kidney was not affected by drug S-130.

Critique

The research hypothesis is whether drug S-130 would affect prostaglandins in the collecting tubules of the rat kidney. The general ANOVA for this experiment is presented in Table 6.1. The specific ANOVA table for this study would be

Source	df	Error term
Group	3	S/Group
S/Group	116	
Total	119	

In this experiment, only 12 animals were used but 120 tissue sample measurements were obtained (i.e., each of the four treatment conditions had 30 observations). Hence, an inappropriate statistical test (a completely randomized between-subject design) was used. In a between-subject design all measurements should be independent observations (4.9, 4.10). In this experiment, the renal physiologist treated each tubule as an independent observation even though more than one tubule was taken from each animal. Because the tubules from each animal were not identified some of these correlated observations (9.2) were nested with drug dose (9.3) and this type of nested design usually produces inflated F-ratios (9.3, 9.4). But, because no significant treatment effects were found it is reasonable to accept the author's conclusions. Note that the author did not say that drug S-130 would not affect prostaglandin synthesis if the dosage was increased.

RESEARCH DESIGN PROBLEM 10

Expiratory neurons in the area of the nucleus retroambigualis were studied in 20 anesthetized cats to determine their responsiveness to the iontophoretic application of the putative neurotransmitter γ–aminobutyric acid (GABA). Twenty phasic expiratory neurons were studied (one from each cat) and the number of spikes/burst was recorded.

The experimental protocol for recording from each neuron was (1) a series of 10 control breaths, application of a resistive-elastic load for one breath, and 10 unloaded recovery breaths; and (2) the same sequence repeated while continuously iontophoresing a given amount of either GABA or vehicle. This entire protocol was repeated four times for each neuron and the order of GABA and vehicle presentation was counterbalanced.

Before statistical analysis multiple measures for each condition were averaged to get a single value for each condition for each neuron (i.e., 10 control breaths averaged to get 1 value). Because the entire protocol was repeated four times the single (loaded breath), and averaged control and recovery values were averaged again.

A mixed factorial ANOVA revealed a significant group effect, $F(1, 28) = 7.80$, $p < .01$, and a significant breath effect $F(2, 120) = 5.12$, $p < .01$, but no significant Group $\times$ Breath interaction, $F(2, 120) = 1.34$. From these data, the authors concluded that GABA significantly increases the number of spikes per burst (because GABA values were higher than either control or recovery values, Newman-Keuls test, $p < .05$, and the control and recovery values did not differ significantly, Newman-Keuls test, NS).

Critique

The research hypothesis is whether GABA application would affect the firing rate of expiratory neurons in the nucleus retroambigualis of the anesthetized cat. A diagram of the experimental design of this respiratory experiment is shown in Figure 14.1.

The general ANOVA for the design used is presented in Table 6.3. There are three levels of factor A (treatment): control (no infusion), vehicle, and GABA

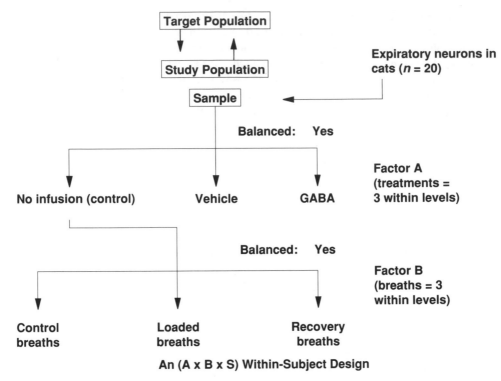

Figure 14.1 Experimental design for research problem 10.

and three levels of factor B (trials): control breath, loaded breath, and recovery breath. The specific ANOVA table for this experiment is

Source	df	Error term
Treatment (T)	2	Treatment × S
Breath (B)	2	Breath × S
Subject (S)	19	
T × B	4	T × B × S
Treatment × S	38	
Breath × S	38	
T × B × S	76	
Total	179	

Because each neuron was exposed to all three treatments (no drug, GABA, and vehicle) and for each condition three breath trials (control, loaded, recovery) were run, the appropriate design would be a complete within-subject design (4.16, Table 6.3). The mixed factorial ANOVA used by the authors was inappropriate (see 4.21). Also, the authors misinterpreted their inappropriate data analysis as they compared the GABA treatment value with control and recovery condition values instead of the vehicle treatment value.

RESEARCH DESIGN PROBLEM 11

A neurophysiologist wanted to determine if changes in neuronal function occurred during aging. Using the marine snail, *Aplysia*, L_7 (a motoneuron innervating the gill) was impaled by a microelectrode in both mature ($n = 6$) and old ($n = 6$) animals. Electric current sufficient to produce spikes in L_7 could be passed through the electrode. Gill contraction and synaptic junction facilitation were measured under nine different stimulating conditions of L_7. Nine separate spike trains of 3-sec duration were delivered to L_7 (i.e., 1–4, 5–8, 10–14 . . . , 35–39, and 40–44). A 2-min rest period was given between each spike train, that is, 1–4 Hz for 3 sec, then a 2-min rest, followed by 5–8 Hz for 3 sec, another 2-min rest, and so forth. Because a reduced preparation was used the neurophysiologist recording the data did not know when an old or mature ganglion was being tested. Also, because only one preparation could be done each day, old and mature *Aplysia*, surgically prepared, were delivered to the neurophysiologist in a counterbalanced order.

A mixed factorial design was used and statistical analysis indicated a significant spike train (frequency) effect, $F(8, 80) = 11.01, p < .001$, and a significant Age $\times$ Spike Train interaction, $F(8, 80) = 14.09, p < .001$, for the contraction data. The same statistical results were found for the facilitation data, that is, a significant spike train effect and a significant Age $\times$ Spike Train interaction. The main effect of age was not significant for either the contraction or the facilitation data.

Appropriate multiple comparison tests of each of the significant interactions found significant differences between the two age groups only at the two highest spike rates (i.e., 35–39 and 40–44) with the mature animal having greater contraction and facilitation values compared with the old animal. The neurophysiologist concluded, therefore, that L_7 from an old *Aplysia* was not as responsive to high-frequency stimulation as was L_7 from a mature *Aplysia*.

Critique

The research hypothesis is whether significant differences in gill contraction and synaptic facilitation would occur in mature and old *Aplysia* as the spike train frequency delivered to L_7 was increased. The general ANOVA for the design used is presented in Table 6.4. The specific ANOVA table for this experiment would be

Source	df	Error term
Age (A)	1	S/Age
Spike Train (T)	8	Spike Train $\times$ S/Age
S/Age	10	
A $\times$ T	8	Spike Train $\times$ S/Age
Spike Train $\times$ S/Age	80	
Total	107	

The statistical tests selected were appropriate, but the author's interpretation cannot be accepted because of a time-related confound (4.19). The two highest frequencies of stimulation were always presented at the end of a long series of stimulations (stimulation occurred in order of increasing frequencies) and, therefore, the high-frequency data are confounded with time. Counterbalancing (4.20) the different stimulation rates and increasing the length of the rest periods may have controlled for any general fatigue processes in the old animals. The old animals may be able to respond to high frequencies just as well as the mature animals but the old animals may fatigue quicker than the mature animals.

RESEARCH DESIGN PROBLEM 12

Physicians have long used anteroposterior (AP) diameter of the chest to diagnose emphysema, yet until recently no empirical studies had tested the validity of this diagnostic procedure. In an initial study, chest AP diameters of hospitalized emphysema patients were measured and compared to the same measurements in a group of health professionals without respiratory symptoms. The mean chest AP diameter for the health professionals ($n = 30$) was 21.0 cm, and for the emphysema patients ($n = 36$) the value was 22.3 cm. A single factor ANOVA with unequal n's indicated no significant group effect, $F(1, 64) = 1.20$.

In a follow-up study at another hospital, chest AP measurements were taken in a group of hospitalized emphysema patients ($n = 31$), a group of patients hospitalized for other illnesses ($n = 48$), and a group of health professionals ($n = 34$): the mean chest AP diameters for these three groups were 23.2, 22.0, and 21.9 cm, respectively. A single factor ANOVA with unequal n's indicated no significant group effect, $F(2, 110) = 1.68$. Therefore, the authors of this latter study concluded that taken together the results of these studies indicate that patients do not show a significant increase in chest AP diameter when they have emphysema.

Critique

The research hypothesis is whether a greater chest AP diameter occurs in patients who have emphysema compared with individuals who do not have emphysema. The groups that were used in this study were based upon classification variables (4.2) and the study was not an experimental study (4.1) but rather a retrospective study (4.3). For both studies the general ANOVA for the design used is presented in Table 6.1. If you indicated that an ANOVA test was inappropriate for a two-group between-subject design see 5.18. The specific ANOVA tables for the two studies are

Study 1

Source	df	Error term
Group	1	S/Group
S/Group	64	
Total	65	

Study 2

Source	df	Error term
Group	2	S/Group
S/Group	110	
Total	112	

The statistical tests selected were appropriate but the authors may only conclude that they were not able to find a significant condition effect. By stating that patients do not show an increase in AP diameter when they have emphysema is actually proving the null hypothesis (1.2, 5.5). If the authors had concluded that ". . . an increase in chest AP diameter is not a useful clinical sign of emphysema" then their conclusion would be appropriate. A complete within-subject design might be sensitive to pre- and postdisease AP differences (4.16), but the results of this type of design would be of limited value to physicians (6.21) who would not normally have the predisease AP measurements of their patients.

If the authors had remembered the research hypothesis the comparison being made would have been clear. The research hypothesis was *not* whether a significant increase in AP diameter occurs in patients when they have emphysema. Rather, the research hypothesis was whether a greater chest AP diameter occurs in patients who have emphysema compared with individuals who do not have emphysema.

RESEARCH DESIGN PROBLEM 13

Exercise blood flow in rat muscles after training was determined in two groups of animals. One group of male Sprague-Dawley rats ($n = 8$) was *trained* (T) for 1 h/day for 13–17 weeks at 30 m/min on a treadmill at a 5° incline. A second *undertrained* group (UT) of male rats ($n = 8$) was conditioned for 10 min/day for 4 weeks at the same speed and incline as the T group. After this differential training, blood flows (BFs) in 48 hindlimb muscles were measured with labeled microspheres during preexercise (PE) and while the rats ran for 30 sec, 5 min, and 15 min at 30 m/min. Single factor ANOVA's indicated no significant differences in total hindlimb muscle BFs between UT and T rats before or during exercise, but T rats had higher PE BFs in the deep red extensor muscles, suggesting a greater anticipatory response for exercise demand ($p < .05$). Also, T rats had higher BFs in red extensor muscles during exercise ($p < .03$) whereas UT rats had higher BFs in white muscles ($p < .04$). The authors concluded that these findings demonstrate that differential exercise training causes significant changes in the distribution of BF within and among muscles both before and during exercise.

Critique

The research hypothesis is whether exercise training causes significant changes in the distribution of blood flow in the hindlimb muscles of rats. A single factor ANOVA (Table 6.1) was used to analyze the results but repeated measures were taken on the two groups. Therefore, the statistical analysis should have been a mixed factorial ANOVA (4.21) supplemented with post hoc multiple comparisons tests (6.9, Chapter 10) which would have controlled for familywise error rate. Given the number of analyses performed and the p values obtained for the significant comparisons, the likelihood of making a Type I error (5.10) would be high. Because the df's associated with the statistic were not given (5.17), the number of independent (4.9) and correlated (9.2) observations in each comparison cannot be determined. Because blood flows in the hindlimbs of a given rat are probably correlated ignoring this correlation would result in an error term that is numerically less than it should be, thereby leading to inflated F-ratios (9.3).

This research design illustrates a common problem when only probability levels (i.e., $p < .05$) are given to support major conclusions (A.5). When only probability levels are given you cannot determine whether correct comparisons were made or whether appropriate statistical tests were used to analyze the data. To evaluate a paper you should be able to reconstruct the experimental design used, the experimental protocol for animals in the different groups, and the analysis of variance table used (when appropriate) to determine significance levels (3.2, 6.3).

RESEARCH DESIGN PROBLEM 14

Crushing chest pain (angina pectoris) is associated with an inadequate supply of blood to the heart because of clogged arteries. Although some drugs will bring fast relief, it is usually only temporary; consequently, many surgical procedures have been proposed to reduce angina pectoris.

One suggestion was that tying off the mammary arteries (a relatively simple operation requiring only a local anesthetic) might shunt more blood to the heart muscle through the smaller vessels. In a clinical trial study 50 clinically similar angina patients were randomly assigned to a treatment ($n = 25$) and a control ($n = 25$) group. Before treatment all patients were given a reliable stress test during which they informed a physiologist of the degree of their chest pain during different exercise conditions. After this test, all patients were informed of the expected benefits of the operation as well as possible aversive effects (e.g., some postoperative pain). The 25 patients in the treatment group consented to the operation which was performed within one week. One month later all 50 patients were again given the identical stress exercise test by the same physiologist (the physiologist did not know the patient's treatment history nor was the surgeon present when these tests were done).

A mixed factor ANOVA was performed on the pain-exercise test data and a significant group effect, $F(1, 48) = 4.08$, $p < .05$, a significant pre-post test effect, $F(1, 48) = 4.09$, $p < .05$, and a significant Group $\times$ Pre-Post interaction, $F(1, 48) = 52.6$, $p < .0001$ were found. Newman-Keuls post hoc tests revealed no significant difference between the two groups on the pretreatment test but on the posttreatment test the surgery patients had significantly lower pain scores than the control patients ($p < .01$). Furthermore, although the control patients did not differ on their pre- and posttreatment tests, the experimental patients showed a significant decrease in their reported pain scores from the pre- to post-treatment test ($p < .01$). From these findings the surgeon concluded that a shunting of blood to the heart muscle by tying off the mammary arteries produces a significant reduction in angina pectoris.

Critique

The research hypothesis is whether tying off the mammary arteries in angina patients would reduce perceived chest pain (angina pectoris). The general ANOVA for the $2 \times (2 \times 25)$ mixed factorial design used is presented in Table 6.4. The specific ANOVA table for this experiments is

Source	df	Error term
Group (G)	1	S/Group
Pre-Post Test (T)	1	T × S/Group
S/Group	48	
G × T	1	T × S/Group
T × S/Group	48	
Total	99	

The data obtained in this study were confounded by a placebo effect. By informing both groups of patients that the operation should decrease angina pectoris, requesting consent, and doing the operation only on the experimental group confounds expectation with the data obtained. Indeed, the pain experienced by the experimental patients may have affected only their perception of their pain. Ethical considerations might prevent a control group of patients from receiving a sham operation. On the other hand, a positive (significant) outcome implies that many subsequent patients may receive a useless operation for angina pectoris. (This surgical procedure was used in patients suffering from angina pectoris, but subsequent clinical trials showed no significant benefits from this operation.) Another potential problem with this study is that the dependent variable (perceived pain) may have been measured as an ordinal variable (5.3) and a nonparametric statistical method may have been appropriate for this ranked data. However, the instructions to the patients could have asked them to evaluate their pain perception on a ratio scale, that is, on a scale from 0 to 10, regard 5 as 5 times the minimal amount of pain (1) perceived. Fischer's exact probability test (11.2) could have been used in the data analysis using only the posttreatment data, that is, in the two groups of 25 patients how many felt less pain during the exercise test than they felt on the pretreatment exercise test. But again any change in the experimental groups' pain perception (because of pain associated with recovery from the operation) would have biased these data. In this experiment, a one-tailed test could also have been used to evaluate the data (5.20) as the surgeon would not have been interested in an operation which would increase angina pectoris.

RESEARCH DESIGN PROBLEM 15

A cardiovascular physiologist was interested in whether experimentally induced congestive heart failure or right ventricular hypertrophy in cats produced significant cardiovascular functional changes as measured by heart rate. Therefore, 30 cats were randomly assigned equally to three groups: (1) a control group, (2) a group with induced congestive heart failure (CHF), and (3) a group with induced right ventricular hypertrophy (RVH). Data were analyzed by performing t-tests for each pair of treatments using as a critical value that for the t-statistic with degrees of freedom $n_i + n_j - 2$, where n_i and n_j were the sample sizes for groups i and j. This data analysis indicated that cats in the CHF group had significantly lower heart rates than either cats in the control ($p < .01$) group or the RVH group ($p < .001$). Furthermore, the cats in the RVH group had significantly higher heart rates than cats in the control group ($p < .01$). The physiologist concluded that both CHF and RVH produce significant changes in cardiovascular functioning as measured by heart rate.

Critique

The research hypothesis is whether experimentally induced congestive heart failure or right ventricular hypertrophy in cats produces significant functional cardiovascular changes as measured by changes in heart rate. The general ANOVA for the single-factor design used in this experiment is presented in Table 6.1. The specific ANOVA table for this experiment is

Source	df	Error term
Group (G)	2	S/Group
S/Group	27	
Total	29	

Even though a single-factor between-subject ANOVA (4.10) and a post hoc multiple comparison test (6.9, Chapter 10) would have been the expected statistical tests to use, *given the* significance of the three t-test comparisons which the physiologist made, the increase in Type I error (5.11) that occurs when multiple uncorrected t-tests are used would not have significantly affected the author's conclusions (5.19). Three t-test comparisons were made, the lowest p was less than .01 which means that the familywise error rate would be about $p < .03$, that is, $3(.01) = .03$. Hence, the comparisons were at least significant at $p < .03$ and the physiologist's conclusions should be accepted. Because the physiologist was only interested in whether CHF or RVH produced significant changes in heart rate compared to a control group, the Dunnett test would have been the more appropriate test to use (10.6). Although the physiologist did compare the

CHF and RVH groups, the research hypothesis and conclusion did not include this comparison. Indeed, this comparison would not make biological sense and the physiologist was wise in not trying to interpret this statistically significant result (6.21). For the same reason, an ANOVA would not be the most sensitive statistical test to use (6.8) as the overall F-ratio includes the probability of making the CHF and RVH comparison.

RESEARCH DESIGN PROBLEM 16

The mammalian hippocampus has been proposed to be an important brain region for memory processing; consequently, interfering with hippocampal functioning should produce a greater effect on complex tasks (requiring extensive memory processing) than on simple tasks. To test this hypothesis, a neurophysiologist implanted bilateral stimulating electrodes in the hippocampi of 20 male rats (90 days old), and 20 other male rats of the same age served as controls by having electrodes implanted in the same brain region but no current delivered during testing. After surgery, all rats were tested on a simple two-choice T-maze and on a complex radial arm (RA) maze with multiple choice points. The order of maze testing was counterbalanced so that one-half of the rats in each group was trained first on the T-maze and subsequently on the RA maze. The other 10 rats in each group were trained in the reverse order. Food reward was used in both tasks and all rats were maintained at 85 percent of their pretraining weight. During each trial a low-voltage, high-frequency stimulation was delivered through the implanted electrodes in the experimental rats, and the number of trials to reach 90 percent correct responding on each task for both groups was recorded.

A mixed factorial ANOVA indicated a significant group effect, $F(1, 38) = 8.35, p < .01$, and a significant test effect, $F(1, 38) = 8.95, p < .01$. The Group $\times$ Test interaction was not significant, $F(1, 38) = 1.20$. Both the hippocampus-stimulated and control rats required more trials to learn the RA maze than the T-maze. Also, the hippocampus-stimulated rats required more trials to learn the two mazes compared to the control rats. From these findings, the neurophysiologist concluded that stimulation of the hippocampus during maze learning has a greater effect on the learning of complex than simple tasks, a conclusion which supports the hypothesis that the hippocampus is involved in memory processing.

Critique

The research hypothesis is whether disruption of normal hippocampal neural activity would interfere more with a rat's performance on a radial arm maze than on a T-maze. The general ANOVA for the 2 $\times$ (2 $\times$ 20) mixed factorial design used in this experiment is presented in Table 6.4. The specific ANOVA for this experiment is

Source	df	Error term
Group (G)	1	S/Group
Test (T)[a]	1	Test × S/Group
S/Group	38	
Group × Test	1	Test × S/Group
Test × S/Group	38	
Total	79	

[a]The order of when each of the two tests was given could have been included as an additional factor.

The statistical test selected was appropriate but the neurophysiologist's conclusions were wrong. If the neurophysiologist's conclusions were correct, a significant Group × Test interaction (6.12, 6.13) would have been obtained. Subsequent analyses of this interaction should also have indicated that for the hippocampus-stimulated animals the difference in errors made on the complex and simple tasks was greater than the trial error difference between these two behavioral tests for the sham-operated controls. But, the Group × Test interaction, $F(1, 38) = 1.20$, was not significant; consequently, the only conclusions the neurophysiologist could make would be interpretations based upon the two significant main effects, namely that the stimulated rats required more trials to learn the two mazes compared with the control rats and that both groups required more trials to learn the complex than the simple maze. Therefore, there was no evidence that hippocampal stimulation affected the rat's performance more on complex than on simple tasks.

RESEARCH DESIGN PROBLEM 17

White blood cell counts from 10,000 virally infected patients and 10,000 bacterial-infected patients were compared to determine whether these counts could be a useful clinical procedure to differentiate between viral and bacterial infections. Viral infection patients had an average white count of 7513 ($\pm$ SD 212) whereas those with bacterial infections had an average count of 8102 ($\pm$ SD 282). A single-factor between-subject ANOVA revealed a significant group effect, $F(1, 19,998) = 3.89, p < .05$. The authors concluded, therefore, that the white blood cell count would be a significant clinical procedure to differentiate between viral- and bacterial-infected patients.

Critique

The research question is whether differences in white blood cell counts would be a useful clinical procedure to differentiate between patients with viral infections and patients with bacterial infections. The general ANOVA table for this study is presented in Table 6.1. The specific ANOVA table for this study is

Source	df	Error term
Group	1	S/Drug
S/Group	19,998	
Total	19,999	

The statistical test selected was appropriate. The t-test is a special case of the F-ratio (5.18); consequently, either a t-test or the F-test can be used for a single-factor between-subject design with two groups. Although a statistically significant difference existed in white blood cell counts between the two infected groups, this information would not be a useful clinical procedure. Many people in the two groups would have the same values with the means and standard deviations presented. With a very sensitive statistical test (5.14) extremely small differences among groups may be statistically significant but these differences may not have any functional significance given the large sample sizes that are necessary (6.21). In the biological sciences, samples are usually relatively small; therefore, the insensitivity of the statistical test is a more common problem (5.12, 5.15).

RESEARCH DESIGN PROBLEM 18

Phenylketonuria (PKU) is a rare genetic disorder (one out of every 10,000 caucasian births) that affects the infant's ability to metabolize a class of amino acids (phenylalanine) which may result in mental retardation. If the child's diet is corrected early, mental retardation does not occur. Unfortunately mothers, treated successfully for PKU as infants, have a very high risk of having children with mental retardation, microcephaly, and heart defects.

A biomedical scientist wanted to determine whether this high offspring risk was associated with the PKU mother's current diet. A random sample of 500 PKU females (25 to 45 years old) was obtained from a total population of 10,000 files from a national PKU clinic. Telephone interviews with these females indicated that 300 had given birth to children within the past ten years and were willing to answer an extensive questionnaire regarding their eating habits prior to and during their pregnancy. A questionnaire was prepared, sent to these women, and all were returned. Sixty percent of the women (180) reported that their children had no particular problems and most of these women (140) indicated that they had continued their special PKU diet prior to and during their pregnancy. The other 40 percent of the women (120) reported that their children had a variety of health problems (retardation, microcephaly, heart defects). Most of these women (90) also indicated that they had not followed the restricted PKU diet prior to and during their pregnancy. From these data, the biomedical scientist concluded that the birth defects found in children of some PKU mothers are related to the probable high phenylalanine levels *in utero* of PKU mothers who had not continued on their special PKU diet.

Critique

The research hypothesis is whether birth defects found in the children of PKU mothers are related to the diet of the mother prior to and during her pregnancy. Because a cause-and-effect relation is not postulated the author's conclusion is appropriate given the design of the study and the data obtained.

RESEARCH DESIGN PROBLEM 19

A biomedical scientist wanted to determine whether social bonding would reduce stress and thereby produce longer survival in patients with prior coronary occlusions. Two groups of coronary patients were used in this study, one group of patients (n = 120) had owned a dog or cat for at least one year before their coronary occlusion; whereas, the control group of patients (n = 120) were not prior pet owners. The patients in the two groups were matched for age, weight, sex, and severity of their coronary disease. Two years after their occlusions, 97 percent of the pet owners were still alive but only 63 percent of the non-owners were alive, a difference in survival that was statistically significant ($p < .001$). The biomedical scientist concluded from this study that pet owners were more likely to survive coronary occlusions for two years than patients who did not have pets.

Critique

The proposed research question is whether social bonding would reduce stress and thereby produce longer survival in patients with prior coronary occlusions. The research question tested was whether pet owners are more likely to survive coronary occlusions than patients who did not have pets. The author's conclusion is that pet owners differ from nonpet owners and this difference (whatever it may be) affects survival following coronary occlusions. Therefore, the conclusion of the biomedical scientist is correct but the study did not test the research question proposed. If the biomedical scientist had concluded that giving pets to coronary patients would increase their chances of being alive two years later, this conclusion would be wrong. Indeed, making nonpet owners take care of a pet after coronary occlusions may have increased stress for these individuals which might have resulted in even lower survival times for these patients.

RESEARCH DESIGN PROBLEM 20

Some evidence exists that the body's natural analgesics, the endorphins, might cause infant-apnea syndrome (near-miss sudden infant death syndrome). In an experiment, β-endorphin levels were obtained from the cerebrospinal fluid of a random sample of 100 infants whose prior medical history indicated a substantial risk for sudden infant death syndrome. Sixty of the infants stopped breathing for a period of at least 20 sec during a 1-h observation period and these infants had a mean endorphin level of 62.0 pmol/mL, SD = 6.7. The other 40 infants did not show any breathing irregularities during their 1-h observation period and their mean endorphin level was 45.0 pmol/mL, SD = 10.6. A double-blind procedure was used during the experiment, that is, neither the physician who took the sample of cerebrospinal fluid from each infant nor the neuropharmacologist who measured endorphin levels were aware of the breathing patterns of the infants. The mean endorphin levels between the two groups of infants were significantly different, $F(1, 98) = 96.4, p < .001$, and the investigators concluded that high levels of β-endorphin produce significant infant apnea.

Critique

The research hypothesis is whether high levels of endorphins cause infant-apnea syndrome. The general ANOVA table for this study is presented in Table 6.1. The specific ANOVA table for this study is

Source	df	Error term
Group	1	S/Group
S/Group	98	
Total	99	

The statistical test selected was appropriate. However, this study used classification variables (4.2) as the infants were divided into the two groups by the extent of their breathing irregularities during a 1-h observation period (self-selection into the two groups). Cause-and-effect statements cannot be made when only classification (correlation) variables are used (4.1). Also, the direction of an association cannot be determined by a correlation. The infants who stopped breathing for at least 20 sec may have had high CNS levels of endorphins because of their breathing irregularities.

RESEARCH DESIGN PROBLEM 21

A research specialist wanted to determine whether interferon would decrease tumor size in mice. Eighty young mice of an inbred strain that spontaneously developed tumors later in life were divided randomly into two equal groups. One-half of the mice (group 1) were given weekly injections of interferon for 3 months, whereas the other 40 mice (group 2) were given weekly injections of the vehicle for 3 months. When 120 days old, all mice were sacrificed and the number and size of their tumors were measured by a technician who did not know the prior history of the mice. Average total tumor volumes for the mice in the drug and control groups were 1.90 cm^3 and .65 cm^3, respectively, group effect, $F(1, 78) = 12.02, p < .001$. The researcher concluded that weekly interferon treatment for 3 months significantly decreased tumor volume in this particular inbred strain of mice.

Critique

The research hypothesis is whether mice given weekly injections of interferon would have reduced tumor size. The general ANOVA design for this experiment is presented in Table 6.1. The specific ANOVA for this experiment is

Source	df	Error term
Group (G)	1	S/Group
S/Group	78	
Total	79	

The statistical test selected was appropriate (see 5.18), but the conclusion should have been that interferon treatment significantly increased tumor volume as the interferon-injected mice had an average total tumor volume of 1.90 cm^3 whereas the vehicle controls had an average total volume of only .65 cm^3.

RESEARCH DESIGN PROBLEM 22

A neurophysiologist wanted to determine whether glutamate was the neurotransmitter at the neuromuscular junction between motor neuron L_7 and the medial smooth muscle of the *Aplysia*'s gill. The medial muscle of the gill was surgically removed from 12 *Aplysia*, slightly stretched, and connected to a very sensitive force transducer in an enclosed temperature-controlled seawater bath chamber. The chamber was perfused with either a control solution (100 M KCl) to measure the amplitude of contraction or different concentrations of glutamate (10^{-8}, 10^{-6}, 10^{-4}, and 10^{-2} M glutamic acid in distilled water).

For the first muscle sample, the control solution (100 M KCl) was first infused for 2 min, followed by a 2-min recovery period with normal seawater infused, 10^{-8} M glutamic acid infused for 2 min, followed by a 2-min washout with seawater, 10^{-6} M glutamic acid infused for 2 min, and so forth. For the second muscle sample, the treatment order (following the control solution) was started with 10^{-6} M glutamic acid and ended with 10^{-8} M glutamic acid. For the third muscle sample, the treatment order was started with 10^{-4} M and ended with 10^{-6} M. Hence, the treatment order was counterbalanced across the 12 muscle samples. Tension/muscle weight values were calculated for each muscle and a complete within-subject ANOVA was performed. Mean tension muscle values for the five treatment conditions were

	Treatment (glutamate)			
100 M KCl	$10^{-8}M$	$10^{-6}M$	$10^{-4}M$	$10^{-2}M$
45	2	10	44	60

Because the 100 M KCl treatment was used only to determine whether the muscle was damaged during surgery, that is, not capable of showing a contraction, the ANOVA was performed using only the four glutamic acid doses. There was a significant treatment effect, $F(3, 33) = 5.60$, $p < .01$, with a significant linear component, $F(1, 11) = 8.90$, $p < .01$. The neurophysiologist concluded that these results support the view that glutamate was the transmitter at the L_7–smooth muscle junction in *Aplysia*. But, the neurophysiologist emphasized that presynaptic release experiments and postsynaptic receptor experiments would have to be done to confirm this hypothesis.

Critique

The research hypothesis is whether glutamic acid (in different concentrations) applied to the medial smooth muscle of *Aplysia*'s gill would produce muscle contraction. The general ANOVA table for a single-factor complete within-subject ANOVA is presented in Table 4.5. The specific ANOVA table for this experiment is

Source	df	Error term
Treatment (T)	3	T × S
Subject (S)	11	
T × S	33	
Total	47	

The statistical test selected was appropriate. The problem with this experiment, however, is that proper vehicle control groups were not used. The control solution used was $100\ M$ KCl and it was applied to determine whether the smooth muscle was capable of contracting after its surgical removal. But as the amount of glutamic acid is increased (from $10^{-8}\ M$ to $10^{-2}\ M$) the pH of the infused solution would also change. Hence, the treatment conditions are systematically confounded with another potential independent variable (4.4). Proper counterbalancing of treatment order (4.20) would not solve this treatment confound problem.

RESEARCH DESIGN PROBLEM 23

Adenosine, a breakdown product of adenosine triphosphate, has been suggested to be responsible for coupling coronary blood flow to myocardial O_2 demand. The aim of the present study was to determine if the coronary circulation develops tachyphylaxis (a desensitization) to adenosine while remaining sensitive to other metabolically linked vasodilator mechanisms. Experiments were conducted in eight pentobarbital-anesthetized, open-chest dogs whose blood flow in the left anterior descending coronary artery (LAD) was measured electromagnetically during a 3-h infusion of adenosine into the LAD. Measurements of regional myocardial blood flow (radioactive microspheres), myocardial O_2 consumption (Fick principle), and percent segment shortening (ultrasonic crystals) were also obtained. Adenosine was infused into the LAD at a rate of 27.0–72.0 μmol/min, depending on blood flow rate. Calculated concentration of adenosine in LAD blood averaged .484 ± .111 μmol/mL, which was in excess of that required for maximal coronary vasodilation. A single-factor within-subject ANOVA was used, $F(2, 14) = 9.07, p < .01$, and Student-Newman-Keuls tests were done to determine significant differences among three treatment means. LAD blood flow averaged 21.5 ± 2.2 mL/min during the preadenosine control condition. LAD blood flow after 3 h of adenosine (123.3 ± 23.0 mL/min) was not significantly higher from that after 1–3 min of adenosine (105.8 ± 17.9 mL/min) but LAD blood flows for both adenosine times were significantly higher compared with the control condition ($p < .01$). There was no significant transmural variation in LAD blood flow during adenosine infusion. Adenosine had no significant effect on myocardial O_2 consumption or percent segment shortening. The authors concluded that their data demonstrate persistent transmural vasodilation in the canine coronary circulation during long-term, supramaximal doses of adenosine and are consistent with a role for endogenous adenosine in maintenance of coronary vasodilation during sustained elevations in myocardial energy demands.

Critique

The research hypothesis is whether the coronary circulation develops tachyphylaxis to adenosine but not to other metabolically linked vasodilator mechanisms. The general ANOVA table for the design used is presented in Table 4.5. The specific ANOVA for this single-factor within-subject study is

Source	df	Error term
Time (T)	2	T × S
Subject (S)	7	
T × S	14	
Total	23	

The statistical tests selected were appropriate. No significant differences in LAD blood flow occurred between 3 min and 3 h of adenosine infusion; consequently, the coronary circulation did not appear to develop a desensitization to adenosine within this time period. Notice, however, that the authors only concluded that a persistent transmural vasodilation in coronary circulation during long-term, supramaximal doses of adenosine was obtained *in their experiment*. The authors do not indicate whether the values following the mean blood flows for the three conditions are standard deviations or standard errors of the mean (5.2).

RESEARCH DESIGN PROBLEM 24

After surgical removal of one adrenal gland, the cortex of the remaining adrenal gland increases in size. This compensatory adrenal growth is characterized by increased weight and DNA content of the remaining adrenal 72 hours after unilateral adrenalectomy, and has been found to be mediated by a neural reflex rather than by pituitary hormones. Therefore, a neuroscientist wanted to determine whether the compensatory adrenal growth response was dependent on the integrity of the sympathetic nervous system.

Newborn rats were sympathectomized by subcutaneous injections of quanethidine or 6-hydroxydopamine every other day for the first 2 weeks of life (both drug procedures eliminated sympathetic neural activity). Littermate controls received injections of vehicle solutions on the same schedule ($n = 16$ in each of the four groups). At 40 days of age, etherized rats underwent either left adrenalectomy ($n = 8$ in each of the four groups) or sham operations (where the adrenal was exposed but not touched, $n = 8$ in each of the four groups). All rats were killed by decapitation 72 h later and the removed right adrenals were collected on ice, cleaned, weighed, and frozen at $-60°C$ until assayed for DNA, RNA, and protein content. Plasma was also collected from all rats for subsequent radioimmunoassay of corticosterone. A drug (4) × operation (2) between-subject ANOVA was used to determine significance levels. No significant differences in corticosterone levels existed among the four groups. However, for adrenal weights there was a significant drug effect, $F(3, 56) = 6.70, p < .001$, and a significant operation effect, $F(1, 56) = 7.31, p < .01$, but no significant Drug × Operation interaction, $F(3, 56) = 2.20$. Also, significant drug and operation effects but no significant Drug × Operation interactions were found for DNA/adrenal and RNA/adrenal. Because the chemical sympathectomy animals had significantly lower mean adrenal values than their vehicle controls (Tukey's HSD test, $p < .05$) and the operated rats had higher adrenal weights than their sham-operated controls the author concluded that the sympathetic nervous system mediates the adrenal cortical cell proliferation that occurs normally after unilateral adrenalectomy.

Critique

The research hypothesis is whether the compensatory adrenal growth response after unilateral adrenalectomy would be found in young rats sympathectomized by subcutaneous injections of quanethidine or 6-hydroxydopamine during the first 2 weeks after birth. A diagram of the experimental design of this developmental pharmacological experiment is shown in Figure 14.2.

The general ANOVA table for this experiment is presented in Table 6.2. The specific ANOVA table for this experiment is

Source	df	Error term
Drug (D)	3	S/Drug × Operation
Operation (O)	1	S/Drug × Operation
Drug × Operation	3	S/Drug × Operation
S/Drug × Operation	56	
Total	63	

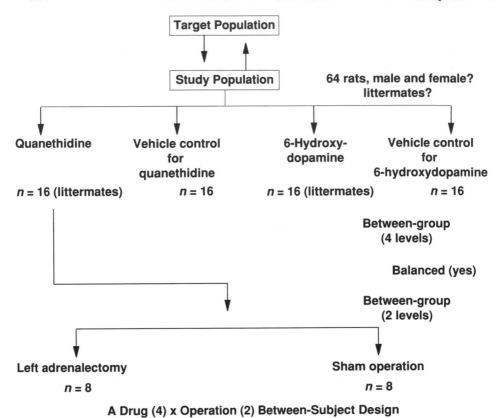

A Drug (4) x Operation (2) Between-Subject Design

Figure 14.2   Experimental design for research problem 24.

The statistical test selected was appropriate. However, to answer the neuro-scientist's research question a significant Group × Operation interaction (6.12, 6.13) is required followed by appropriate post hoc comparison tests (6.9). The significant main effect of drug is collapsed across both operated and nonoperated rats for the four drug groups (see experimental diagram and A × B matrix). Dif-ferences among these four means, therefore, would not determine whether the sympathetic nervous system mediates the adrenal cortical cell proliferation that occurs normally after unilateral adrenalectomy. Similarly, the significant main effect of operation is collapsed across the four drug groups (see experimental dia-gram and A × B matrix). A difference between these two means, therefore, only indicates that the operation had an effect (increased adrenal weights). For exam-ple, the values in Table 14.2 would be consistent with a significant main effect of drug and a significant main effect of operation but no significant Drug × Operation interaction. Indeed, the values were constructed by first having all means set at 20 mg/kg and then subtracting 5 mg for a drug effect and adding 5 mg for an operation effect to the means of each appropriate cell. If the DNA and RNA values followed the same pattern as adrenal weights then a reasonable

Table 14.2 Mean Adrenal Weights for the Eight Groups

	Drug-Q	Vehicle-Q	Drug-6H	Vehicle-6H	M
Operation	20	25	20	25	22.5
Control	15	20	15	20	17.5
M	17.5	22.5	17.5	22.5	

interpretation would be that unilateral adrenalectomy increases adrenal weight and chemical sympathectomy decreases adrenal weight.

The experimental description does not indicate whether both male and female rats were used and whether littermates were used across all conditions. It is doubtful that a randomized-blocks design (littermates = blocks) was used in the experiment as eight littermates would be needed to be assigned to the different groups (9.4).

A × B Matrix (6.13)

		Levels of factor A					
		a_1	a_2	a_3	a_4		
Levels of factor B	b_1	a_1b_1	a_2b_1	a_3b_1	a_4b_1	Mb_1	Main effects of factor B
	b_2	a_1b_2	a_2b_2	a_3b_2	a_4b_2	Mb_2	(operation)
		Ma_1	Ma_2	Ma_3	Ma_4		
		Main effect of factor A (drug)					

RESEARCH DESIGN PROBLEM 25

Across some species, a negative correlation between length of life and metabolic rate per unit of metabolic (lean body) mass has been reported. In short-term dietary programs, reducing food intake tends to lower the metabolic rate per unit of metabolic mass. In rats, food restriction retards the aging process and prolongs life by apparently slowing the metabolic rate per unit of metabolic mass. To determine whether the same metabolic reduction effect could be maintained over a significant portion of the life span, metabolic rate was determined by measuring O_2 consumption in two groups of 9-month-old male rats fed *ad libitum* (group 1) for 7.5 months or maintained for the same length of time on a life-prolonging food-restriction regimen (group 2). Fifty young rats, 30 days old, were randomly assigned in an equal number to the two treatment groups. When the rats were 9 months old, O_2 measurements were made continuously for 23.75 h under conditions nearly identical to those of the daily life of the rats. The metabolic rate per kilogram body weight was greater for the rats on a food-restriction regimen (124 Kcal/kg) than for rats fed *ad libitum* (113 Kcal/kg), $F(1, 48) = 4.04$, $p < .05$. However, when the data were expressed on a per kilogram lean body mass basis, no significant difference existed between the two groups (group

1, 137 Kcal/kg; group 2, 142 Kcal/kg). Also, when the data were expressed body weight to the two-third or three-quarter power (commonly used scaling factors in expressing metabolic rate) no significant difference existed between the two groups. Therefore, the authors concluded that reducing food intake over a significant portion of the life span of a rat did not significantly lower the metabolic rate per unit of metabolic mass.

Critique

The research hypothesis is whether reduced food intake for 7.5 months would lower the metabolic rate per unit of metabolic mass in rats. The general ANOVA table for this single-factor two-group experiment is presented in Table 6.1. The specific ANOVA table for this experiment is

Source	df	Error term
Group	1	S/Group
S/Group	48	
Total	49	

The statistical test selected was appropriate (5.18). The authors' conclusion was actually a brief summary description of their data; that is, in their experiment reducing food intake over a significant portion of the life span of a rat did not significantly lower the metabolic rate per unit of lean body mass. If the authors had concluded that reducing food intake over a significant portion of the life span *does not* significantly lower the metabolic rate per unit of lean body mass then they would have made the mistake of proving the null hypothesis (1.3, 5.4, 5.5). When the present tense is used the conclusion normally indicates a general effect. When the past tense is used, the conclusion is just a summary (description) of what was found in the experiment (sample). This distinction is now being blurred in many articles because of the current shift in scientific writing from the past to the present tense.

RESEARCH DESIGN PROBLEM 26

Mammals normally show an increase in pulmonary arterial blood pressure (PAP) in response to acute exposure to hypoxia. This increase in PAP is due, at least in part, to an increase in pulmonary vascular resistance elicited by vasoconstriction. The purpose of this experiment was to determine whether bar-headed geese who fly at altitudes up to 9000 m have an unusual hypoxic pulmonary pressor response. Therefore, PAP was measured in unanesthetized bar-headed geese and Pekin ducks (nonflying birds) during exposure to hypoxia. After preparations for measurement of arterial blood pressure (and withdrawal of arterial blood samples), of pulmonary arterial blood pressure, and of body temperature, the birds were placed individually in a dark Plexiglas box where they sat throughout the experiment while gas mixtures of known composition flowed through the box at 25 L·min^{-1}. Experiments were performed at ambient temperatures of 23–25°C and at a barometric pressure of 732 ± 5 (SD) mmHg.

Ducks (n = 6) and geese (n = 6) were randomly exposed to 21% O_2 [142 torr inspired pO_2 (pIO_2)], 10% O_2 (68 torr pIO_2) or 5% O_2 (34 torr pIO_2), with the balance made up of N_2. The birds were exposed to the test gas for at least 15 min before measurements were made. The relationship between PAP and arterial pO_2 (PaO_2) for the two groups was as the PaO_2 decreased from 95–100 to about 34 torr, PAP increased about 4 mmHg in ducks, $t(10) = 2.96$, $p < .05$, but was unchanged in geese. With further decreases in PaO_2 to about 28 torr, PAP was about 11 mmHg above normal in ducks, $t(10) = 3.54$, $p < .01$, but only 3 mmHg above normal in geese. From these results, the authors concluded that bar-headed geese, compared with Pekin ducks, have a significantly diminished pulmonary pressor response to hypoxia and, therefore, may provide a unique animal model in which to study control mechanisms in the pulmonary circulation.

Critique

The research hypothesis was to determine whether bar-headed geese have a significantly diminished pulmonary pressor response to hypoxia compared with Pekin ducks. The general ANOVA table for this 2 × (3 × S) mixed factorial experiment is presented in Table 6.4. The specific ANOVA table for this experiment is

Source	df	Error term
Group (G)	1	S/Group
Exposure (E)	2	E × S/Group
S/Group	10	
Group × Exposure	2	E × S/Group
Exposure × S/Group	20	
Total	35	

The statistical tests used (t-tests) were not appropriate for the mixed factorial design. However, although the authors used multiple t-test comparisons (5.19) the increase in familywise error rate (6.9) would have made it more likely for a significant pulmonary pressor response to hypoxia to be found for the bar-headed geese. The experimental methodology was sensitive enough for significant differences to be observed for the Pekin ducks. Hence, a small size of 6 was sufficient for this species. With an appropriate mixed factorial analysis the Group × Exposure interaction would be expected to be significant. A trend analysis (5.28) could then be used to further analyze the significant Group × Exposure interaction.

A potential problem in this experiment could be the random exposure of the birds to the three treatment conditions. Given the small sample sizes used, a counterbalancing of the treatment conditions across the two groups would have been a more efficient procedure (4.20). No direct statistical tests were reported for determining differences between the two groups of birds. The experimental description does not indicate whether the two groups of birds were tested at the same time. Perhaps one group was tested first and then the other group was tested and the authors did not compare across species because of a possible time confound.

RESEARCH DESIGN PROBLEM 27

In Brattleboro rats (BR) homozygous for diabetes insipidus (DI), the paraventricular nucleus (PVN) and supraoptic nucleus (SON) of the hypothalamus show morphological indications of hyperactivity. Differences in metabolic activity of these hypothalamic nuclei in DI rats would be expected because the magnocellular neurons in the PVN and SON are the primary sites of arginine vasopressin (AVP) production in normal rats, and DI rats are unable to synthesize AVP. Histochemical localization of cytochrome oxidase (COX) has been used to study functional activity (increased metabolic activity in cell body) of neurons. The purpose of the present study was to determine whether increases in COX activity occur in the PV and SO nuclei of the BR's hypothalamus and, if so, whether this increase in COX activity could be eliminated by the administration of exogenous AVP.

Male Brattleboro rats (270–300 g), homozygous for DI, were allowed to adapt to metabolic cages for 2 weeks, and body weight, water intake, urine output, and urine osmolality were then measured daily for 3 days in all rats. At the end of this 3-day control period, pairs of rats were matched and one animal of each pair was randomly assigned to the experimental group ($n = 12$) and the other to the control group ($n = 12$). Both groups had 1-week osmotic minipumps implanted subcutaneously at the back of the neck under light anesthesia. In the experimental group, the minipumps delivered [Arg^8]vasopressin in saline at the rate of 1.6 μg · 100 g body wt^{-1} · day^{-1} (1 μL · h^{-1}), and in the control group the minipumps delivered saline at the rate of 1 μL · h^{-1}. The same measurements taken during the control period were obtained daily during the 7 days the pumps were operative. At the end of this period, all rats were killed and their brains were removed, frozen, and sectioned for localization of COX.

Four 2 (group) by 7 (days) ANOVAs with repeated measures on the last factor were used to determine significant levels for body weight, water intake, urine output, and urine osmolality. As expected, continuous infusion of AVP for 7 days corrected the polyuria and hypoosmolality found in DI rats. For example, for urine osmolalities, the control group averaged 201 mOsm/kg across the 7-day experimental period whereas the experimental group averaged 1701 mOsm/kg, group effect, $F(1, 22) = 15.01, p < .001$. The Group × Day interaction was also significant, $F(6, 132) = 4.06, p < .001$. After 2 days of treatment and for the duration of the AVP infusion osmolalities in the experimental group were significantly higher than those in the control group, Newman-Keuls tests, $p < .05$. Likewise, continuous infusion of AVP resulted in significantly lower COX in the brain than did saline infusion, (t-test, $p < .001$ for both nuclei). The author concluded that the increase in COX activity in the PV and SO nuclei of the BR's hypothalamus can be eliminated by the administration of exogenous AVP.

Critique

The research hypothesis was to determine whether increases in COX activity occur in the PV and SO hypothalamic nuclei of the BR rat and whether any increase in COX activity could be eliminated by giving exogenous AVP. The general ANOVA for the $2 \times (7 \times 12)$ mixed factorial design used is presented in Table 6.4. The specific ANOVA for this experiment is

Source	df	Error term
Group (G)	1	S/Group
Days (D)	6	D × S/Group
S/Group	22	
Group × Days	6	D × S/Group
D × S/Group	132	
Total	167	

This analysis would be used to determine whether there were any significant differences across days for the two groups in body weight, water intake, urine output, and urine osmolality. For this purpose, the statistical test selected was appropriate. A significant group effect and a significant Group × Day interaction (6.12, 6.13) were reported. This significant interaction and subsequent post hoc tests were used to evaluate differences between the two groups which occurred as a function of time (days). The group data indicated that there were differences in urine osmolalities between the two groups. A trend analysis (6.16), rather than multiple post hoc comparisons (10.1), could have been used to evaluate the significant Group × Day interaction.

None of these analyses, however, would answer the proposed research question. The general ANOVA for evaluating changes in COX activity is presented in Table 6.1. The specific ANOVA table is

Source	df	Error term
Group	1	S/Group
S/Group	22	
Total	23	

Because the t-test is a special case of the general F-test (5.18) the statistical test reported is appropriate and correct. Significant differences in COX activity in the PVN and SON of the hypothalamus between the two groups were reported. But, the conclusion of the authors should be rejected because an appropriate control group was not used in the study. The experiment did not show that an increase in COX activity in the PV and SO nuclei of the BR's hypothalamus occurred. Animals not homozygous for DI would have to be used as controls for this comparison. This experiment could not determine whether increases in COX activity occurred in the PV and SO nuclei of the BR's hypothalamus but only that *exogenous AVP would decrease* COX activity in the BR's hypothalamus. The authors should have concluded that exogenous AVP decreases COX activity in the PV and SO nuclei of the BR's hypothalamus.

RESEARCH DESIGN PROBLEM 28

Arginine vasopressin (AVP), like angiotensin II, is a very potent pressor hormone (i.e., its vasoconstrictor activity increases vascular resistance which increases blood pressure). The role of angiotensin II in maintaining blood pressure of normal subjects and hypertensive patients has been well defined using specific inhibitors of the renin-angiotensin system. In contrast the extent to which AVP actively participates in human cardiovascular homeostasis remains unclear. The present experiment was designed to evaluate the role of AVP in maintaining blood pressure of normally hydrated normotensive volunteers with or without an intact renin-angiotensin system. An effective AVP antagonist was administered to four healthy normally hydrated volunteers and blood pressure, heart rate, and skin blood flow measurements were taken. The renin system of each volunteer was then acutely blocked by 25 mg of captopril PO (by this blocking procedure the pressor sensitivity to AVP might be enhanced), and the same measurements were taken. No significant changes in any of the measurements occurred during the experiment (paired t-tests). The authors concluded that circulating arginine vasopressin, even in the face of a blocked renin-angiotensin system, does not actively contribute to maintenance of cardiovascular homeostasis.

Critique

The research hypothesis was to determine whether an AVP antagonist would produce blood pressure changes in normally hydrated normotensive individuals when their renin system was acutely blocked by captopril. The general ANOVA table for this complete within-subject design is presented in Table 4.5. The specific ANOVA table for this study is

Source	df	Error term
Treatment (T)	1	T × Subject
Subject (S)	3	
T × Subject	3	
Total	7	

Several problems exist in this experiment. The statistical test selected was appropriate; however, the power of the statistical test (5.12), given the small sample size, must be considered. With only 1 and 3 degrees of freedom (5.17), an F-value of 10.13 would be required for the .05 level of significance. To obtain the MS error the total variance associated with the error estimate is divided by the number of degrees of freedom available. With a larger number of degrees of freedom the MS error would tend to be lower. Hence, an increase in the df's associated with the error term decreases the F-value required for significance and tends to increase the F-value by decreasing the MS error term. Mean and standard deviations for the treatment conditions would have helped in evaluating the power of the statistical tests used.

No control group (captopril only) is available to compare with the experimental group (AVP antagonist-captopril). Apparently no control group for AVP administration was included unless baseline control measures were taken for the volunteers before drug administration. Also, because the treatment conditions were not counterbalanced (4.20) it is possible that the effective vasopressin antagonist may have lost its potency before the renin-angiotensin system was blocked. With these latter two problems if a significant effect had been observed the basis for the effect could not be determined.

RESEARCH DESIGN PROBLEM 29

In many species including humans the platelet-activating factor is a phospholipid (AGEPC) produced by white cells and platelets. The purpose of this study was to determine the cardiovascular action of AGEPC by examining its effects on coronary blood flow (CBF) and other hemodynamic parameters in six anesthetized open-chest domestic pigs. Mean arterial blood pressure (MBP), electrocardiogram, heart rate (HR), left ventricular pressure, and CBF were continuously recorded. AGEPC was injected (bolus, 0.1 mL) into the left anterior descending coronary artery at increasing doses of .03–10 nmol.

After each injection, all parameters were continuously monitored for 10–15 min or until the complete return of parameters to baseline (whichever was longer). Intracoronary AGEPC produced biphasic changes in CBF: a dose-dependent increase in CBF (up to 50%) followed by a decrease (up to 92%) in CBF. The two-tailed Student's t-test was used for statistical analysis of the data, and dose-response curves for CBF were drawn by a curve-fitting program. The changes in CBF were not directly related to any systemic effect, although MBP was reduced consistently after a dose higher than 1 nmol of AGEPC. The authors concluded that AGEPC release from aggregating platelets may play an important role in modulating CBF and cardiac function in situations involving platelet-coronary interaction.

Critique

The research hypothesis is whether acute injection of AGEPC would affect cardiovascular functioning in domestic pigs. The general ANOVA for this complete within-subject design is presented in Table 4.5. The specific ANOVA table for this experiment is

Source	df	Error term
Dose	?	Dose × Subjects
Subjects	5	
Dose × Subjects	?	
Total	?	

The appropriate statistical test was not used (multiple t-tests were done) and the ANOVA table cannot be reconstructed because the levels of factor A were not given (the number of doses given). Hence, the inadequate description of the experimental protocol (4.5) makes it difficult to evaluate this experimental report. The number of t-tests that were used (given the number of measurements taken) and possible carry-over effects (doses were increased not counterbalanced) are not considered in the interpretation of the results (4.16, 4.19). A major question is whether the return of parameters to baseline means that carry-over effects would not be important. In spite of these potential problems, given the size of the dose-dependent changes in CBF reported, the relatively weak conclusion of the authors that AGEPC release from aggregating platelets may play an important role in modulating CBF appears reasonable. This experimental report would have been easier to evaluate if the values of the statistic and the significance levels for the reported comparisons had been given. Unfortunately, many experimental reports in the biological literature do not provide adequate information on the statistical analysis done (A.5).

RESEARCH DESIGN PROBLEM 30

The development and mineralization of bone is greatly impaired in diabetes mellitus. In diabetic patients, the forearm mineral content is decreased in comparison with age- and sex-matched controls. In animal models, encephalomyocarditis (EMC) virus normally produces both early metabolic changes and some of the long-term complications of diabetes mellitus. The purpose of the present experiment was to determine the effect of EMC on bone mineralization. Forty male mice (6 weeks old) were randomly assigned equally to two groups, an infected treatment group and an uninfected control group. At both 30 and 180 days after infection with EMC virus, 10 experimental mice were compared with 10 control mice. A 2 (infection) $\times$ 2 (time) factorial design was used in the statistical analysis. In the infected mice although the concentration of calcium and phosphate in the serum were not significantly different from controls, the alkaline phosphate activity and the rate of mineralization in the proximal tibial epiphysis were both significantly decreased in the 30- and 180-day infected mice compared with those of the age-matched uninfected mice, infection effect, $F(1, 36) = 9.17$, $p < .001$ and $F(1, 36) = 10.02$, $p < .001$, respectively. For these measures neither the main effect of time nor the Infection $\times$ Time interaction were significant. To determine whether the decrease in bone formation and mineralization might be secondary to virus-induced cell damage, sections of the mouse proximal tibial epiphysis were also stained with FITC-labeled anti-EMC viral antibody at 30 and 180 days after infection. Viral specific antigens were not found in the tissue in any of the intervals. The authors concluded that endochondral bone formation and mineralization are greatly impaired in EMC virus-induced mice, and that the decreased bone formation and mineralization are not due to virus-induced tissue damage but to the persistent metabolic alterations associated with diabetes mellitus.

Critique

The research hypothesis is whether mice infected with EMC would show changes in bone mineralization compared with noninfected controls. The general ANOVA table for the 2 × 2 factorial design used in this experiment is presented in Table 6.2. The specific ANOVA table for this experiment is

Source	df	Error term
Infection (I)	1	S/I × T
Time (T)	1	S/I × T
Infection × Time	1	S/I × T
S/I × T	36	
Total	39	

The statistical test selected was appropriate. The authors' first conclusion that endochondral bone formation and mineralization are greatly impaired in EMC virus-induced mice is a restatement of the significant results obtained and is appropriate. The magnitude of these effects, however, is not presented and perhaps the authors are confusing statistical significance ($p < .001$) with biological significance (6.21) when they use the term "greatly" impaired. The second conclusion of the authors is not appropriate given the data presented. No evidence was obtained in this study that EMC virus produced persistent metabolic alterations associated with diabetes mellitus (hyperglycemic and hypoinsulinemic) in the strain of mice used.

RESEARCH DESIGN PROBLEM 31

Conditioned place preference (CPP) is a behavioral technique used to assess drug reinforcement in rats. During conditioning, experimental animals are given a reinforcing drug in a distinctive environment and on alternate days are given saline in a different distinctive environment. Using the same training schedule, control animals are given saline in *both* environments. A rectangular box made with two compartments separated by a removable door is normally used during conditioning and testing—one compartment is painted white and the other compartment is painted black. Because rats are nocturnal animals, when given a choice, they will spend more time in the black part of the box. Therefore, researchers pair the reinforcing drug with the initially nonpreferred white side of the apparatus. Following conditioning, animals are given a preference test in which they have free access to both compartments simultaneously. With this paradigm, the drug-treated experimental animals show CPP if they spend more time in the white side of the box relative to saline-treated controls.

Morphine and heroin (opiate agonist drugs) are highly reinforcing in animals and humans and both of these drugs produce CPP in rats. A neuroscientist wanted to determine whether opiate antagonist drugs, which block the effects of opiate agonists, would have an opposing action on drug reinforcement when a

CPP procedure was used. Three groups of animals ($s = 10$ per group) were used: One group received the opiate agonist morphine (5 mg/kg) paired with the white compartment; the second group received the opiate antagonist naloxone (5 mg/kg) paired with the white compartment; and the third group received saline paired with the white compartment. All drug injections were given subcutaneously. On alternate days, all three groups received saline paired with the black compartment. This sequence of pairings continued until all rats had been given five placements in each compartment. The following day the rats were given a 15-min (900-sec) preference test during which they had free access to either compartment. The neuroscientist predicted that because morphine is reinforcing, morphine-treated rats would spend more time in the white compartment relative to saline controls and because naloxone is aversive (opposing effect to morphine) naloxone-treated rats would spend less time in the white compartment relative to saline controls.

The mean seconds spent in the white compartment for each group were morphine-treated rats (510 sec, SD ± 118), the naloxone-treated rats (140 sec, SD ± 56), and saline controls (166 sec, SD ± 61). A one-way analysis of variance on the time spent in the white compartment revealed a significant main effect of group, $F(2, 27) = 7.86$, $p < .01$. The morphine-treated rats spent significantly more time in white than either of the other two groups, Newman-Keuls test, $p < .05$, but no significant difference occurred between the naloxone- and saline-treated rats. From these results, the neuroscientist concluded that equal doses of morphine and naloxone do not have opposing effects on drug reinforcement because although morphine produced a strong conditioning place preference, naloxone did not produce a significant aversive place preference.

Critique

The research hypothesis is whether naloxone, an opiate antagonist, would produce an aversion to the environment in which rats were placed after receiving the drug. The general ANOVA for this experiment is presented in Table 6.1. The specific ANOVA table for this experiment is

Source	df	Error term
Drug (D)	2	S/Drug
S/Drug	27	
Total	29	

The statistical test selected is appropriate given that a one-way ANOVA is a very robust test (5.23). Because of the variance differences among the groups the latency data (time in seconds) could have been transformed into logarithm time in seconds to satisfy the assumptions of ANOVA (5.24). But, the major problem in this experiment is that the measurements of place preferences and place aversions were not equally sensitive. Because rats normally prefer the dark compartment, an aversion to the white side by pretreatment with naloxone would be difficult to demonstrate because the saline rats (controls) would be expected to spend most of their time in the dark compartment. With such a ceiling effect (5.25) it would be impossible to demonstrate an aversive effect of naloxone. To determine place aversion, naloxone should be paired with the initially preferred black compartment and time spent in this black compartment compared to controls who received saline in the black compartment. Bottom effects (and ceiling effects) may occur even when derived measures are not used (5.25).

RESEARCH DESIGN PROBLEM 32

Depressive illness has been related to changes in the biological rhythms of patients who suffer from this illness. These changes may include alterations in the patient's normal sleep patterns, activity patterns, and eating patterns. Recently, a decrease in the serotonin uptake of the platelets of depressive patients has been reported. Because serotonin levels show a marked diurnal rhythm in healthy people a decrease in serotonin uptake by platelets in depressive patients may be caused by an alteration of a normal circadian rhythm of platelet serotonin uptake. To test this latter hypothesis measurements of the serotonin uptake by platelets of normal, healthy subjects were taken during a 24-h period to determine if a circadian rhythm of serotonin uptake existed.

Thirty healthy, drug-free men (range of 21 to 55 years old) were selected after a rigorous screening procedure (drugs can affect biological rhythms; consequently, drug-free subjects must be selected). A blood sample was drawn from each man at 0800 h on the first test day, and every 4 h (1200, 1600, and so forth) until the final sample was taken at 0800 h on the following test day. During the day the men continued their everyday physical activities with the exception of refraining from strenuous physical labor. During the night they slept in the laboratory so they could be awakened at the proper time for samples to be taken.

Platelet rich plasma was prepared from each blood sample and these samples were stored on ice until the end of the experiment. Serotonin uptake (V_{max} and K_m) values were obtained for each sample. All samples were run at the same time by the same laboratory technician. All samples were also coded so that the technician did not know the time the blood sample was taken.

A complete within-subject ANOVA indicated that a significant time effect existed for serotonin uptake, $F(6, 174) = 4.03$, $p < .001$. Post hoc Newman-Keuls tests indicated that serotonin uptake at 0400 was lower than any other time values ($p < .05$) and these other time values did not differ significantly among themselves. The researchers concluded that normal males have a diurnal rhythm of platelet serotonin uptake with a minimum at 0400 h.

Critique

The research hypothesis is whether a circadian rhythm of serotonin uptake by platelets exists in normal healthy individuals. The general ANOVA for this experiment is presented in Table 4.5. The specific ANOVA table for this complete within-subject design is

Source	df	Error term
Time (T)	6	Time × Subject
Subject (S)	29	
Time × Subject	174	
Total	209	

The statistical test selected was appropriate; however, an ANOVA would not be the *best* statistical procedure available to identify a circadian rhythm (a time series analysis would probably be a more sensitive procedure). The statistical tests that were used, ANOVA and post hoc testing, would only indicate significant differences among the seven means and not be very sensitive to a gradual change in mean values across time.

Only one mean was significantly different from all the other means. But, a potential confound exists in the protocol in that men were required to sleep in the laboratory for the night measurements. The stress of sleeping in a novel laboratory setting may have affected serotonin uptake (4.4) and the blood sample taken at 0400 would have been the most stressful as the majority of men would probably have been sleeping when this measurement was scheduled. To assess a circadian rhythm in serotonin uptake the subjects should be monitored over a longer period under controlled laboratory conditions to permit acclimatization to the laboratory, and a chronic blood sampling procedure should be used which would not require waking the subjects. The early blood samples were kept on ice for a longer period of time than the later ones which might also have affected the serotonin values obtained for the early times. Given all these potential confounds the author's conclusion that normal males have a diurnal rhythm of platelet serotonin uptake with a minimum at 0400 h should not be accepted.

RESEARCH DESIGN PROBLEM 33

Samorin is an effective agent against several trypanosomal (parasitic protozoans) infections in domestic animals. However, samorin's safety (toxicity) in different species has not been extensively studied. Therefore, a veterinarian wanted to determine the safety of samorin in domestic camels.

Twenty healthy camels (10 male, 10 female) were randomly assigned to four groups (5 each): two groups (A, B) were injected with *Trypanosoma evasi* (a common infection among camels) and the other two groups were injected with saline (groups C, D). Twenty-four hours later groups B and C were injected with 1 mg/kg Samorin (the expected therapeutic dose). Group A was injected with .5 mg/kg Samorin and group D was injected with saline.

Acetylcholinesterase activity (AChE) was measured in all animals 24 h after the first set of injections and 24 h after the second set of injections (AChE activity is used as one measure of a drug's or chemical's toxicity). All camels were observed for 1 week postinjection and no animals showed any clinical signs of drug toxicity.

A mixed factorial ANOVA was performed and AChE activity was not significantly affected by any factor: group effect, $F(3, 16) = 2.21$, time of measurement, $F(1, 16) = 3.16$, Group × Time interaction, $F(3, 16) = 2.61$. The veterinarian concluded that Samorin (at 1 mg/kg) was completely safe to use in domestic camels and at this dosage was an effective agent against *Trypanosoma evasi*.

Critique

The research hypothesis is whether Samorin (1 mg/kg) is a safe therapeutic drug against *Trypanosoma evasi* in domestic camels. The general ANOVA table reported for this experiment is presented in Table 6.4. The specific ANOVA table reported for this experiment is

Source	df	Error term
Group (G)	3	S/Group
Pre-Post Measurement (M)	1	M × S/Group
S/Group	16	
G × M	3	M × S/Group
M × S/Group	16	
Total	39	

The statistical test selected was appropriate; however, no appropriate control group exists in this study, that is, a group which is injected with *Trypanosoma evasi* and then saline. To answer the research question the infection and drug combination must be shown to be not harmful to the animals because Samorin would be given to infected *not* normal animals. If the *Trypanosoma evasi* was not potent, only the effects of Samorin were being studied. The design used in this study was not balanced; hence, a 2 × 2 × (2 × 5) factorial ANOVA could not be used to analyze the data (4.21).

The treatments of the four groups reported in this experiment were

	Injection (0 h)	Injection (24 h)
Group A	*Trypanosoma evasi*	.5 mg/kg Samorin
Group B	*Trypanosoma evasi*	1 mg/kg Samorin
Group C	Saline	1 mg/kg Samorin
Group D	Saline	Saline

If group A had received saline (instead of .5 mg/kg Samorin) at the 24-h injection then the experimental design would have been balanced and the question of whether the *Trypanosoma evasi* used was potent would have been answered.

A balanced $A \times B \times (C \times S)$ mixed factorial design is present in Table 6.7. The specific ANOVA table for a balanced $2 \times 2 \times (2 \times S)$ mixed factorial design is

Source	df	Error term
Infection (I)	1	S/ID
Drug (D)	1	S/ID
Time (T)	1	T × S/ID
S/Infection, Drug (ID)	16	
Infection × Drug	1	S/ID
Infection × Time	1	T × S/ID
Drug × Time	1	T × S/ID
I × D × T	1	T × S/ID
Time × S/ID	16	
Total	39	

In this balanced design the overall variance and 3 df associated with groups in the unbalanced design have been partitioned into three sources of variance with 1 df each. Likewise the overall variance and 3 df associated with the Group × Measurement interaction have been partitioned into three interaction sources of variance with 1 df each. Although single-df post hoc comparisons could also be made using the original design none of these comparisons could answer the question of whether the *Trypanosoma evasi* used in the study was potent.

Other potential problems with the reported design and analysis are (*a*) the random assignment of the camels to the four groups might have resulted in more males or females in some of the groups, (*b*) extrapolation of results would be questionable as only one drug toxicity test (AChE) was used, and (*c*) the author must be concerned with the power of the statistical test used as the conclusion (no significant toxicity of drug) is actually proving the null hypothesis (5.12).

RESEARCH DESIGN PROBLEM 34

Aquatic invertebrates are commonly used in "water quality" toxicity tests because they are very sensitive to toxic chemicals. To determine the effect of cadmium on the reproduction and survival of *Ceriodaphnia dubia* (a water flea), an experiment was designed using five cadmium concentrations (5, 10, 20, 40, and 80 μg/L) and a control water ($< .01$ μg/L) with 10 fleas per treatment condition. To obtain *Ceriodaphnia* neonates, 60 adult females were separated and placed into individual beakers. Four hours later the beakers were examined and those having broods with five or fewer neonates were discarded. Ten beakers of those remaining were then randomly selected. From each of these beakers (broods of six or more) six neonates were randomly selected and placed individually in a counterbalanced order into one of the six treatment conditions (10 beakers per concentration). Each day the *Ceriodaphnia* were fed and the solutions were changed in all beakers. Because neonates become reproductive females within a few days, mortality and reproduction were recorded daily until the toxicity test was terminated after 7 days.

Statistical analyses were performed on the weekly totals for each treatment condition. Fischer's Exact Probability test indicated that the mortality for the two highest cadmium concentrations was significantly higher than the control ($p < .01$). A single-factor ANOVA on the reproduction data (number of neonates per beaker) indicated a significant concentration effect, $F(5, 54) = 3.82$, $p < .01$, and multiple comparison tests using Dunnett's method indicated that reproduction was significantly lower from the control only at the two highest cadmium concentrations. The toxicologist concluded that only cadmium concentrations of 40 and 80 μg/L had a significant effect on the survival and reproductive ability of *Ceriodaphnia*; hence, a water quality criterion of 20 μg/L would be appropriate for the protection and propagation of this species.

Critique

The research hypothesis is whether cadmium in various concentrations differentially affects the reproduction and survival of *Ceriodaphnia dubia*. The general ANOVA table for this experiment, as reported, is presented in Table 6.1. The specific ANOVA table for this study is

Source	df	Error term
Group	5	S/Group
S/Group	54	
Total	59	

This ANOVA would be a rather insensitive statistical test and a concentration of 20 μg/L of cadmium might not be an appropriate criterion for the protection and propagation of this species. Because neonates from each brood were randomized across concentrations (9.4), the variance attributed to broods could be estimated and eliminated both from the error term used to calculate the F-ratio (9.4) and the error term for subsequent multiple comparison tests (6.9, 10.1). Note that the ANOVA used had an error term with 54 df (6.5) indicating that brood variance was not estimated.

The general ANOVA table which would estimate brood variance is presented in Table 9.3. The specific ANOVA table for this analysis would be

Source	df	Error term
Between Broods	9	
Within Treatments	5	Broods × Treatments
Broods × Treatments	45	
Total	59	

Notice that the total variance and degrees of freedom (59) available has been partitioned into three estimates: broods (9), treatments (5), and interaction (45). The variance and degrees of freedom for the treatments remain the same in both ANOVAs but in the second, randomized-blocks ANOVA, the previous error variance and its associated degrees of freedom are divided into two components: a variance estimate of brood with 9 df's and a variance estimate of the interaction of Broods × Treatments (error) with 45 df's. If the variance estimate associated with broods was significant, the reduction in error variance *and* df's would provide a more sensitive test. If broods did not contribute a significant amount of variance to the error estimate, losing the 9 df's would not be advisable.

At the two highest cadmium concentrations reproduction was also confounded with mortality because flea loss due to death would also result in decreased reproduction. Reproductive data were the number of neonates per beaker. If a substantial number of fleas had died within 2 days they would not have reproduced, a zero would be the score for these beakers, and at the highest concentrations there would have been minimal variance (5.22). The ANOVA should have been done on those concentrations where mortality was not significantly different from controls. There is also a question as to why the Dunnett test (10.6) was used. This test would have been appropriate by itself if the only question was how the cadmium groups differed from the control group (6.10). Given the number of statistical problems with the data analysis the researcher's conclusions should be rejected particularly because a more sensitive analysis might have shown that 20 μg/L of cadmium would affect the reproduction and survival of the water fleas.

If the doses of toxicants are transformed into logarithms, often the tolerances of many organisms to these poisons are approximately normally distributed. These transformed doses are called dosages and increasing dosages lead to a cumulative normal distribution of mortalities, called *dosage-mortality curves*. An entire field of biometric analysis called bioassay is concerned with these kinds of curves. The most common technique in bioassay is *probit analysis*. For a detailed discussion of current statistical techniques in bioassay see Govindarajulu (1987).

RESEARCH DESIGN PROBLEM 35

In most desert lizards "panting" is a thermoregulatory response to high body temperatures. Lizards begin to pant at a certain body temperature, referred to as the panting threshold, and under water stress (dehydration) they also adjust their water expenditure to minimize the amount of water lost from the body. Because panting increases water loss, a zoologist predicted that desert lizards when dehydrated would show an elevation in panting threshold compared with when they were fully hydrated.

Thirteen adult lizards of the same species, collected from the field, were laboratory-housed for several weeks with food and water available *ad lib*. From these well-hydrated lizards, head and cloacal panting thresholds were measured during heat stress, and after these control measurements the lizards were denied both food and water for a few weeks to induce dehydration. Head and cloacal panting thresholds were remeasured in each lizard under the same heat stress conditions when progressive body weight loss (a reliable measure of water loss) was 3 percent (Category I), between 3 and 7 percent (Category II), and greater than 7 percent (Category III) of initial body weight.

Mann-Whitney nonparametric tests were performed comparing panting thresholds in the three different body weight categories. Both head and cloacal panting thresholds were significantly greater in Category II than in Category I ($p < .05$) and in Category III than in Category I ($p < .05$). Category II and Category III were not significantly different ($p > .05$). From these results, the zoologist concluded that in this lizard species panting thresholds during heat stress are elevated from control levels during dehydration to minimize water loss at the expense of effective thermoregulation.

Critique

The research hypothesis is whether lizards would have a higher panting threshold during heat stress when dehydrated than when fully hydrated. The general ANOVA table for the reported experiment is presented in Table 4.5. The specific ANOVA table for the complete within-subject design reported in this experiment is

Source	df	Error term
Treatment	2	Treatment × Subject
Subject	12	
Treatment × Subject	24	
Total	38	

In the experimental report, three Mann-Whitney tests (11.5) were done which would increase the familywise error rate (6.9). The same type of problem occurs when multiple t-tests are used leading to an increase in Type I errors (5.10). A complete within-subject ANOVA could have been used with body temperature at the beginning of panting as the dependent variable (ratio scale). Why a nonparametric instead of a parametric test was selected is not clear. More important, control data were not presented and control panting threshold temperatures were not compared with dehydrated-state panting thresholds. Without this control comparison it cannot be concluded that the panting threshold increases with increased dehydration levels because the hydrated panting threshold (control) may have been higher than any of the dehydration thresholds, particularly that of Category I. The specific ANOVA table for an experiment including the control hydrated measurement would be

Source	df	Error term
Treatment	3	Treatment × Subject
Subject	12	
Treatment × Subject	36	
Total	51	

A significant treatment effect would have to be further evaluated with appropriate post hoc multiple comparison tests (6.9, Chapter 10). Unfortunately, a time confound also exists in this experiment as Category III was always the last panting threshold measurement taken and some lizards may have become ill when their body weight loss was over 7 percent. Remember the lizards would have been given three heat stress tests before Category III's test. Any cumulative effects of body weight loss and heat stress would appear during the later tests. Any unhealthy lizards may have affected comparisons involving Category III. A partial answer to this time confound problem could be obtained by examination of the individual data to see whether all animals had a similar relationship between panting temperature threshold and body weight loss.

RESEARCH DESIGN PROBLEM 36

Glucose transport from the small intestine is a first-order, sodium-coupled process. Identifying specific reversible inhibitors of this sodium-coupled process would provide a valuable research tool. In this research, a synthetic compound's effect on the first-order elimination rate constant (K_e) is measured (K_e is the slope of the line when the log of the amount of glucose in the lumen is plotted against time). An *in situ* procedure for measuring glucose elimination in rat intestine was used to test the properties of a promising new synthetic drug, R216. The experimental protocol was measuring K_e for glucose at 10 mM with only vehicle present, then measuring K_e for glucose at 10 mM with the drug R216 at a total concentration of 50 μM, and finally remeasuring K_e for glucose at 10 mM with only vehicle present following a complete washout of the glucose-drug solution. During each treatment condition, five data points from each rat were used to calculate the elimination rate constant (K_e) and the process remained first-order throughout all measurements.

The following mean results were obtained for the 12 male adult rats used in the experiment: K_e before drug was .092 SD $\pm$ .003, K_e with drug was .045 SD $\pm$ .002, K_e after washout was .096 SD $\pm$ .004. Because every rat was used in all treatment conditions, a complete within-subject ANOVA was performed. A significant treatment effect was found, $F(2, 22) = 10.73$, $p < .001$, and the pharmacologist concluded that the drug at a total concentration of 50 μM does decrease the K_e, and the drug effect is reversible (does not permanently inhibit the sodium-coupled glucose elimination process) when 10 mM of glucose is used.

Critique

The research hypothesis is whether the drug R216 will significantly reduce the first-order rate constant (K_e) for glucose elimination in the adult male rat's intestine and whether K_e will return to normal after the drug is removed. The general ANOVA table for this experiment is presented in Table 4.5. The specific ANOVA table for the complete within-subject ANOVA used in this experiment is

Source	df	Error term
Treatment	2	Treatment $\times$ Subject
Subject	11	
Treatment $\times$ Subject	22	
Total	35	

A significant treatment effect indicates that the means of the conditions differ but does not indicate which means are significantly different from others (6.8); hence, post hoc multiple comparison tests (6.9, Chapter 10) normally must be done to determine which pair-comparisons are significant. In this experiment, however, the mean and SD values for the three treatment conditions indicate that the drug treatment condition is significantly different from the two control conditions (pre- and postdrug) and these control conditions do differ significantly from each other. Consequently, even though post hoc tests were not done, the pharmacologist's conclusions are appropriate given the data presented. Usually, the means and SDs are not as clear-cut as the data obtained in this experiment and post hoc tests would be necessary. The two procedures of the control measurements are identical (pre- and postdrug) and the same control outcome indicates that the drug effect is reversible, that is, does not permanently inhibit the sodium-coupled glucose elimination process.

RESEARCH DESIGN PROBLEM 37

Experiments with humans and rats have shown that enkephalins (ENK) and catecholamines (CA) are released during emotional stress. An exercise physiologist wanted to determine whether ENK and CA are also released during physical activity in fit and normal men. Twenty males (21–40 years old) were pretested for VO_2 max and then divided equally into 2 groups: fit (F), VO_2 max being greater than 54 mL·kg^{-1}·min^{-1}, and normal (N), VO_2 max being less than 44 mL·kg^{-1}·min^{-1}. The exercise test was 6 min on an ergometer with the first 4 min at 70 percent VO_2 max and the last 2 min at 120 percent VO_2 max. Before testing an indwelling catheter was placed in a right arm vein of each man and a basal blood sample (6 mL) was drawn (0 min blood sample) after a 1-h relaxation period. Blood samples were divided into separate tubes for RIA analysis of CA and ENK using sensitive methods. The testing of the fit and normal men was counterbalanced during the day. During testing, blood samples were drawn at 4 min, 6 min, and 7 min (1-min postexercise). CA and ENK data were analyzed separately using mixed factorial ANOVAs. The results of these ANOVAs were

CA

Group	$F(1, 18) = 8.56$	$p < .01$
Time	$F(3, 114) = 8.72$	$p < .001$
Group $\times$ Time	$F(3, 114) = 3.85$	$p < .01$

ENK

Group	$F(1, 18) = 8.95$	$p < .01$
Time	$F(3, 114) = 7.76$	$p < .001$
Group $\times$ Time	$F(3, 114) = 4.01$	$p < .01$

Subsequent post hoc multiple comparison tests revealed the following significant mean differences ($p < .05$). All comparisons not given were not significant ($p > .05$):

CA

Group	F > N
Time	All times different with 6 > 4 > 7 > 0 min
Group $\times$ Time	N > F at 4 min, F > N at 6 min

ENK

Group	F > N
Time	All times different with 4 > 6 > 7 > 0 min
Group $\times$ Time	N > F at 4 min, F > N at 6 min

Based upon these analytical comparisons the major conclusions of the exercise physiologist were that (*a*) both ENK and CA are released during exercise, (*b*) the length of exercise produces an attenuation of the ENK response and potentiation of the CA response, and (*c*) the fit and normal men show the same pattern of release of ENK and CA as a function of exercise length.

Critique

The research hypothesis is whether enkephalins and catecholamines are released during physical activity in both fit and normal men. A diagram of the experimental design of this exercise experiment is shown in Figure 14.3. The general ANOVA table for this experiment is presented in Table 6.4. The specific ANOVA table for this $2 \times (4 \times 10)$ mixed factor design is

Source	df	Error term
Group (G)	1	S/Group
Time (T)	3	Time $\times$ S/Group
S/Group	18	
Group $\times$ Time	3	Time $\times$ S/Group
Time $\times$ S/Group	54	
Total	79	

The statistical test was appropriate but calculations of F-ratios are not correct. The number of degrees of freedom associated with the error term for the F-ratios for time and the Group $\times$ Time interaction is inflated. In the calculation of the

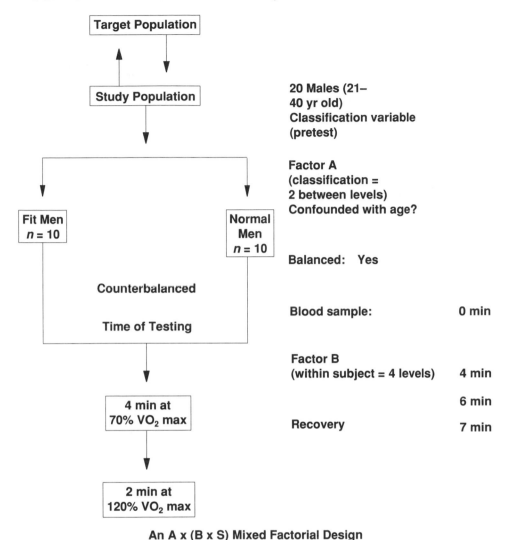

An A x (B x S) Mixed Factorial Design

Figure 14.3   Experimental design for research problem 37.

error term for these comparisons the degrees of freedom are given as 114 which suggests that an incorrect sample size of 20 for each group was used (6.5). For this reason, the conclusions should be rejected. Also, in this experiment, exercise intensity changed at 4 min (from 70% VO_2 max to 120% VO_2 max); consequently, intensity would be the important variable not exercise length as the exercise physiologist concluded. The classification variable (4.2, fit or normal) used may have been confounded (4.23) with the age of the male. Finally, the Group × Time interaction (if correctly performed) would indicate that fit and normal men *do not* show the same pattern of release (6.12, 6.13).

RESEARCH DESIGN PROBLEM 38

Glucose transport in human erythrocytes (red blood cells) is insensitive to insulin, even though the transport protein is very similar (physically and kinetically) to insulin-sensitive glucose transporters located in other places of the body. Human K-562 cells, a leukemic erythrocyte precursor, can be grown in culture and induced to mature to three distinct stages of erythrocyte maturation. By studying glucose transport and insulin effects upon these precursors, a biomedical scientist wanted to determine at which stage erythrocytes become insulin-insensitive during their development.

K-562 cells were grown in standard culture media and when cell density reached 10^{12} cells/mm^3 they were separated equally into three populations (groups). These three groups were then inoculated into culture media containing varying concentrations of a drug (DMSO) known to cause differentiation to stages 1, 2, or 3 (1 being blastic and 3 nearly mature). After reaching 5 generations each group was then divided into 20 subpopulations and allowed to reach 3 generations at which time glucose influx was determined at 1, 2.5, and 5 mM glucose concentrations with and without insulin (1 pM) present and cell density held constant at 10^6 cells/mm^3. K_m and V_m were determined by Haynes plot for each subpopulation and the mean and standard deviation for each group were

| | Number of cell | Insulin $\pm$ SD | | No insulin $\pm$ SD | |
Stages	population	K_m(mM)	V_m	K_m(mM)	V_m
1	20	1.24 $\pm$ .02	18 $\pm$ 2	1.25 $\pm$ .01	4 $\pm$ 1
2	20	1.26 $\pm$ .01	6 $\pm$ 1	1.24 $\pm$ .02	6 $\pm$ 1
3	20	1.25 $\pm$ .02	5 $\pm$ 1	1.26 $\pm$ .01	5 $\pm$ 1

For both K_m and V_m a 3 $\times$ 2 mixed factorial design with repeated measures on the last factor was done. For K_m neither the two main effects nor the Group $\times$ Insulin interaction were significant. For V_m there was a significant group effect, $F(2, 57) = 3.20$, $p < .05$; a significant insulin effect, $F(1, 57) = 4.12$, $p < .05$; and a significant Group $\times$ Insulin interaction, $F(2, 57) = 3.31$, $p < .001$. A Newman-Keuls post hoc test of the significant interaction revealed that cells in stage 1 given insulin had significantly higher V_m values than all the other cell groups ($p < .05$), and these other five groups did *not* differ significantly among themselves. The author concluded that human erythrocytes become insulin-insensitive following their blastic stage of development.

Critique

The research hypothesis is whether erythrocytes become insulin-insensitive at a particular stage of development (differentiation). The general ANOVA for this experiment is presented in Table 6.4. The specific ANOVA table for this experiment is

Source	df	Error term
Group (G)	2	S/Group
Insulin (I)	1	I × S/Group
S/Group	57	
Group × Insulin	2	I × S/Group
Insulin × S/Group	57	
Total	119	

The statistical analysis was appropriate and correct. But, the author's conclusion is an inappropriate extrapolation of the outcome of the experiment because data were obtained from cancerous cells not normal erythrocytes (3.3, 4.25). It is reasonable to expect that cells derived from leukemic erythrocyte precursors would show different developmental characteristics than normal erythrocytes. Hence, biological considerations would restrict the generalization of the data obtained (3.3, 4.25).

RESEARCH DESIGN PROBLEM 39

A major aim of preventive medicine is to identify good predictors of health problems. A medical research team wanted to determine what variables would be the best predictors of cardiovascular problems. The medical team randomly selected 100 medical charts on males between the ages of 45–65 obtained from each of 1000 randomly selected physicians in Chicago (i.e., $n = 100,000$). The correlations between incidence of cardiovascular problems and 20 other variables taken from the medical charts were calculated. Of these variables, weight had a correlation of .81 ($p < .001$) and caloric intake/day had a correlation of .63 ($p < .01$). All the other variables considered had correlations of less than .40. The report of the medical research team concluded, therefore, that of the variables considered, the best prediction of cardiovascular problems for males 45–65 living in Chicago would be made using weight and caloric intake/day rather than a combination of any other two variables.

Critique

The aim of the study is to determine what variables recorded on medical charts are correlated significantly with cardiovascular problems. A research hypothesis cannot be specified as the study is an attempt to find possible predictors of cardiovascular problems. Although weight and caloric intake/day are both correlated with cardiovascular problems, these two correlations probably provide redundant information. That is, when squared (r^2), they both "explain" the same variance in cardiovascular problems (5.27). A variable that provides more "unique" or independent information (even with a lower correlation with cardiovascular problems) when combined with either caloric intake/day or weight would probably provide a more accurate prediction of cardiovascular problems. A stepwise multiple regression procedure could be used to determine which variables would be the best predictors of cardiovascular problems (5.26). In principle, there is no limit to the number of independent variables which may be included in a multiple regression equation, but the number of variables should be kept at a manageable level. Various methods are available to choose the "best" set of independent variables for inclusion in the equation. Stepwise inclusion methods evaluate all the possible independent variables not already in the equation and enter into the equation, at each step, the variables that increase the coefficient of multiple correlation to the greatest extent. The validity of these predictors, however, would have to be determined in another study because the stepwise multiple regression procedure is a *post hoc* method of analysis.

RESEARCH DESIGN PROBLEM 40

Low doses of morphine (i.e., 1–3 mg/kg) induce hyperactivity in rats presumably by stimulating dopaminergic neurons. If dopaminergic neurons are involved in this behavior then pretreatment of rats with a dopamine antagonist (pimozide) should block hyperactivity induced by morphine. Twenty-four adult male rats were divided randomly into two groups ($n = 12$ per group). The rats in the first group were pretreated with pimozide (.25 mg/kg, IP) 4 h before testing (the effect of pimozide is strongest 4 h after IP injection). Ten minutes before testing, these same rats were injected with morphine (2 mg/kg, SC) and these rats were called the P-M group. Rats in the other group were injected with the pimozide vehicle 4 h before testing, and injected with saline 10 min before testing (the V-S group of rats). All rats were tested in an observation chamber and were scored at 5, 10, 20, and 30 min according to a 9-point activity rating scale ranging from asleep (1), through normal alert activity (4), up to stereotyped activity (8), and dyskinetic movement (9). Ratings were made by two trained observers who did not know the treatment conditions. The apparatus was also equipped with two photobeams that divided the chamber into four equal quadrants. Each time a rat crossed the path of the photobeam, a count was registered. The total number of counts at the end of the 30-min test provided another measure of the rat's activity.

The mean activity rating of each group at each test time was analyzed using Mann-Whitney U tests with an adjusted alpha level for multiple comparisons. Results of these tests showed that group P-M was significantly more active at each test time than group V-S. The mean number of activity counts was analyzed using a t-test. The results showed that group P-M was significantly more active than group V-S, $t(22) = 2.89$, $p < .01$. Because group P-M was significantly more active than group V-S on both a qualitative (ranking) and a quantitative (counts) measure of activity, the pharmacologist concluded that a dose of .25 mg/kg pimozide does not affect morphine-induced activity.

Critique

The research hypothesis is whether pretreatment of rats with pimozide, a dopamine antagonist, would block morphine-induced hyperactivity. An ordinal scale of measurement (9-point activity rating scale) was used (5.3) and, therefore, a nonparametric rather than a parametric test would be appropriate for this measure (11.1). The Mann-Whitney U-test (11.5) is a nonparametric test for two independent means and because more than one test was done the alpha level (5.9) was adjusted for the multiple comparisons (6.9).

The total number of photocell counts at the end of the 30-min test was evaluated by a t-test. The general ANOVA table for this parametric measure is presented in Table 6.1. The specific ANOVA table for this activity measure is

Source	df	Error term
Group	1	S/Group
S/Group	22	
Total	23	

Because the t-test is only a special case of the F-test (5.18), the statistical tests used were appropriate and correct. But, there is no proper control group to conclude that .25 mg/kg pimozide does not affect morphine-induced activity. To make this conclusion, a significant difference between the group of rats pretreated with pimozide (P) and then given morphine (M) and a group of rats not pretreated with pimozide (V) and given morphine (M) must be obtained. The control group of rats in this study was not pretreated with pimozide (V) and was not given morphine.

RESEARCH DESIGN PROBLEM 41

The increase in body temperature that occurs during exercise may act as a fever and prevent viral infections in people who exercise 4 or more days a week. Indeed, many exercise enthusiasts report that they are now healthier than before they began exercising. To determine whether exercise-induced hyperthermia prevents viral infections, exercised and nonexercised rats were infected with a pyrogen (which causes fever in healthy rats) and body temperatures of these infected rats were then monitored.

Forty male rats were randomly assigned equally to two groups. Experimental rats were placed on an exercise regimen that involved running on a treadmill at 60 percent VO_2 max for 45 min 6 days a week for 3 weeks (within 3 weeks physiological responses to exercise have reached a steady state). The other 20 rats served as nonexercised controls. After the 3-week training period, five rats from each group were randomly assigned to one of four drug groups: vehicle control, low, medium, and high pyrogen doses. Chronic rectal temperature probes were implanted, the pyrogen and control rats were injected, and body temperatures were recorded continuously for 72 h after the injection. The exercised rats were maintained on their normal exercise regimen during the measurement period. In both the nonexercising medium- and high-dose groups two rats died and were replaced. One rat from the exercising high-dose group died and was also replaced.

An ANOVA using the highest rectal temperature recorded from each rat revealed a significant exercise effect, $F(1, 32) = 7.81$, $p < .01$ and a significant dose effect, $F(3, 32) = 3.61$, $p < .05$. The Exercise $\times$ Dose interaction was not significant, $F(3, 32) = 1.43$. The exercised rats had significantly higher rectal temperatures than their controls, $p < .01$. The vehicle and low-dose rats did not differ significantly from each other but had lower rectal temperatures than rats in the medium- and high-dose groups (Newman-Keuls test, $p < .05$). Rats in these two highest-dose groups did not differ in rectal temperatures.

The biologist concluded that a daily exercise regimen does prevent infection by destroying viruses before they reach a critical level of production and that exercise also minimizes the effectiveness of viruses because fewer rats from the exercised group died.

Critique

The research hypothesis was to determine whether exercise-induced hyperthermia will prevent viral infections in rats. The general ANOVA table for this experiment is presented in Table 6.2. The specific ANOVA table for this 2 $\times$ 4 factorial experiment is

Source	df	Error term
Exercise	1	S/Exercise $\times$ Dose
Dose	3	S/Exercise $\times$ Dose
Exercise $\times$ Dose	3	S/Exercise $\times$ Dose
S/Exercise $\times$ Dose	32	
Total	39	

The statistical test selected (using one data point) was correctly calculated. But, numerous problems exist in this research report. The first is a conceptual problem of how to measure viral infection. Body temperature was used as an indirect measure of viral infection but both exercise and the pyrogen injected would produce an increase in body temperature. Hence, the research hypothesis tested would be that exercise-induced hyperthermia prevents pyrogen-induced hyperthermia. A test of this hypothesis might be that the normal hyperthermia induced by pyrogen should be reduced in exercised rats compared with nonexercised rats. Thus, lower body temperatures *during rest periods* could be expected for the exercised rats when compared with the nonexercised rats. If exercise had a significant effect on body temperature, given the experimental design, a significant Group $\times$ Dose interaction would also be expected (6.12).

The highest rectal temperature recorded was used to evaluate the research hypothesis. Besides the conceptual confusion, a confound exists when this particular data point is used, namely, the highest rectal temperature for the animals in the exercised group should occur during their daily 45-min exercise period. Hence, the fact that the exercised rats had higher rectal temperatures than their nonexercised controls should be expected and does not support the biologist's conclusion. Neither, of course, does the data presented regarding significant dose differences because the significant main effect of dose is collapsed across the exercised and nonexercised rats (6.12).

On the other hand, the loss of rats in the various subgroups does provide some evidence for the research hypothesis. A selective loss of animals occurred in a few of the treatment conditions, that is, 40 percent of the animals (two out of five in each group) died and were replaced in the nonexercising medium- and high-dose groups; whereas, only one animal died in the high-dose exercised group and was replaced. Therefore, 4 out of 10 animals died in the two highest-dose groups of nonexercised rats and only 1 out of 10 animals died in the corresponding groups of exercised rats. A chi-square test (11.2) for a 2×2 contingency table indicated the following results, $X^2 = 1.07$, $p < .30$. If the cause of these deaths was the pyrogen treatment (4.12) then the exercise regimen may have protected the rats from fever and death. Unfortunately, this post hoc examination of the data for the two highest doses across groups is not conclusive (see 5.19).

A more sensitive data analysis would evaluate body temperature changes across time. For example, a selection of the body temperature measurements of the rats immediately after pyrogen injections and then every 6 h during a 72-h monitoring period would provide 13 body temperature measurements for each rat. The specific number of measurements selected for analysis should avoid measurements taken immediately before, during, or immediately after the daily exercise period. This analysis would avoid the exercise-temperature confound and the general ANOVA table for this $2 \times 4 \times (13 \times S)$ mixed factorial is presented in Table 6.7.

RESEARCH DESIGN PROBLEM 42

The molluscan neuropeptide SCPb (Small Cardioactive Peptide "B") increases heart rate and heart muscle contractility in several species of molluscs. A neurobiologist wanted to determine if this neuropeptide had similar functional effects in the opisthobranch mollusc, *Aplysia californica*, as SCPb had been found recently in this species. Ten healthy *Aplysia*, randomly selected from a common holding tank, were used. The heart of each *Aplysia* was dissected and placed quickly in a microperfusion chamber. Each heart was attached to a sensitive force transducer and solutions were delivered intraventricularly by a peristaltic pump. Heart rate (bpm) and heart contractility (mg force/g dry weight) were measured for each heart.

When each heart was first placed in the chamber, rate and contractility were measured for 20 min during which time the heart was perfused with *Aplysia* saline. This initial perfusion was followed by a 20-min treatment period during which the heart was perfused with saline plus $2 \times 10^{-15}\,M$ SCPb and then a 20-min recovery period during which the heart was once again perfused with saline alone. This testing order was repeated with a sequential increase in SCPb concentrations (2×10^{-14}, 2×10^{-13}, 2×10^{-12}, 2×10^{-11}, 2×10^{-10}, 2×10^{-9}, 2×10^{-8}, 2×10^{-7}, 2×10^{-6}, 2×10^{-5}, $2 \times 10^{-4}\,M$ SCPb). Each treatment period was immediately preceded by a saline control perfusion.

A complete within-subject ANOVA with repeated measures was performed. A significant dose effect was found for heart rate, $F(11, 99) = 3.54$, $p < .001$. Newman-Keuls multiple comparison tests indicated that the values for $2 \times 10^{-15} M$, 2×10^{-14}, M and $2 \times 10^{-13} M$ SCPb were not significantly different from control but all other doses were different from control, and the values of $2 \times 10^{-4} M > 2 \times 10^{-5} M > 2 \times 10^{-6} M > 2 \times 10^{-7} M > 2 \times 10^{-8} M > 2 \times 10^{-9} M > 2 \times 10^{-10} M > 2 \times 10^{-11} M > 2 \times 10^{-12} M$ SCPb. The same pattern of significant results was obtained for heart contractility using a complete within-subject ANOVA and Newman-Keuls multiple comparison tests. From these results the author concluded that both heart rate and contractility increase in a dose-dependent manner upon application of SCPb and that the threshold for SCPb effects on *Aplysia* heart is near $2 \times 10^{-12} M$ SCPb.

Critique

The research hypothesis is whether the molluscan neuropeptide SCPb increases heart rate and heart muscle contractility in *Aplysia californica*. The general ANOVA table for the experiment is presented in Table 4.5. The specific ANOVA table for this experiment is

Source	df	Error term
Dose	12	Dose × Subject
Subject	9	
Dose × Subject	108	
Total	129	

The statistical analysis selected was appropriate but is not correct as reported. In the reported experiment 12 doses of SCPb were used and *at least* one control (saline?) dose. Unfortunately it is not clear what data were used as control values. The df's reported for the two mean squares of the F-ratio were incorrect if control data were incorporated in the overall analysis (see specific ANOVA table).

This control data problem is apparent because the experimental design is not balanced. A saline-treatment only condition (20 min) needs to be added, that is, saline (20 min) and saline-treatment only (20 min). In a balanced design, an (A × B × S) or a treatment (13) by measurement (2) complete within-subject ANOVA could be used. The two levels of measurement are prior and during treatment. If there were no significant differences among the saline control periods (prior to treatment), these values could be averaged for each heart to provide values for a control saline period, an (A × S) design. Although a saline control period immediately preceded each treatment period, there is no evidence presented that a return to baseline occurred before each treatment condition. In the study design a saline control period followed each treatment period but this recovery saline control was also the prior saline control for the next treatment condition. Furthermore, the order of administration of the peptide was not counterbalanced; hence, the author cannot conclude that the threshold is near $2 \times 10^{-12} M$ SCPb as the effect at this dose could be because of some cumulative dosage (4.19, 4.20) or slight changes in the functional state of the heart. A simple counterbalancing procedure for the various doses would have eliminated these potential problems.

If the neuroscientist had only concluded that SCPb increases heart rate and heart muscle contractility (the research hypothesis), the significant F-ratio and the pattern of significant means would have made this limited conclusion appropriate.

RESEARCH DESIGN PROBLEM 43

Dopamine has been shown to protect chicks from strychnine-induced seizures, but this protective effect has not been observed in mammals. The purpose of this study, therefore, was to determine whether levodopa (L-DOPA), a dopamine precursor, would affect strychnine seizures in mice.

Albino male mice were randomly assigned to a control (vehicle) and five treatment groups (6.25, 12.50, 25.00, 50.00, and 100.00 mg/kg L-DOPA), with 12 mice in each group. All mice weighed between 20 and 25 g, and food and water were available during the experiment. Each mouse was used only once to test its seizure response which was defined as a tonic extension of the hindlimbs (a sign of powerful convulsive state in the mouse).

The mice were pretreated with the appropriate dose of L-DOPA or vehicle IP 15 min prior to administration of strychnine. All doses were prepared to give an injected volume of .2 mL, and all solutions were prepared fresh daily. The dose of strychnine used was 1 mg/kg SC which had been shown previously to produce profound tonic extension of the hindlimbs in adult mice. Also, L-DOPA injected IP produces optimal brain dopamine levels in adult mice within 15 min.

Each mouse was observed for 1 h after the strychnine was given to record any seizure activity, and was kept for an additional 2 h to record any strychnine-induced deaths. Animals were run throughout the day (treatment conditions were counterbalanced) in a temperature-controlled room and the results obtained are shown in Table 14.3.

Student's t-tests on seizure time onset data found all doses of L-DOPA compared with the control to cause a significant delay in the onset of seizures at $p <$

Table 14.3 Effects of L-Dopa on Tonic Seizure and Mortality

L-DOPA (mg/kg)	Number of mice convulsed ($n = 12$)	Time of tonic seizure onset (Mean ± SEM)	% Mortality
Control	12	9.8 ± 1.4 min	50.0
6.25	8	18.3 ± 1.8	25.0
12.50	8	12.8 ± 1.6	12.5
25.00	7	11.9 ± 2.7	25.0
50.00	7	12.7 ± 2.7	37.5
100.00	6	15.0 ± 2.2	12.5

.001 levels. Chi-square tests on the mortality data and the occurrence of seizures were not significant ($p > .05$). Based upon the latency of seizure onset, the author concluded that levodopa does have an anticonvulsant effect in albino adult mice treated with strychnine.

Critique

The research hypothesis is whether pretreatment with L-DOPA would affect strychnine seizures in mice. The general ANOVA table for this experiment is presented in Table 6.1. The specific ANOVA table for this experiment is

Source	df	Error term
Dose	5	S/Dose
S/Dose	66	
Total	71	

Although multiple t-tests were used to evaluate the latency data, only five comparisons were reported, each significant at $p < .001$; therefore, the increase in familywise error (6.9, 10.1) would be around .005 as estimated by 5(.001). If the control-treatment comparisons were the only ones of interest then the Dunnett test would have been appropriate (10.6). From the report it is not clear whether a dose-response question was being tested. If so, then comparisons among the different drug groups would be expected. The conclusion of the author is very restrictive as comparisons among drug groups were not made. A significant dose effect in the ANOVA would require subsequent multiple comparison tests (Chapter 10) or a trend analysis (6.16).

RESEARCH DESIGN PROBLEM 44

In many animals pinealectomy produces changes in temperature regulation. In lizards, as well as in most animals, melatonin is a principal product of the pineal gland, and normal circulatory levels of melatonin are disrupted by pinealectomy. Hence, circulating melatonin levels and behavioral thermoregulation may be related. The aim of the present study was to determine whether modification of melatonin levels would affect behavioral thermal selection in lizards.

Twelve adult lizards were housed in an environmental chamber in which they were acclimated to an ambient temperature cycle of 30°C during the light period (photophase) and 15°C during the dark period (scotophase). A light-dark cycle of 12 hours of light (30°C) and 12 hours of dark (15°C) for one week prior to testing was used. (Lizards are fully acclimated to temperature and light-dark cycles within one week.) After this acclimation phase, all lizards were placed in a linear thermal gradient long box. In a temperature gradient box lizards spend more time within a well-defined thermal region which is termed the preferred body temperature of the animal. During this temperature testing phase, the photoperiod was the same as that during acclimation. For each lizard core temperature was recorded automatically every 30 min by a chronic indwelling thermocouple inserted into the intestine via the cloaca.

Before behavioral testing, the 12 lizards were randomly assigned to two groups: a control ($n = 6$) and an experimental ($n = 6$). The experimental group received an intraperitoneal injection of 1 μg melatonin per g of body weight and the control group received an equivalent injection of vehicle solution. After injection the lizards were placed in the thermal gradient box. The identical procedure was used for two more days. Means of body temperatures were calculated for each hour of the day (time) and for each day. A mixed factorial ANOVA revealed the following sources of variance, F-values, and probability levels:

ANOVA of Temperature Experiment

Source of variance	df	F	p
Time of day	47	4.42	<.001
Day	2	12.05	<.001
Treatment	1	0.15	NS
Time × Day	94	0.44	NS
Time × Treatment	47	2.61	<.001
Day × Treatment	2	54.75	<.001
Time × Day × Treatment	94		NS

Analysis of the data revealed that the experimental lizards selected higher body temperatures than the controls on day 1 and day 2, but a lower temperature on day 3. Also, the Time × Treatment interaction indicated that the experimental animals selected higher mean body temperatures during photophase and lower mean body temperatures during scotophase than did controls. The cause of the significant main effect of day was due to an increase in the mean daily body temperature by approximately 1°C with each succeeding day for the controls and for days 1 and 2 for the experimental animals.

Thermal selection with time of day was also significant with higher temperatures preferred from mid-day to late photophase and lower temperatures preferred in late scotophase and early photophase. Control animals reached maximum and minimum body temperatures later in the day than did experimentals. The zoologists' main conclusion was that melatonin clearly affects thermal selection and its effect differed depending on the time of day and the day that body temperatures were recorded. They also concluded that both control and experimental lizards had significant day to day changes in thermal selection and experienced significant changes in thermal selection with time of day, and that melatonin altered these time-dependent responses.

Critique

The research hypothesis is whether an increase in circulatory levels of melatonin would affect behavioral thermal selection in lizards. A general ANOVA table for this multiple factor study has not been previously presented. A diagram of the experimental design of this thermoregulatory experiment is shown in Figure 14.4.

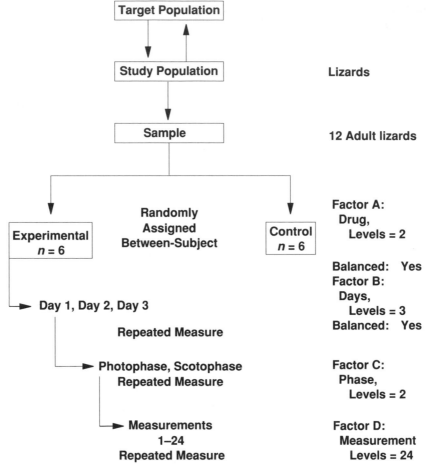

A 2 x (3 x 2 x 24 x S) Mixed Factorial Design

Figure 14.4   Experimental design for research problem 44.

The specific design described is actually an A × (B × C × D × S) mixed factorial or a 2 (group) × 3 (day) × 2 (phase, photo or scoto) × 24 (measurements). However, the author used a 2 (treatment) × 3 (day) × 48 (measurement, called time) ANOVA to analyze the data.

This brief is an excellent example of overdesigning an experiment (4.24) and illustrates the difficulty of attempting to interpret three-way (6.14) and four-way (6.15) interactions. The first step in an analysis of this data probably would be to reduce the amount of data analyzed. For example, even though measurements were taken every 30 min, it may be beneficial to obtain an hourly average (12 per phase period). Calculation of the expected degrees of freedom should be used to make sure that the appropriate error terms (when small number of subjects are used) remain good estimators of variance (see Tables 6.6 and 6.7). Another possibility would be to do separate ANOVAs on each day's data. In this situation, the ANOVA used would then be a 2 (group) $\times$ 2 (phase, photo or scoto) $\times$ 12 (measurements), that is, an A $\times$ (B $\times$ C $\times$ S) mixed factorial design (see Table 6.9).

Because this experiment was not analyzed properly, the authors' conclusions should be rejected. The authors used a 2 (treatment) $\times$ 3 (day) $\times$ 48 (time) ANOVA to analyze the data, and then appeared to interpret a significant day effect by using the means involved in a significant Day $\times$ Treatment interaction. The significant Time $\times$ Treatment interaction was difficult to interpret, perhaps, because 96 means were being compared. A trend or time series analysis (6.16) would probably be a more sensitive and appropriate procedure to evaluate any significant outcome with measurement as a factor.

The data from day 1 would answer the proposed research question. It is not clear, therefore, why the experimental data from days 2 and 3 were included. Other factors (e.g., habituation, conditioning, change in melatonin levels by repeated injections) would probably affect behavioral thermal selection on these latter two days. Just because measurements are easy to obtain does not mean that they must be reported.

RESEARCH DESIGN PROBLEM 45

A relatively new belladonna alkaloid, mythicalamine, was isolated from a rare plant in South America. Previous studies indicated that mythicalamine when given acutely was a strong, long-acting appetite suppressant and might be an effective chronic diet aid. To determine mythicalamine's effect on body weight 16 male rats (90–110 days old) ranging from 200–300 g were randomly divided into two groups of eight. The control group of animals received IP injections of vehicle, and the experimental group received IP injections of mythicalamine in vehicle (.005 mg/kg). The injections were given daily for eight weeks and all rats had free access to food and water all the time. The weight of each rat was measured at the beginning of the first week and again at the end of each week for the next eight weeks. A mixed factorial ANOVA showed a significant main effect of drug, $F(1, 14) = 5.26$, $p < .05$, but the main effect of week, $F(8, 112) = 1.02$, or the Drug $\times$ Week interaction, $F(8, 112) = 1.76$, were not significant. The pharmacologist concluded that because a significant drug effect on body weight was found mythicalamine was an effective chronic diet aid at least in the male rat.

Critique

The research hypothesis was whether mythicalamine given daily would significantly reduce the body weights of rats. The general ANOVA table for this experiment is presented in Table 6.4. The specific ANOVA table for the 2 $\times$ (9 $\times$ 8) mixed factorial used in this experiment is

Source	df	Error term
Group	1	S/Group
Week	8	Week × S/Group
S/Group	14	
Group × Week	8	Week × S/Group
Week × S/Group	112	
Total	143	

The statistical test selected was appropriate. However, the direction of weight change is not presented, that is, the drug may have actually increased body weights. Hence, the author's conclusion should be rejected. Also, given the wide range of body weights for the rats at the beginning of the experiment, group body weights probably were not the same before treatment conditions were introduced. Random assignment of animals to groups (1.4) does not, particularly with small samples, ensure that the groups will be the same. A significant drug (group) effect reported in this experiment may only reflect an initial body weight difference. Also, the fact that the Drug × Week interaction was not significant suggests that mythicalamine was not an effective weight suppressant. Weight differences between the two groups should have increased as time on the drug increased (normal rats continue to gain weight as they mature). In this experiment the rats could have been matched in blocks of two for initial body weight and then one member of each block randomly assigned to either the experimental or control condition (4.8). With this procedure, the groups would not have had significant differences in initial body weight. Also, by the introduction of another factor, from an A × (B × S) design to an A × B × (C × S) design a comparison of the effects of this drug on rats with low and high body weight could have been done. But the sample size of the groups would have to be increased to make these latter comparisons meaningful (5.15).

Considering the research question, the use of daily IP injections would not be the best method for drug delivery. Although both groups of rats received injections, the trauma associated with daily IP injections would likely affect food intake in both groups. Oral administration or the chronic implantation of minipumps would appear to be more reasonable procedures to determine whether mythicalamine might be an effective chronic diet aid.

RESEARCH DESIGN PROBLEM 46

Cribbing, a reflexive biting response of stabled horses, forces air into the stomach and may result in colic. Because cribbing might be caused by boredom and mediated by endogenous opiates, an experiment was performed to determine whether different opioid antagonists (naloxone, nathrexone, nalmefene, and diprenorphine) would eliminate cribbing behavior. Fifteen horses (known cribbers) were divided randomly into 5 groups (3 each). All the horses were put in stalls and monitored for cribbing behavior. The data were recorded as responses per 5 min. After 1 h, the groups were injected with one of five treatments: saline (10 mL), naloxone, naltrexone, nalmefene, or diprenorphine (all 1 mg/kg) and monitored for an additional 2 h. All four groups receiving a narcotic antagonist showed a decrease in cribbing behavior initially, but by 2-h postdose had returned to baseline. No change in the saline group was observed. A mixed factorial ANOVA was performed with the following results: treatment effect, $F(4, 70) = 2.58, p <$ .05; time effect, $F(3, 210) = 2.60, p < .05$; Treatment × Time interaction, $F(12, 210) = 1.20$, NS. The researchers concluded that narcotic antagonists are a viable treatment for cribbing in stabled horses.

Critique

The research hypothesis is whether opioid antagonists would eliminate cribbing in stabled horses. The general ANOVA table for the A × (B × S) mixed factorial design is presented in Table 6.4. The specific ANOVA table for the data analysis reported is

Source	df	Error term
Group	4	S/Group
Time	3	Time × S/Group
S/Group	10	
Group × Time	12	Time × S/Group
Time × S/Group	30	
Total	59	

The wrong number of degrees of freedom (df) was used in the statistical analysis (5.17, 6.5). In calculation of sample size (s), the researchers used 15 rather than the correct individual group sample size of 3. Even if the correct df's had been used, the design of this experiment was not very efficient given the small number of animals in each group and the fact that the repeated-measures factor (time) was probably confounded with pretreatment, treatment, and perhaps recovery effects (4.19). From the df given for time, measurements during four time periods were used in the ANOVA; however, these particular time periods cannot be identified. The conclusion of the researchers was that narcotic antagonists are a viable treatment that could be used effectively for a chronic condition. Repeated doses of the drugs would be necessary to eliminate cribbing and repeated doses of narcotic antagonists were not used in the reported study. Constant medication with these antagonists would probably not be a viable treatment for cribbing given the length of effective suppression of cribbing (2-h postdose), the number of daily doses that would have to be given to be effective, and the changes induced in receptors and behaviors from chronic administration.

RESEARCH DESIGN PROBLEM 47

A significant research problem is to determine the developmental mechanisms that produce synaptic connections within the vertebrate central nervous system.

Because of the difficulty of using embryonic nervous systems (small size, delicate nature of the material, and so forth), vertebrate studies have focused on the regeneration of adult neurons (after lesions) to understand some processes that might be involved in formation of functional synaptic connections during development. A major problem with this latter approach, however, is that most central neurons in adult vertebrates will not regenerate following CNS lesions. Consequently, invertebrates whose central neurons do regenerate functional connections following lesions are being used as research preparations. In addition to its regenerative properties, the CNS of most invertebrates is a collection of distinct ganglia with discrete paths of connection, or commissures, between them. Hence, a lesion to the commissures of a ganglion will completely isolate it from the rest of the CNS and eliminate any interganglionic connections.

To determine the regeneration of central cholinergic neurons within the CNS of the snail, *Helisoma trivolvis*, lesions were made in the cerebro-pedal commissure (a connection between the cerebral and pedal ganglia which when lesioned completely isolates the cerebral ganglion). In this study the regeneration of synaptic connections between two groups of cholinergic neurons, one within the cerebral ganglion and one within the pedal ganglion, was determined. Because these two groups of neurons made connections only via the cerebro-pedal commissure, a study of their connectivity following complete lesion of this commissure should identify the regeneration of their axons through this commissural pathway.

Twenty snails were randomly assigned equally to two groups, a sham lesion control group and an experimental group. The 10 experimental animals were cold anesthetized and the cerebro-pedal commissure was lesioned. The sham animals were also cold anesthetized and the cerebro-pedal commissure exposed but not lesioned. Twenty days after surgery, half of the animals in each group were dissected, the CNS was removed, and the neural tissue placed in a electrophysiological recording chamber. Simultaneous recordings were made from neurons in the pedal ganglion and neurons in the cerebral ganglion to test for synaptic connections. Forty days after surgery the other half of the animals in each group was tested electrophysiologically using the same procedures. Of the 60 neurons (30 cerebro-pedal pairs) tested from the control animals at 20 days, 59 showed connection defined as reciprocal neural activity whereas only 2 of the 50 neurons tested from the lesioned animals at 20 days showed a connection. In contrast, 48 of the 52 neurons from the lesioned group at 40 days showed a connection, and 38 of the 40 neurons from the control animals at 40 days showed connections.

An arcsin transform of the proportional data was done so that it would more nearly approximate a normal distribution, and a 2×2 factorial ANOVA was performed with the following results: a significant treatment effect, $F(1, 198) = 5.21$, $p < .05$; a significant time effect, $F(1, 198) = 4.52$, $p < .05$; and a significant Treatment $\times$ Time interaction, $F(1, 198) = 6.87$, $p < .02$. Post hoc Newman-Keuls tests revealed that the experimental 20-day value was significantly lower than all other values and no significant differences existed among the values of the other three groups. Therefore, the author concluded that central cholinergic neurons in *Helisoma* can regenerate and that this process takes between 20 and 40 days.

Critique

Although not stated explicitly the research hypothesis is whether central cholinergic neurons within the CNS of the snail regenerate functional synaptic connections after commissural severance of their axons. Apparently, the neurobiologist used more than one neuronal pair from some snails and treated each pair of neurons as an independent observation (4.9). Although independent and dependent measurements may have been confounded in this experiment, the conclusion of the researcher is correct based upon the individual numbers presented. Hence, even though the statistical treatment of the data may have been inappropriate (probably a nesting of neurons within animals per group because of the unequal number of neurons sampled from some snails), the conclusion can be judged to be correct by the numerical counts of connected cells in the two groups at the two different times. In each of the groups, only one animal could have supplied all the group data but this outcome does not appear likely. The dependent variable used in the ANOVA performed was not identified but a parametric statistical test would not be appropriate as the number of neurons is the only unit of measurement presented (5.3). Comparisons using Fisher's Exact Probability test (11.2) would have been a more appropriate statistical test. The neurobiologist, therefore, was sloppy in data presentation, was wrong in analysis of the data, but was probably correct in the interpretation of the experimental data.

RESEARCH DESIGN PROBLEM 48

Acute psychological stress is believed to cause disturbances of metabolic control in patients with Type I diabetes. To examine the validity of this assumption, nine healthy persons (mean $\pm$ SEM, blood glucose level, 74 $\pm$ 2 mg/dL), nine patients with Type I diabetes who had normoglycemia (130 $\pm$ 10 mg/dL), and nine diabetic patients with hyperglycemia (444 $\pm$ 17 mg/dL) were exposed to two acute psychological stresses: mental arithmetic and public speaking. Subjects in the three groups were matched for age, weight, sex, and socioeconomic status. All subjects were studied, without stress, on the first day (control), arithmetic stress on day 2, and public speaking on day 3. On each day the duration of each session was 140 min and was divided (for the two stress test days) into a baseline period of 10 min, a stress period of either 15 or 45 min (public speaking or arithmetic), and a recovery period of 105 or 75 min, respectively. Measurements of heart rate (12 for each subject), blood pressure (12), epinephrine and norepinephrine (10), and glucose (10) were made on each subject during each daily session. For statistical analysis a three-factor analysis of variance with repeated measures was used. Post hoc analyses of significant main effects and interactions were done using Tukey's test.

The analysis of variance did not reveal differences among the three groups in either heart rate or blood pressure. For all groups during the stress periods there were marked increments in blood pressure [$F(2, 48) = 65.5, p < .001$] and increases in heart rate [$F(2, 48) = 40.5, p < .001$]. A significant increase over time also occurred with heart rate [$F(11, 264) = 70.2, p < .001$] and blood pressure [$F(11, 264) = 116.7, p < .001$]. Differences in epinephrine (Epi) and norepinephrine (NE) were not significant among groups, but the two stress situations had significant effects on both variables in all three groups: Epi [$F(2, 48) = 11.8, p < .001$] and NE [$F(2, 48) = 3.3, p < .05$]. A significant time effect for Epi and NE was also found, p's $< .001$. As expected, blood glucose levels differed markedly among groups [$F(2, 24) = 142.2, p < .001$]. Glucose levels remained unaffected by both stress situations [$F(2, 48) = 1.8$, NS]. A time-dependent change in the glucose levels was found [$F(10, 240) = 38.3$, p $< .001$]. This effect differed among groups as indicated by the Group $\times$ Time interaction [$F(20, 240) = 12.6, p < .001$].

The authors concluded that short-lived psychological stimuli which cause marked cardiovascular responses and moderate elevations in catecholamines did not disturb metabolic control in patients with Type I diabetes.

Critique

The description of the experimental design and the presentation of the statistical analysis makes it impossible to evaluate adequately the authors' conclusion. The experimental design, as described, is not a balanced design. Consequently, a three-factor ANOVA would not be appropriate to analyze the data.

The design appears to be an A $\times$ (B $\times$ C $\times$ S) mixed factorial design (4.21) and the general ANOVA table for this design is presented in Table 6.9. The design in this specific experiment would be a 3 (groups: healthy, Type I diabetic-normoglycemia, and Type I diabetic-hyperglycemia) $\times$ 3 (days: control, arithmetic stress, and public speaking) $\times$ 3 (measurement: baseline, stress, recovery). Unfortunately, for the different dependent variables (heart rate, blood pressure, Epi, and so forth) 10 or 12 measurements per day were taken but from the experimental protocol it is impossible to determine under which of the three conditions (baseline, stress, recovery) these measurements were obtained. Furthermore, the authors' choice of labels for the various factors does not provide sufficient information to reconstruct an ANOVA table. The factor labeled time is difficult to evaluate because both a significant time-dependent change in glucose levels and a significant Group $\times$ Time interaction for this dependent variable are reported. In short, the result section of this report is incomprehensible. For these reasons, the authors' conclusions should be rejected.

Another problem may exist in this experiment. The hyperglycemic group had significantly higher blood glucose levels compared with the other two groups before treatment conditions were introduced. This initial blood glucose difference was used to classify the Type I diabetics into two groups (classification groups, 4.2). If these initial differences affected baseline measurements of some of the other dependent variables (blood pressure, Epi, and so forth), an interpretation problem regarding treatment effects on these variables may exist.

RESEARCH DESIGN PROBLEM 49

A neurobiologist wanted to determine the effects of food aversion learning on synaptic efficiency (ease with which current may be passed) of an identified synapse between two neurons known to be involved in the generation of feeding movements within the brain of the mollusc *Pleurobranchia californica*. The neurobiologist predicted that a significant increase in synaptic efficiency at this synapse would occur as a result of food aversion learning.

Animals of about the same weight were matched for feeding responsiveness to a highly palatable squid homogenate and then randomly assigned to one of two groups. In the experimental group, animals were presented the squid homogenate and if the animals did not withdraw from the food source within 60 sec, a very aversive shock was delivered for 90 sec. Control animals were presented with the squid homogenate for 60 sec but were given the same shock .5 h after food presentation. This daily training procedure was repeated until all animals in the experimental group showed a withdrawal from the food source within 60 sec on four consecutive trials. When an experimental animal reached criterion, its matched control animal was used for simultaneous neurophysiological testing.

Each animal's brain was dissected, the two specified neurons were impaled with microelectrodes, and the frequency of stimulation needed to just pass current from one neuron to another was determined. An animal from the experimental group was used for further testing if a criterion of less than 20-Hz stimulation (20 current pulses per sec) was required to just pass current, and a control animal was used for further testing if a criterion below 30-Hz stimulation was met (these were the normal ranges for learning versus control stimulation frequencies and were used to ensure that the impalement had not damaged the synapse). The experiment continued until 10 animals from each group completed neurophysiological testing. If the neurons of either animal in the matched pair were damaged, *both* animals were eliminated from the study.

The frequency needed to not only pass current across the synapse but also to elicit an action potential (AP) in the second neuron was determined. The synapse from each brain was tested four times and the averaged value of these measures was used in a between-subject ANOVA. The frequency of stimulation necessary to elicit an AP was significantly different between the two groups with the experimental animals having lower frequencies compared with their controls, $F(1, 18) = 8.90, p < .01$. The neurobiologist concluded that food aversion learning resulted in an increase in efficiency of a specific synapse in the mollusc, and proposed that this model system would be useful for understanding synaptic mechanisms underlying aversion learning.

Critique

The research hypothesis is whether food aversion learning of the mollusc *Pleurobranchia californica* will increase the efficiency of a central synapse involved in feeding movements. The general ANOVA table for this experiment is presented in Table 6.1. The specific ANOVA table for this experiment is

Source	df	Error term
Group	1	S/Group
S/Group	18	
Total	19	

The statistical test selected was appropriate because the more commonly used t-test is a special case of the F-test (5.18). But, the selection of animals on the basis of their synaptic efficiency produces an initial self-selection confound between the groups. The two groups differed in the frequency needed to just pass current across the synapse (the experimental animals having a lower frequency) which *must be* correlated with the amount of current needed to elicit a postsynaptic action potential. Consequently, the experimental animals would be expected to have lower stimulation frequencies for APs compared with their controls.

A reexamination of the data could provide an answer to the proposed research question. If relatively few animals were eliminated from the study then the initial criterion difference between the two groups could be caused by the treatment conditions. If only one or two animals were eliminated from each of the two groups then the neurobiologist's conclusion would be correct, that is, food aversion learning results in an attenuation at a given synapse. However, this conclusion would only be appropriate if the experimental and control animals received the same number of aversive shocks. In the experimental protocol the experimental animals could avoid the aversive shock and to reach criterion they had to avoid the shock on four consecutive trials. If the control animals continued to receive shock on these trials, the number of shocks would have been different in the two groups. If the neurobiologist had used "yoked" controls (controls receiving shock only if their matched experimental animal did) then there would be no treatment confound related to general stress effects.

RESEARCH DESIGN PROBLEM 50

Leucine aminonaphthylamidase (LAN) is a lysosomal enzyme that appears in the blood after cell death. Elevated levels of plasma LAN (PLAN) in mammals have been used to diagnose liver damage and wasting disorders. For these reasons, PLAN activity has been proposed to be a nonspecific indicator of toxicant stress in vertebrates. To test this hypothesis 180 laboratory-raised rainbow trout (80–100 g) were anesthetized and then injected (30 fish per dose × 6 doses) intraperitoneally (IP) with the toxin p-methylphenol (PMP) at doses of 0 (vehicle only) to .75 of the 96-hour (h) IP LD50 (lethal dose to kill 50% of the fish). The fish were held for 96 h in control tanks and blood samples were then collected, stored on ice, and assayed within 1 h. Another 60 fish were exposed to a water-borne exposure of either 0 or .028 mM PMP (.41 of the 96-h LD50 of .069 mM). Ten fish from each treatment ($n = 30$) were randomly sampled after 48, 96, and 192 h and their plasma assayed under identical procedures.

There was a significant correlation, $r = .76$, $p < .05$, between dose and PLAN activity after PMP injection. The PLAN levels of fish injected with PMP at doses of .075–.75 of the 96-h IP LD50 were elevated by 27 to 63 percent relative to controls. A complete factorial ANOVA of the PLAN data of the water-borne exposure experiment indicated a significant group effect, $F(1, 54) = 7.31$, $p < .01$; a significant time effect, $F(2, 54) = 3.23$, $p < .05$; and a significant Group $\times$ Time Interaction, $F(2, 54) = 5.16$, $p < .01$. Newman-Keuls tests of the significant interaction indicated that exposure of fish to water-borne PMP significantly increased PLAN activity ($p < .05$) after 48, 96, and 192 h; activities increased by 38 to 87 percent relative to controls. In addition, the 96-h and 192-h experimental groups differed significantly from each other ($p < .05$) and both of these groups had significantly higher activity than the control groups ($p < .05$). None of the control groups differed significantly from each other. The toxicologist concluded that increased PLAN activity would be useful for estimating toxicant stress in laboratory trout populations if the response to PMP was indicative of the response for other toxicants.

Critique

The research hypothesis is whether PLAN activity is a reliable nonspecific indicator for estimating toxicant stress in laboratory trout populations. Two completely separate experiments were run. In the first experiment, it is not clear why a correlation, rather than a linear regression, analysis was reported (5.26, 5.27). Correlation analysis indicates that an association exists between two random variables; whereas, a regression analysis permits cause-and-effect conclusions to be made. The amount of toxin injected was the independent variable and was under the control (manipulated) by the researcher (5.26, 5.27). But, the conclusion from this first study was only that a significant correlation, $r = .76$, $p < .05$, existed between the dose of toxin and PLAN activity and this weak conclusion is correct.

The second experiment was a 2 (group) $\times$ 3 (time) factorial design. The general ANOVA table for this experiment is presented in Table 6.2. The specific ANOVA table for this experiment is

Source	df	Error term
Group	1	S/Group $\times$ Time
Time	2	S/Group $\times$ Time
Group $\times$ Time	2	S/Group $\times$ Time
S/Group $\times$ Time	54	
Total	59	

The ANOVA selected was appropriate and the post hoc multiple test evaluation of the significant Group $\times$ Time interaction supported the toxicologist's

Table 14.4   Mean Bile Flow ($\mu l \cdot$ BS per min) and Standard Deviations (SD) for Female and Male Rats

Time (min)	Female ($\pm$ SD)	Male ($\pm$ SD)
0	5.0 (.8)	5.5 (.9)
15	2.6 (.5)	4.2 (.4)
30	1.3 (.2)	3.7 (.5)
45	2.1 (.4)	4.4 (.5)
60	2.8 (.4)	5.1 (.6)
75	4.2 (.6)	5.0 (.7)
90	4.8 (.7)	5.2 (.8)
105	5.2 (.8)	5.4 (.7)
120	5.1 (.7)	5.6 (.8)

conclusion that increased PLAN activity is useful for estimating toxicant stress in laboratory trout populations.

RESEARCH DESIGN PROBLEM 51

The effect of a natural estrogen metabolite, estradiol-17-glucuronide (E2-17G), on the capability of the liver to produce bile was studied in both male and female rats. E2-17G is cholestatic in amounts less than tenfold normal and E2-17G was expected to have a greater effect in females than males because females normally have greater amounts of E2-17G in their blood than do males. To determine if a gender-dependent effect existed, 16 Sprague-Dawley 90-day-old rats, eight male (350-400 g) and eight female (310-345 g) had separate cannula placed in the bile duct and portal vein. Postoperative bile flows were measured and were used for control bile flow (time 0). Following these control measurements, E2-17G (1 mg in 1 mL vehicle) was injected into the portal vein of each rat. Quarter hourly bile flow measurements were then taken for 2 h (see Table 14.4).

A mixed 2×9 factorial ANOVA with repeated measures on the last factor was used to determine significance levels with the following outcomes: sex, $F(1, 14) = 4.93, p < .05$; time, $F(8, 112) = 2.25, p < .05$; Sex $\times$ Time interaction, $F(8, 112) = 1.08$, NS. Because the Sex $\times$ Time interaction was not significant, the authors concluded that the time course of cholestasis was similar for both male and female rats. More important, the authors concluded that the significant difference in the response of female rats to E2-17G compared with male rats indicated that this differential gender response was probably related to the increased normal levels of estrogen in the female rat.

Critique

The research hypothesis is whether a natural estrogen metabolite, E2-17G, would produce a greater effect on bile flow in female than in male rats. The general ANOVA for this experiment is presented in Table 6.4. The specific ANOVA for this $2 \times (9 \times 8)$ mixed factorial design is

Source	df	Error term
Sex	1	S/Sex
Time	8	Time × S/Sex
S/Sex	14	
Sex × Time	8	Time × S/Sex
Time × S/Sex	112	
Total	143	

The statistical test selected was appropriate. However, the experimental design did not control for the normal body weight differences between male and female rats. As may be seen, the male rats had heavier body weights and showed less of an effect on bile flow when injected with 1 mg of E2-17G compared with the same dose given to the smaller female rats. The dose of E2-17G should have been adjusted for body weight which would have exposed all rats to the same effective dose independent of body weight (X mg/kg). Exposing all female and all male rats to the same effective dose should also reduce within-subject experimental error (5.16). Because of the range of body weights *within* each group, the animals in each group were also receiving different physiological doses which would produce greater variability within each group (i.e., increasing experimental error).

RESEARCH DESIGN PROBLEM 52

Cadmium contamination of many aquatic environments has already occurred and significant concentrations of cadmium (> 32 ppm) are being detected in many plants and animals. Because of its widespread contamination, cadmium may affect the survival behavior of many species. To determine if cadmium affected the avoidance behavior of young black ducks, 48 breeding pairs of adult black ducks were placed in individual outdoor pens. These breeding pairs were randomly assigned to three treatment groups ($s = 16$) which were fed diets containing either 0, 4, or 40 ppm cadmium (as cadmium chloride). The cadmium chloride was dissolved in distilled, deionized water and added to duck breeder mash in a ratio of 1 part water to 99 parts mash. Hens began to lay eggs about 4 months after dietary treatments began. For 1 week after hatching, the ducklings were housed with their parents and were also fed a diet of duck starter mash containing the same cadmium concentration that their parents were fed. At the end of the first posthatch week, 144 ducklings from 27 hens were tested for their response to a fright stimulus (spinning black and white pattern with accompanying noise). To eliminate isolation distress all ducklings from a given hen (a brood) were tested together. The distance each duckling ran from the stimulus during a 20-sec exposure was recorded (see Table 14.5).

A single-factor between-subject ANOVA indicated a significant group effect, $F(2, 24) = 9.34, p < .001$, and a Tukey multiple comparison test revealed that ducklings given 4 ppm cadmium were significantly different from the other two groups which did not differ between themselves. The toxicologist's concluded

Table 14.5   Distance Traveled By the Broods of the Three
Diet Groups

Cadmium added to diet (ppm)	Number of broods[a]	Distance traveled (cm) Mean ± SE
0	9	31 ± 8.3
4	9	69 ± 8.9[b]
40	9	23 ± 8.7

[a]A mean distance was calculated for each brood using all the ducklings from that brood, this mean value/brood was then averaged across the nine different broods to obtain the mean value for the particular treatment group.
[b]Significantly different from the other two groups at $\alpha = 0.05$ using Tukey's test.

that cadmium has a critical dose effect on avoidance responding in young ducks in that a low dose (4 ppm cadmium) results in hyperresponsiveness and a high dose (40 ppm) does not significantly affect the duckling's behavior. Because hyperresponsiveness could be harmful to a wild bird the biologist also suggested that increasing cadmium exposure from 4 to 40 ppm may actually be beneficial to some species like the black duck.

Critique

The research hypothesis is whether cadmium affects the avoidance behavior of young black ducks. The general ANOVA table for this experiment is presented in Table 6.1. The specific ANOVA table for this experiment is

Source	df	Error term
Group	2	S/Group
S/Group	<u>24</u>	
Total	26	

The statistical test selected was appropriate. However, potential treatment and animal confoundings (4.12) exist in this experiment. Although 48 pairs of ducks were randomly assigned to the three groups, only 27 broods were used in the avoidance testing phase. Consequently, a selection bias (4.12) probably occurred as cadmium affected either the ability of the hens to lay eggs or the hatchability of eggs. If, by chance, seven breeding pairs in each treatment condition did not reproduce, the general experimental conditions for successful reproduction were not adequate and the generalization of any conclusion from this study would be restricted. Most likely, the highest-dose group had only nine available broods and for comparison only nine broods were selected from the other two groups.

A more subtle selection bias is also involved in the use of averaged responses from broods. No evidence is given that the average number of chicks in each brood is about the same in the three groups and fewer chicks may be in the broods of the highest cadmium group. The decrease in avoidance scores for the

40 ppm cadmium chicks may only reflect the weakened condition of the surviving chicks in this group, that is, some of these chicks may not have been capable of running away from the stimulus. In summary, the number of successful breeders in each treatment condition, the number of chicks per brood, and average body weight of the broods in each treatment condition should have been reported. Without these data, the toxicologist's conclusion that "increasing cadmium exposure from 4 to 40 ppm may actually be beneficial" should be rejected.

RESEARCH DESIGN PROBLEM 53

The drug furosemide is used to control pulmonary bleeding in racing horses. Furosemide is a controversial drug because it also appears to act as a stimulant in healthy horses. Therefore, a study was done at a major training track just outside of Lexington, Ky., to determine if furosemide decreases thoroughbred running times. Thirty thoroughbred horses, on normal training schedules, were shipped to and housed in stalls at the track. All 30 horses were exercised at the track at their normal morning times by professional jockeys. Each horse was allowed to gallop ½ mile, then was urged to sprint 3 furlongs (⅜ of a mile). The 3-furlong sprint times were clocked and recorded by professional clockers. After a week of only galloping 2 miles per day (rest period), the sprint schedule was repeated with all horses receiving a therapeutic dose of furosemide 4 h prior to their workout on the track (furosemide is normally given 4 h before posttime to control pulmonary bleeding during a race). The 3-furlong times were again recorded and compared with the previous times using a complete within-subject ANOVA. Sprint times were significantly lower when furosemide was used, $F(1, 29) = 13.61, p < .001$, and because the 3-furlong times were significantly lower following furosemide pretreatment, the researchers concluded that this drug acts as a stimulant and should be banned as a medication for racing horses.

Critique

The research hypothesis is whether furosemide decreases thoroughbred running times. The general ANOVA table for this study is presented in Table 4.5. The specific ANOVA table for this study is

Source	df	Error term
Treatment	1	Treatment × Subject
Subject	29	
Treatment × Subject	29	
Total	59	

The statistical test selected was appropriate. In this study, a one-tailed test (5.20) could have been used because the researchers would not have been interested in whether furosemide increased thoroughbred running times. However, treatment (furosemide) and time were confounded (4.19) in this complete within-subject design (4.16). The decrease in 3-furlong times may be because of the horses adapting to the local track conditions during their 2-week rest period. A control group of horses should have been used in this study. If one-half of the horses ($s = 15$) had been given a vehicle injection during the second training phase, a $2 \times (2 \times 15)$ mixed factorial design (4.21) would have been used and a significant Group $\times$ Training interaction would have been predicted (see Table 6.4).

RESEARCH DESIGN PROBLEM 54

During amphibian development most organ systems progressively increase in complexity until metamorphosis into the adult form occurs. The cardiovascular system may be an exception to this general developmental-complexity rule. In the bullfrog, chronic cardiac vagal inhibition produces a low resting heart rate early in larval development which persists through the older larval stages. However, this vagal tone at rest disappears during metamorphosis. Because the vagal tone in bullfrogs is mediated by acetylcholine (ACh), the purpose of this study was to determine whether changes in cardiac response to ACh causes the normal heart rate changes which occur during amphibian development.

Three larval stages (VII-IX, X-XIV, XVI-XIX) and one adult bullfrog group each consisting of 10 animals were used. The pericardial chamber was opened and heart rate was continuously recorded during the experiment. ACh was directly applied to the ventral surface of the heart and changes in heart rate were measured with the following dosages: 10^{-8}, 10^{-7}, 10^{-6}, 10^{-5}, 10^{-4}, and 10^{-3} M. As a control measure the heart was flushed with bullfrog Ringer's solution between these ACh doses. Another application of ACh did not occur until the resting heart rate returned to control levels.

A mixed factorial ANOVA revealed a significant stage effect, $F(3, 36) = 2.92$, $p < .05$; a significant dose effect, $F(5, 180) = 2.29$; and a significant Stage $\times$ Dose interaction, $F(15, 180) = 2.30, p < .01$. Subsequent post hoc comparisons (Tukey's test) revealed that the magnitude of heart rate reduction mediated by ACh increased with larval development. The heart rate responses at 10^{-5}–10^{-3} M ACh were significantly larger ($p < .05$) at stages XVI-XIX than at stages VII-IX. When the effect of ACh on heart rate in adults was compared with the intermediate and late larval stages the adults had a significantly smaller response than either of the larval stages ($p < .01$). The response of the adults was not significantly different from that of the earlier larval stage ($p > .05$).

The zoologists concluded that during larval development up to metamorphosis the sensitivity of the heart to ACh increases. They speculated that this increase may reflect changes either in ACh receptor number or affinity or increased sensitivity of the pacemakers cells to ACh. Furthermore, they concluded that the large decrease in sensitivity of the heart to ACh following metamorphosis supports the view that the development of the cardiovascular system in amphibians is neither linear nor progressive.

Critique

The research hypothesis is whether changes in cardiac response to ACh produce the normal heart rate changes which occur during amphibian development. The general ANOVA table for the mixed factorial design used in this experiment is presented in Table 6.4. The specific ANOVA table for the 4 (group) × 6 (dose × 10) mixed factorial design used in this study is

Source	df	Error term
Stage	3	S/Stage
Dose	5	Dose × S/Stage
S/Stage	36	
Stage × Dose	15	Dose × S/Stage
Dose × S/Stage	180	
Total	239	

The statistical test selected was appropriate, but the statistical analysis of the data and its presentation are confusing. The zoologists begin by interpreting the significant Dose × Stage interaction with post hoc tests but then switch and interpret the significant stage effect. Their conclusions, which are relatively weak, appear to be correct given the minimal information presented. A more informative statistical approach would have been to do a trend analysis of the significant Dose × Stage interaction (6.16). Although the dose of ACh was increased (10^{-8}, 10^{-7}, to 10^{-3} M), the authors indicated that resting heart rate returned to control levels between ACh applications; hence, there was apparently no significant carry-over effect (4.19). Also, there was apparently no time-related effect as control heart rates did not apparently increase or decrease during the course of the experiment (4.19).

RESEARCH DESIGN PROBLEM 55

A sodium-restricted diet may increase the risk of heat illness; therefore, the aim of this study was to specify the effects of moderate and severe sodium depletion on heat tolerance. Fifty male Sprague-Dawley rats, 475–525 g, were randomly and equally assigned to two heat stress groups: a moderate and a severe group. Both groups were placed on a 4-day sodium depletion regimen which consisted of a sodium-free diet and deionized water. Rats in the severe group also received the diuretic furosemide (10 mg·kg^{-1}·day^{-1}) which induced further sodium depletion. Sodium balance after 4 days was $-1.6 \pm .1$ mEq for the moderate group and $-5.0 \pm .2$ mEq for the severe group, resulting in plasma sodium levels of 129 and 125 mEq/L, respectively. On the fifth day all rats were exposed to a 42°C environment. Rectal temperature of each rat was monitored continuously until 42.0°C was reached and then the rat was removed from the heat, placed in a 26°C environment, and rectal temperature monitored until a return

Table 14.6   Mean (M) Temperature Rate Changes for the
Two Groups

Groups	Heating (M ± SD)	Cooling (M ± SD)
Moderate	.048 ± .003	.088 ± .015
Severe	.095 ± .010	.055 ± .013

to normal level occurred. Time in the heat, a measure of thermoregulatory performance, was 113 ± 10 and 181 ± 8 min for the severe and moderate groups, respectively, a difference significant at $p < .001$. Heating and cooling rates (°C/min · kg body weight) for the two groups are presented in Table 14.6.

An analysis of variance indicated that the heating rate of the severe group was significantly greater than that of the moderate group, $F(1, 48) = 7.31, p < .01$. Conversely, the cooling rate of the moderate group was significantly greater than that of the severe group, $F(1, 48) = 7.62, p < .01$.

The authors concluded that severe sodium depletion results in a physiologically important decrement in thermoregulatory performance in the heat. Therefore, individuals on a sodium-restricted diet should be advised of the increased risk of heat illness when exposed to a hot environment.

Critique

The proposed aim of the study is to specify the effects of moderate and severe sodium depletion on heat tolerance. A more explicit research hypothesis is whether diuretic-induced sodium depletion affects the thermoregulatory ability of the rat. The general ANOVA table for this study is presented in Table 6.4. The specific ANOVA table for this experiment is

Source	df	Error term
Group	1	S/Group
Rate	1	Rate × S/Group
S/Group	48	
Group × Rate	1	Rate × S/Group
Rate × S/Group	48	
Total	99	

In this study the authors decided to use two separate ANOVAs to analyze the data—an ANOVA for heating rate and another ANOVA for cooling rate. For this analysis the general ANOVA table is presented in Table 6.1. The specific ANOVA for these two ANOVA cases would be

Source	df	Error term
Group	1	S/Group
S/Group	48	
Total	49	

Using a mixed factorial ANOVA would permit conclusions regarding any significant differences between heating and cooling rates (rate as a factor) and any significant group differences in these two rates (Group × Rate interaction). With separate ANOVAs these types of questions cannot be answered (4.13). In this situation, using the mixed factorial ANOVA would not have changed significantly the authors' conclusions.

Proper control groups were not used in this experiment. No control group exists to evaluate the effects of sodium depletion by diet on thermoregulatory ability. Also, no control group to evaluate the effects of furosemide per se was included in the design. Being a diuretic, furosemide would have altered blood volume and a decrease in blood volume would have an effect on thermoregulation. Also, the severe group probably differed from the moderate group in body weight. Diuretics are commonly used in fast weight loss diets and a 4-day treatment with a diuretic would affect body weight. Body weight differences between the two groups would affect passive heat and cooling mechanisms. The severe group would also be approaching the cutoff temperature of 42°C at a faster rate (113 ± 10 min) than the moderate group (181 ± 8 min) which means the severe group would be at a slightly higher body temperature when removed from the heat stress. The cooling rate data, therefore, would be contaminated by this initial difference in body temperature between the two groups. A control group of rats maintained on a normal diet would have allowed the effects of the sodium diet per se on thermoregulatory ability to be evaluated. A control group of rats maintained on a normal diet and given furosemide would have allowed the effects of only furosemide on the thermoregulatory ability to be evaluated. A mixed factorial design (4.21, 4.22) in which two drug groups (saline, furosemide) were exposed to the same temperature conditions under normal and sodium-restricted diets may have provided a more efficient and sensitive design.

RESEARCH DESIGN PROBLEM 56

A pharmacologist wanted to determine the effects of perfusion duration of a calcium channel blocker on an isolated heart preparation. Eight rats were randomly obtained from a university rat colony, killed, and their hearts rapidly removed and placed in perfusion apparatuses in which beats per minute (bpm) could be measured (calcium channel blockers decrease bpm). Heart rate was measured for each heart and a calcium channel blocker or vehicle was then added to the perfusate and bpm measured again. Following this treatment each heart was perfused with fresh buffer until heart rate returned to predrug or vehicle levels (bpm for the vehicle did not change but the heart preparation was also washed with fresh buffer). The drug or vehicle was then given depending on what was the prior treatment condition (if drug was given first then vehicle was given second and vice versa). Four hearts were selected randomly to receive the calcium channel blocker first (hearts 1–4) and the other four hearts (5–8) were given the vehicle. Four time measurements (0, 5, 10, and 15) were taken during each treatment condition.

The data collected were analyzed using a complete within-subject ANOVA for a $(2 \times 12 \times 8)$ design. The main effect of drug was significant, $F(1, 7) = 5.89$, $p < .05$, but neither the main effect of time, $F(11, 70) = 1.88$, or the Drug $\times$ Time interaction, $F(11, 70) = 1.79$, were significant. No other effect was found to be significant. The pharmacologist concluded that the time of perfusion of a calcium channel blocker has no significant effect on the beats per minute of an isolated rat heart.

Critique

The research hypothesis is whether the duration of perfusion of a calcium channel blocker affects the spontaneous firing rate (beats per minute) of an isolated heart preparation. The general ANOVA table for the described study design is presented in Table 6.11. Essentially, in the experiment three within-subject (4.16) factors are presented: drug-vehicle (2) $\times$ predrug-postdrug (2) $\times$ time of measurement (4) $\times$ subjects (8). Usually with three factors the design would be an $(A \times B \times C \times S)$ or a $(2 \times 2 \times 4 \times 8)$ complete within-subject design. But a $(2 \times 12 \times 8)$ complete within-subject design was used to analyze the data. An $(A \times B \times S)$ ANOVA with the A factor being drug (2) and the B factor being time (12) was used (the reported degrees of freedom for the time factor, 11, indicates that 12 time values per animal were used). However, it is not possible to have 12 measurements for each heart and have two treatment conditions.

The design, as reported, was not balanced (no pretreatment measurements taken before the vehicle for hearts 1–4 and before the drug for hearts 5–8). The pharmacologist indicated that heart rate returned to predrug and vehicle levels after perfusion with fresh buffer. If so, then a complete within-subject ANOVA could be used to analyze the data, a $(3 \times 4 \times S)$. The isolated hearts 1–4 received the schedule: pre-, drug, wash, vehicle; whereas, hearts 5–8 received the schedule: pre-, vehicle, wash, drug. Four measurements were taken during the pre-, drug, and vehicle periods. Hence, three treatment conditions (control, drug, and vehicle) and four measurements under each treatment condition (0, 5, 10, and 15) across the eight hearts would be the $(A \times B \times S)$ ANOVA used in analyzing the data (see Table 6.3). This within-subject design (4.16, 4.17) would only be appropriate if there were no differential carry-over effects caused by the drug condition (4.19). From the analysis presented, the time measurements are nested within the drug condition (6.2) and the statistical analysis used is not appropriate; consequently, the pharmacologist's conclusions should be rejected. To answer the research question a significant Treatment $\times$ Time interaction is required if the suggested $(A \times B \times S)$ design and analysis were used. Furthermore, post hoc comparisons tests should reveal a significant time-dependent effect during treatment with the calcium channel blocker but not during pretreatment or during treatment with the vehicle. A significant Treatment $\times$ Time interaction could be evaluated with a trend analysis (6.16). Because the reported statistical analysis was not correct, the conclusion of the pharmacologist cannot be evaluated; hence, the conclusion should be rejected. If descriptive statistics had been presented (means and standard deviations) it might have been possible to evaluate the pharmacologist's conclusions (5.1).

Table 14.7 Mean Arterial Blood Flows for Treatment Groups

Treatment	Blood flow (mL/min) (M ± SD)		
	Carotid	Coronary	Renal
Control	135 ± 14	55 ± 7	109 ± 13
Hydrolozine	161 ± 21	82 ± 13*	41 ± 14*
Indomethacin	131 ± 28	71 ± 9	53 ± 14*
Hydrolozine + Indomethacin	107 ± 25	48 ± 8	105 ± 16

RESEARCH DESIGN PROBLEM 57

An experiment was done to determine if the vasodilatory effects of hydrolozine on the regional circulations of the carotid, coronary, and renal arteries of conscious dogs were mediated by prostaglandins. Mongrel dogs, 19–24 kg body weight, were surgically instrumented for monitoring blood flows. During a 10-day recovery period, hemodynamic functions were monitored daily. Twenty instrumented dogs were randomly assigned to four treatment groups: control, hydrolozine, indomethacin, and hydrolozine plus indomethacin ($s = 5$ per group). Indomethacin is a potent inhibitor of cyclooxygenase, which is an enzyme necessary for the synthesis of prostaglandins. Hydrolozine was given at an effective vasodilatory dose (1 mg/kg PO), and indomethacin was given (2 mg/kg IV) 15 to 20 min prior to hydrolozine when both drugs were used. Animals were stabilized for 30 min, hydrolozine was given, and after 90 min the readings presented in Table 14.7 were recorded.

An analysis of variance indicated a significant main effect of artery, $F(2, 32) = 5.40, p < .01$; and a significant Treatment × Artery interaction, $F(6, 32) = 3.47, p < .01$. Post hoc multiple comparisons using the Dunnett test indicated that the starred values were significantly different from control values at $p < .05$. As may be seen hydrolozine increased coronary blood flow and indomethacin blocked this vasodilatory effect. On the other hand, hydrolozine decreased renal blood flow and indomethacin also blocked this effect. But, indomethacin alone also significantly decreased renal blood flow. None of the three drug values were significantly different from the control value for carotid blood flow. From these data the authors concluded that the vasodilatory effect of hydrolozine in renal vessels is mediated by prostaglandins; whereas, the coronary vasodilation is independent of prostaglandin activity.

Critique

The research hypothesis is whether the vasodilator effects of hydrolozine on the regional circulations of the carotid, coronary, and renal arteries of conscious dogs are mediated by prostaglandins. The general ANOVA table for the experiment is presented in Table 6.4. The specific ANOVA table for the experiment is

Source	df	Error term
Treatment	3	S/Treatment
Artery	2	Artery $\times$ S/Treatment
S/Treatment	16	
Treatment $\times$ Artery	6	Artery $\times$ S/Treatment
Artery $\times$ S/Treatment	32	
Total	59	

The significant Treatment $\times$ Artery interaction (6.13) was not analyzed properly. A comparison of the three drug groups to the control group by the Dunnett test (10.6) *within* each of the blood flow conditions (arteries) is not the appropriate comparison given a significant Treatment $\times$ Artery interaction. The significant Treatment $\times$ Artery interaction indicates that a significant difference exists between *at least* two of the means presented in Table 14.7 that is not because of significant differences in treatment effects or artery effects (6.13).

Dunnett test (10.6) is not as corrective for familywise error rate (6.9) as are other post hoc multiple comparison tests (6.9, 10.1). The Dunnett test considers only a limited number of comparisons, normally the control-experimental contrasts, and should be used when comparing individually a *few* experimental groups with the single control group. The Dunnett test (10.6) should be selected as the statistical test before the data are collected and examined (6.9, 6.10). A comparison between the means reported for coronary blood flow under hydrolozine (82 $\pm$ 13) and indomethacin (71 $\pm$ 9) would not be significant. Likewise the same two-mean comparison would not be significant for renal blood flow. Based upon these descriptive mean comparisons the authors' conclusions should be rejected.

RESEARCH DESIGN PROBLEM 58

Beta blockers that normally lower blood pressure and slow heart rate may, in some people, also relieve severe anxiety. To test this hypothesis, propranolol was given to 30 high school students who did poorly on their initial SAT test. Other academic evaluations and IQ tests indicated that these students should have done better on the SAT and all these students implied that they suffered from test anxiety. When these students retook the SAT after taking propranolol their scores improved an average of 50 points on the verbal section and 70 points on the math section, both changes were significant at the $p < .01$ level of confidence. Normally, students who retake the SAT only increase their verbal scores by 18 points and math scores by 20 points. From these results, the researcher concluded that propranolol is effective in reducing extreme nervousness and thereby permits students to perform close to their maximum potential.

Although propranolol may be harmful to individuals with asthma or with certain heart problems, the only side effect in these healthy students was occasional drowsiness. Therefore, the researchers also recommended that students not drive to the testing place after taking the drug.

Critique

The research hypothesis is whether propranolol increases the verbal and math SAT performance of anxious high school students. The general ANOVA table for the reported study is presented in Table 6.3. The specific ANOVA table for this complete within-subject two-factor design (A $\times$ B $\times$ S) is

Source	df	Error term
Test (Verbal/Math)	1	Test $\times$ Subject
Pre-Post	1	Pre-Post $\times$ Subject
Subject	29	
Test $\times$ Pre-Post	1	Test $\times$ Pre-Post $\times$ Subject
Test $\times$ Subject	29	
Pre-Post $\times$ Subject	29	
Test $\times$ Pre-Post $\times$ Subject	29	
Total	119	

This statistical test would be appropriate. However, no control group existed in the present study and the students were a self-selected group of bright individuals. A placebo control group should be used (4.10) because students receiving any type of medication may be less anxious if they thought the drug was helpful. A time confound also exists in this study (practice effect, 4.19) and the authors do indicate that "students who retake the SAT only increase their verbal scores by 18 points and math scores by 20 points." But the averaged practice performance of this normal population *cannot* be used as a control practice outcome for the self-selected highly anxious students. For these "very nervous" students a simple practice effect (relieving anxiety by knowing what to expect) may produce very high improvement scores on the second test *without* propranolol being given. Therefore, the authors cannot conclude that propranolol is effective in reducing extreme nervousness.

RESEARCH DESIGN PROBLEM 59

Continuous intravenous (IV) administration is not normally used for diazepam but, in some cases, optimal therapeutic efficacy may be achieved with IV diazepam. Unfortunately, diazepam has limited solubility in common IV solutions and interacts with the infusion system, both of which produce variable drug delivery. Therefore, the purpose of the present study was to compare the delivery of diazepam through a polyethylene-lined IV administration set with its delivery through a standard polyvinyl chloride (PVC) IV administration set.

Table 14.8   Mean (M) and Standard Deviations (SD) of Percentage of Diazepam Recovered at Distal Ends of the Two IV Delivery Systems

Time	% Diazepam recovered	
	PVC (M $\pm$ SD)	Non-PVC (M $\pm$ SD)
0	61.2 (10.6)	103.8 (4.5)
.25 h	44.1 (4.6)	102.6 (9.2)
.50 h	49.0 (2.4)	102.6 (5.0)
1 h	56.1 (2.9)	99.3 (7.7)
2 h	60.8 (1.5)	98.8 (8.8)
5 h	70.9 (8.2)	101.3 (5.5)
Total	57.0 (5.0)	101.4 (6.7)

Diazepam was prepared in glass containers at a concentration of 50 mg/500 mL of 5% dextrose injection. Eight bottles were connected to each of the two types of administration sets: a PVC-based set and a non-PVC set (normally used with nitroglycerin and containing no plasticizers). Both sets were 254 cm in length and were threaded through volumetric infusion pumps in the usual manner. The infusion pumps were used to control solution flow rate at 50 mL/h through the administration set.

For each of the 16 preparations (8 per group) four solution samples were taken at each of six time points: two from the glass bottle and two from the distal end of the administration set. Samples were taken at the beginning of flow (time 0), and at 15 and 30 min and 1, 2, and 5 h. The diazepam concentration in the glass bottle was taken as 100% and the diazepam concentration of the solution at the distal end of the tubing was compared with this value, that is, expressed as a percentage of this value (see Table 14.8). All samples were assayed using an appropriate diazepam assay.

An ANOVA indicated the following results: main effect of group, $F(1, 30) = 7.31, p < .01$; main effect of time, $F(5, 150) = 2.00$, NS; Group $\times$ Time interaction, $F(5, 150) = 2.39, p < .05$. The pharmacologists concluded that a difference in diazepam delivery exists between the two types of IV sets and that the magnitude of this difference changes with the duration of infusion. They postulated that the significant Group $\times$ Time interaction was because diazepam concentrations at or in the surface of the PVC tubing may reach a saturation point.

Critique

The research question is whether a significant difference exists in the percentage of diazepam recovered from a polyethylene-lined and a standard polyvinyl chloride IV delivery system. The general ANOVA table for an A $\times$ (B $\times$ S) mixed factorial design is presented in Table 6.4. The specific ANOVA table for a 2 $\times$ (6 $\times$ 8) mixed factorial design is

Source	df	Error term
Group	1	S/Group
Time	5	Time × S/Group
S/Group	14	
Group × Time	5	Time × S/Group
Time × S/Group	70	
Total	95	

The specific ANOVA reported, however, is

Source	df	Error term
Group	1	S/Group
Time	5	Time × S/Group
S/Group	30	
Group × Time	5	Time × S/Group
Time × S/Group	150	
Total	191	

In the analysis of the data the pharmacologists treated the two duplicate samples as independent observations (4.9) and, therefore, the degrees of freedom (5.17, 6.5) for the MS error terms (6.6) are inflated. Because the duplicate samples are correlated values (9.2) the error term variance would also be reduced (from what would have been expected with independent observations), and this error term reduction would result in inflated F-values (5.18).

Despite these statistical problems, the pharmacologists' conclusion that a difference in diazepam delivery exists between the two types of IV set is appropriate and should be accepted. From the data presented in Table 14.8, the total mean percentages of diazepam recovered for the PVC and non-PVC sets were 57.0 and 101.4, respectively, and the averaged standard deviations were between 5.0 and 7.0 percent, $t(14) = 15.02, p < .001$. Consequently, even though the appropriate statistical test was not performed correctly, the reported data indicate the pharmacologists' conclusion regarding the main effect of group was correct. However, conclusions based upon the interpretation of a significant Group × Time interaction cannot be accepted because the reported data for the six time measurements from the two groups do not show a clear trend difference between the two groups.

The descriptive statistics (5.1) given in a report must be carefully examined. Even if the statistical analysis of the data collected and the author's interpretation and conclusions are incorrect, the data presented may permit you to make a correct interpretation.

RESEARCH DESIGN PROBLEM 60

For thoroughbred stallions a positive correlation between testicular diameter and fertility has been found, that is, greater testicular diameter is associated with higher fertility—a relationship which is independent of total body weight. In broodmares increasing artificially photoperiods has been shown to stimulate the reproductive cycle. An experiment was done, therefore, to determine whether stallions placed under artificial light would show an increase in testicular diameter. All testicular measurements were done by the stallion manager of a large thoroughbred breeding farm and measurements were taken at 8:00 A.M. with a standard caliper. Each horse was measured 3 times each day and the average of these measurements was used as the measurement for that day.

Twelve healthy stallions (6 to 17 years old) were first age-matched and then randomly assigned to two groups ($s = 6$); consequently, the groups had equal numbers of young and older horses. The study began on November 15 and terminated on May 15. (The official breeding season for thoroughbreds is February 15 to June 15.) All horses were turned out in paddocks in the morning and in the afternoon were returned to their own stalls. At 7:00 P.M. the six experimental horses had their stall lights turned on until 12:00 A.M. The other six were exposed only to the natural photoperiod. In the colder months, most stallions constrict their testicles close to their body and have to be walked before a proper measurement can be taken. Care was taken to ensure each horse was relaxed and the testicles fully descended before a measurement was taken.

A mixed factorial ANOVA 2 × (24 × 6) was used to analyze the data and a significant increase in testicular diameter was observed. Indeed, the main effects of treatment, $F(1, 10) = 5.23$, $p < .05$; time, $F(24, 240) = 1.72$, $p < .05$; and the Treatment × Time interaction, $F(24, 240) = 1.80$, $p < .05$; were all significant. The researchers concluded that artificial photoperiods may be a valuable management tool which might be used to increase fertility rates in thoroughbred stallions.

Critique

The research hypothesis is whether an increased exposure to light (by artificial lamps) would increase testicular diameter in stallions. The general ANOVA table for this experiment is presented in Table 6.4. The specific ANOVA table for this experiment is

Source	df	Error term
Treatment	1	S/Treatment
Time	24	Time × S/Treatment
S/Treatment	10	
Treatment × Time	24	Time × S/Treatment
Time × S/Treatment	240	
Total	299	

The statistical test selected was appropriate. However, the directions of the reported significant effects are not provided. Stallions exposed only to natural light may have had greater testicular diameters than the stallions exposed to both artificial and natural light. The experimental protocol in this study (how, when, and where measurements were taken) was presented in great detail, yet a major fact was omitted, that is, *which* stallions had the greatest testicular diameters.

The significant Treatment × Time interaction was also not analyzed (6.13). Apparently, the time factor was the averaged weekly measurement from each stallion recorded across the 25 weeks of the experiment. Given the number of means involved in the interaction comparison, a trend analysis of the significant two-way interaction would be more informative than post hoc multiple comparisons among the mean values (6.9, 6.16, 10.1). In summary, the results section of this report is incomplete because only significant F-values are presented. In this case, this researcher found significant F-values, reported them, and assumed their interpretation was self-evident (5.18).

RESEARCH DESIGN PROBLEM 61

Locomotor activity of the golden hamster has been shown to be controlled by an endogenous circadian "clock"; that is, the onset, duration, and endpoint of activity occur at precise times during the 24-h day. Also, this periodic rhythm of locomotor activity can be altered by brief, intense pulses of light presented at specific times during the day. As examples, a pulse of light given between 1:00 and 2:00 P.M. will produce a delay in the onset of locomotor activity on subsequent days, a phenomenon referred to as a phase delay because the cycle timing (phase) has been delayed by the light pulse. In contrast, a light pulse between 6:00 and 7:00 P.M. will result in the onset of locomotor activity occurring earlier on subsequent days (a phase advance). Daily neuroendocrine fluctuations may play a controlling role in these phase effects of light, and the neurotransmitter GABA has been postulated to be involved in the phase-changing effect of light on the locomotor rhythm in golden hamsters. Specifically, bicuculline, a GABA antagonist, has been proposed to block the phase alterations of light pulses in male golden hamsters.

To test this hypothesis, 20 male golden hamsters (range, 8–12 weeks old) were randomly assigned to one of two groups, an experimental group and a control group ($s = 10$ per group). Experimental animals had remote control pumps implanted which could deliver bicuculline intraventricularly in a dose of 2.0 mg/kg paired with light presentation at phase delay times (1:00 to 2:00 P.M.) and phase advance times (6:00 to 7:00 P.M.). Various control animals were also fitted with pumps and were given vehicle infusions paired with light pulses, vehicle infusions without any light pulses, or bicuculline infusions without light pulses. Consequently, the difference between controls and experimentals was that only the experimental animals received a light pulse paired with bicuculline, whereas the controls never received a light pulse paired with bicuculline.

All animals were tested for locomotor activity at the same time of the day. The animals were first allowed to acclimate to the running wheels for two days (a baseline measurement of activity prior to treatment). On the third day each animal was given a light pulse at 1:30 P.M. The experimental animals on day 3 received a 2.0-mg/kg dose of bicuculline paired with the light pulse while the controls received the vehicle paired with the pulse. On day 4 all animals were allowed to run on their wheels without any perturbation. On day 5 the experimental animals were again given 2.0-mg/kg bicuculline paired with the light pulse at 1:30 P.M. whereas the controls received no light pulse and a 2.0-mg/kg dose of bicuculline. On the sixth day all animals were left alone. On day 7 the experimental animals were given a 2.0-mg/kg dose of bicuculline paired with the light pulse at 1:30 P.M. whereas controls received no injection of any kind but did receive the light pulse. Once this first stage was completed the same treatment sequence was used again but with light pulses administered at 6:30 P.M. (Stage II).

Data were analyzed using a repeated-measures ANOVA. A significant treatment effect, $F(6, 54) = 7.86$, $p < .001$, was found, but the other main effects and interactions were not significant. Student-Newman-Keuls post hoc comparisons revealed that the bicuculline-injected animals did not show a phase delay when given a light pulse at 1:30 P.M. whereas all other animals did, and that all animals exhibited a phase advance following administration of light pulses at 6:30 P.M.

The authors concluded that bicuculline blocks phase delays but not phase advances produced by light administration and that these results implicate GABA as a neuroendocrine controller of circadian locomotor rhythm in this species. The authors also emphasized that the effect of GABA was dependent on light administration as application of GABA antagonist without the light (as in some of the control trials) did not affect the rhythm.

Critique

The research hypothesis is whether bicuculline, a specific GABA antagonist, will block the phase alteration of locomotor activity of male golden hamsters normally produced by light pulses. The design used is not a balanced repeated-measures design (4.16) because treatments are nested in animal group (6.2); consequently, neither a general or specific ANOVA table can be presented. Superficially, the design appears to be a mixed factorial with two independent groups and repeated measures within groups (4.21) but the two groups received multiple and different treatments. For example, there is a factor due to treatment, one due to time of light administration (two levels), one due to different days (7 levels), one due to order of administration and all the appropriate interactions. But the control animals were receiving different treatments, hence, the design is not balanced (4.5). Also, the authors did not report a significant interaction, yet an interaction appears to be what the authors were testing in their post hoc tests (6.12). The statistical analysis section of this report does not provide sufficient detail to determine what comparisons were made or whether these comparisons were appropriate (2.4).

Given the design presented, a limited ANOVA might be used to extract some information. For example, on the first four days of the experiment a 2 × (3 × 10) mixed factorial could be used to determine whether 2.0 mg/kg of bicuculline eliminated the normal phase delay in activity produced by a light pulse. During this period, the two groups differ only in whether the drug was given (4.4). The general ANOVA table for this design is given in Table 6.4. The specific ANOVA table for this analysis would be

Source	df	Error term
Drug	1	S/Drug
Time	2	Time × S/Drug
S/Drug	18	
Drug × Time	2	Time × S/Drug
Time × S/Drug	36	
Total	59	

The levels of the two factors in this ANOVA are drug and vehicle control (2) and pretreatment time, treatment time, and posttreatment time (3). Only the last day of the pretreatment time would be used and the data for each individual animal would be the time of day for the onset of activity. Hence, for both groups a baseline day is available; on day 2 both groups receive the same light pulse but the experimental hamsters receive bicuculline and the control hamsters receive the vehicle, and on day 3 the hamsters in both groups ran freely in their wheels. A significant Drug × Time interaction would be the expected outcome if bicuculline had an effect on phase delay times. Notice the protocol changes on day 7; consequently, another experiment is being conducted with experienced animals.

In a within-subject design the possibility of significant carry-over effect from one treatment condition to another must be considered (4.19). Unfortunately, in the reported experiment the effect of bicuculline on the phase advance of locomotor activity (Stage II) cannot be adequately evaluated using the suggested 2 × (3 × 10) mixed factorial. The reason is that the Stage II results are confounded by time. Hence, although a different statistical analysis may provide some important information the design of the experiment restricts the conclusions that can be made.

RESEARCH DESIGN PROBLEM 62

Ozone is a common air pollutant which at high concentrations produces death by pulmonary edema. The effectiveness of arterial blood gas measurements for assessing the toxic effects of ozone on lung function and gas exchange was determined by exposing 120 young adult male Sprague-Dawley rats (80 days old) to either clean filtered air, .75 ppm ozone, or 1.0 ppm ozone for either 1, 3, 7, or 14 days (10 rats in each group). Because of a high mortality rate among rats exposed for 14 days to 1.0 ppm ozone, additional rats were added to this group until 10 survivors were obtained. After its specific treatment, each rat was removed from its exposure chamber and placed in an individual test chamber ventilated with only normal filtered air. After 10 min of this air exposure an arterial blood sample was collected from the rat. The test chamber was immediately flushed with 100% O_2 and after 10 min a second blood sample was collected. The test chamber was then flushed with 9% O_2 and 91% N_2 for an additional 10 min and a final blood sample collected. Each rat was then sacrificed and· its lungs examined for pathological changes. Arterial blood Pa_{O_2} was measured immediately after each blood collection. (Altered oxygen concentrations were used to determine whether the sensitivity of blood gas measurements changed at different O_2 levels.)

Analyses of variance were performed using the Pa_{O_2} values with the following results. In none of the analyses was the Ozone × Day interaction significant. For normal filtered air (following previous exposure) there was a significant day effect, $F(3, 108) = 4.43, p < .01$, and a significant ozone effect, $F(2, 108) = 5.78$, $p < .01$, with Pa_{O_2} decreasing significantly with both exposure time and ozone concentration (Newman-Keuls post hoc test, $p < .05$). When ventilated with 100% O_2 there was neither a significant day or ozone effect. When ventilated with 9% O_2 the main effect of day was not significant, however, there was a significant ozone effect, $F(2, 108) = 3.68, p < .05$ with the Pa_{O_2} values lower at the two ozone levels than at the normal air level (Newman-Keuls test, $p < .05$). The two ozone levels did not have significantly different Pa_{O_2} values. Lung pathology showed that the severity of effects increased with ozone concentration and duration of exposure. The authors concluded that, for young adult male Sprague-Dawley rats, Pa_{O_2} measured after breathing ambient air was a more sensitive indicator of ozone-induced pulmonary dysfunction compared to breathing either increased or decreased oxygen percentages.

Critique

The research question is twofold: (a) Whether changes in arterial blood Pa_{O_2} occur as the length of exposure to different concentrations of ozone is increased and (b) whether altered O_2 concentrations affect the sensitivity of blood gas measurements. The general ANOVA table for this experiment is presented in Table 6.7. The specific ANOVA table for the 3 (air) × 4 (exposure length) × 3 (O_2 exposure) mixed factorial design with repeated measures on the last factor, that is, a 3 × 4 × (3 × 10) design, is

Source	df	Error term
Ozone	2	S/Ozone, Day
Day	3	S/Ozone, Day
O_2 Exposure	2	O_2 × S/Ozone, Day
S/Ozone, Day	108	
Ozone × Day	6	S/Ozone, Day
Ozone × O_2	4	O_2 × S/Ozone, Day
Day × O_2	6	O_2 × S/Ozone, Day
Ozone × Day × O_2	12	O_2 × S/Ozone, Day
O_2 × S/Ozone, Day	216	
Total	359	

Three separate ANOVAs, however, were used to analyze the data, one ANOVA for each O_2 exposure. For each ANOVA used in the study the general ANOVA table is represented in Table 6.2. The specific ANOVA for each analysis would be

Source	df	Error term
Ozone	2	S/Ozone, Day
Day	3	S/Ozone, Day
Ozone × Day	6	S/Ozone, Day
S/Ozone, Day	108	
Total	119	

Given the pattern of significant outcomes for the three separate two-factor factorial experiments, A × B (4.13, 6.13), the three-way interaction (6.14) in an A × B × (C × S) mixed factorial design probably would have been significant. To interpret this significant three-way interaction (A × B × C) the A × B interaction at levels C_1, C_2, and C_3 would be evaluated (6.14). In none of three separate ANOVAs, C_1—normal filtered air, C_2—100% O_2, or C_3—9% O_2 was the A × B interaction significant. As the A × B interaction was not significant (6.13), the simple main effects were assessed and, if significant, were evaluated by subsequent post hoc multiple comparison tests (6.8, 6.9, 10.1). Given the significant main effects observed for each O_2 measurement, the authors' conclusion is acceptable if it is assumed that no significant carry-over effects (4.19) occurred from one test condition (normal filtered air) to another test condition (100% O_2). A simple counterbalancing of test conditions would have eliminated this problem. The data and analysis of the lung pathology indicated that structural changes also increased as the amount of ozone exposure increased.

Fortunately the authors' conclusion was not based on an interpretation of a significant two-way interaction (6.13). The authors reported that the Ozone × Day interaction was not significant in any of the three analyses. But, a high mortality rate occurred for animals exposed for 14 days to 1.00 ppm ozone. Hence, the animals that survived this treatment were a selected group of animals. This confounding of treatment and animal loss (4.12) would be important if the authors had concluded that there was not an interaction effect between the amount of ozone and days of exposure. The lung pathological data were discussed briefly in the report, and no summary statistics were presented (2.4).

RESEARCH DESIGN PROBLEM 63

The effects of two different neonatally administered opioid peptides, morphiceptin and D-Ala-D-Leu-enkephalin (DADL), on maze learning in rats were studied. Three males and three females were randomly selected for the experiment from each of 10 randomly selected litters from a university Sprague-Dawley colony. One male and one female from each litter were then randomly assigned to one of three drug treatments: morphiceptin (73 mg/kg), DADL (80 mg/kg), and saline. For 1 week after birth the neonates were injected subcutaneously daily with their respective drug. At 24 days, the pups were separated from the dams and deprived of food and water. On the next day the rats began testing in a Y-maze for food reward. In the two-choice-point maze a wrong turn would lead to an empty compartment and an entry into this compartment was measured as an error. A correct choice led to the compartment with food (goal box). The rats were given five trials on each of two consecutive days. Latency to find the food reward and number of errors were recorded.

An analysis of variance on the latency data for the first test day indicated that the main effects of drug and of sex were not significant and the Sex × Drug interaction was also not significant. On the second day of testing, there was a significant main effect of sex, $F(1, 54) = 5.78, p < .03$; but neither the main effect of drug nor the Drug × Sex interaction was significant. Females rats injected with either drug ran as fast as the drug-treated males on the first day, and control males ran faster than females. By the second day, males in all groups ran faster than the females.

An analysis of variance for the number of errors per trial on the first day did not yield a significant main effect of either drug or sex, but their interaction was significant, $F(2, 54) = 5.56, p < .01$. The analysis of the interaction revealed significant differences among the three female groups, $F(1, 27) = 7.80, p < .01$, but no significant differences among the male groups. Post hoc analysis indicated that only the comparison between the females treated with morphiceptin and the females treated with saline was significant, $F(1, 54) = 7.03, p < .01$. On the second test day the differences between males and females in the drug groups were not significant: main effect of sex, $F(1, 54) = 5.78, p < .05$, main effect of drug and Drug × Sex interaction were not significant. The females in both drug groups made fewer errors than the males on the first day and the control females made more errors than the males. On the second day, the males in all groups made fewer errors than the females.

The authors concluded that early opioid treatment produced a facilitation of maze performance only in female rats. Moreover, both of the opioid peptides (morphiceptin and DADL) produced this facilitation effect in females.

Critique

The research hypothesis is not explicitly stated. The apparent hypothesis is whether opioid peptides (morphiceptin and DADL) given during the neonatal period will differentially affect subsequent maze learning of male and female rats. The general ANOVA table for this experiment is presented in Table 6.7. The specific ANOVA table for this experiment is

Source	df	Error term
Drug	2	S/Drug, Sex
Sex	1	S/Drug, Sex
Day	1	Day × S/Drug, Sex
S/Drug, Sex	54	
Drug × Sex	2	S/Drug, Sex
Drug × Day	2	Day × S/Drug, Sex
Sex × Day	1	Day × S/Drug, Sex
Drug × Sex × Day	2	Day × S/Drug, Sex
Day × S/Drug, Sex	54	
Total	119	

A more complex analysis would be to also include littermates as a factor in a randomized-blocks design (9.4). However, from the F-ratios presented in the brief the authors did separate ANOVAs for each day; consequently, the within-subject factor (repeated measures over days) was eliminated. The general ANOVA table for the analyses reported in the brief is presented in Table 6.2. The specific ANOVA table for the analyses in the brief is

Source	df	Error term
Drug	2	S/Drug, Sex
Sex	1	S/Drug, Sex
Drug × Sex	2	S/Drug, Sex
S/Drug, Sex	54	
Total	59	

Essentially, two ANOVAs are used to analyze the latency data and another two ANOVAs used for the number of errors. For a significant Drug × Sex interaction, the authors did *two more separate* ANOVAs, one for the male rats and one for the female rats (6.13). The general ANOVA table for these latter two analyses is presented in Table 6.1. The specific ANOVA table for each of the single-factor analyses is

Source	df	Error term
Drug	2	S/Drug
S/Drug	27	
Total	29	

The authors have misinterpreted a two-way interaction (6.12). The authors concluded that both morphiceptin and DADL produced a facilitation in performance of female rats. But the analysis indicated that DADL-treated females *did not* differ significantly from saline-treated females.

RESEARCH DESIGN PROBLEM 64

Sickle cell anemia is a genetic-based disease affecting 1 in 600 blacks. In this disease, hemoglobin (Hb) S differs from the normal Hb A by one amino acid and precipitates upon deoxygenation causing severe distortion of the red blood cell (RBC) membrane. This shape change (sickling) causes occlusion of capillary beds which produces infarction and pain. The rate-limiting step for sickling is the intracellular Hb S concentration. Phlorizin benzyl azide (PhzBAz) has been found to cause normal erythrocytes (RBCs) to increase their volume in a dose dependent function. The purpose of the present experiment was to determine whether PhzBAz would inhibit sickling upon deoxygenation by increasing cell volume thereby decreasing intracellular Hb S concentration.

Blood samples from five known Hb S patients, who had no transfusions over the previous 100 days, were obtained. Each blood sample was washed, brought to a 20 percent Hct, and properly stored. One milliliter of a patient's blood was placed into a cell deoxygenator apparatus and 50, 25, 12.5, 5, 6.25, or 0 M of PhzBAz was added (volumes were the same for each drug treatment condition including the control condition of 0 M PhzBAz). All five patients' blood samples were tested with each of the five concentrations of drug and a counterbalancing procedure was used. The cells were allowed to equilibrate for 5 min to 37°C, then were deoxygenated for 10 min (producing the max. % sickling), and finally a sample was removed under anaerobic conditions and fixed in 1% glutaraldehyde. The fixed cells were observed under phase microscopy and the percent sickling determined (length 2X width, fields of at least 100 cells counted). The data obtained are presented in Table 14.9.

A single-factor within-subject ANOVA was used for statistical analysis and revealed a significant treatment effect, $F(4, 20) = 4.51, p < .01$. Post hoc analysis using a Tukey test indicated a significant difference between all doses and the control dose ($p < .05$) and the PhzBAz groups did not differ significantly among themselves. The authors concluded that PhzBAz was an effective antisickling agent in vitro and the optimal dosage under these circumstances was 6.25 M or less.

Critique

The research hypothesis is whether PhzBAz by increasing cell volume will inhibit sickling upon deoxygenation in red blood cells containing Hb S. The gen-

Table 14.9   Percentage of Sickled Cells in Drug Groups

Drug conc.	Percent sickled ($\pm$ SD)
0	72(3)
6.25	21(4)
12.5	25(3)
25.0	22(3)
50.0	24(4)

eral ANOVA table for this study is presented in Table 9.3. The specific ANOVA for this randomized-blocks experiment is

Source	df	Error term
Blood sample	4	
Dose	5	Blood sample × Dose
Blood sample × Dose	20	
Total	29	

The analysis reported in the brief was a single-factor within-subject ANOVA. The general ANOVA table for this analysis is presented in Table 4.5 The specific ANOVA for this single-factor within-subject ANOVA is

Source	df	Error term
Treatment	5	Treatment × Subject
Subject	4	
Treatment × Subject	20	
Total	29	

It is evident that both ANOVAs are the same, that is, a randomized-blocks design (9.4) is the same as a single-factor *within-subject* design (4.16) which is the same as a single-factor *repeated-measures* design (4.16). Only the source names are different; therefore, the authors' conclusion is appropriate. The assumption that PhzBAz produced its antisickling action by increasing cell volume (research hypothesis) was not determined (1.2). The authors only concluded, however, that the PhzBAz was an effective antisickling agent in vitro and the optimal dosage was 6.25 M or less.

RESEARCH DESIGN PROBLEM 65

After strenuous exercise the body temperature of mammals remains elevated for several hours. Endogenous pyrogens, present in the plasma after exercise, may be responsible for this elevation in body temperature. To determine the involvement of endogenous pyrogens in the increase in body temperature after exercise, an effective dose of an antipyretic drug (sodium salicylate) was injected into dogs prior to exercise on a treadmill and body temperature was monitored before, during, and after exercise.

Ten male dogs (10–12 kg body weight) were randomly assigned equally to the drug or vehicle control group. Body temperatures were continuously measured for 1 h before exercise, for 35 min during exercise on the treadmill, and for 1 h following exercise. The mean body temperature during each measurement period was calculated for each dog and used as its data.

An ANOVA revealed a significant drug effect, $F(1, 4) = 7.81, p < .05$; a significant measurement effect, $F(2, 8) = 4.46, p < .05$; but no significant Drug × Measurement interaction, $F(2, 8) = 3.65$. Post hoc analysis of the data revealed that sodium salicylate significantly lowered body temperature following exercise compared with control temperature. Therefore the researchers concluded that endogenous pyrogens cause body temperature to remain elevated following exercise.

Critique

The research hypothesis is whether an effective antipyretic dose of sodium salicylate will lower the normal body temperature increase found after exercise in dogs. The general ANOVA table for the design used in this experiment is presented in Table 6.4. The specific ANOVA table for the $2 \times (3 \times S)$ mixed factorial design used in the experiment is

Source	df	Error term
Drug	1	S/Drug
Measurement	2	Measurement × S/Drug
S/Drug	8	
Drug × Measurement	2	Measurement × S/Drug
Measurement × S/Drug	16	
Total	29	

Many problems exist in this experiment. The most serious is that no significant Drug × Measurement interaction was observed yet the authors' conclusions are based upon a significant interaction. The reported post hoc analysis is not for the significant drug effect or the significant measurement effect, but is based upon pairwise comparisons of the six means of the Drug × Measurement interaction. Also, the experimental design is a mixed factorial (4.21) but the F-ratios were calculated as if a complete within-subject design was used (4.16). Descriptive statistics were not presented; consequently, differences among the groups cannot be determined. Planned comparisons (6.10) could have been used in this experiment (10.1).

RESEARCH DESIGN PROBLEM 66

O-cresol is widely used as a disinfectant, is an intermediate in several industrial chemical reactions, and is also a component of phenolic wastes; hence, as a general environmental contaminant it poses a threat to many species. A study was conducted to determine the dietary toxicity of O-cresol to mink (*Mustela vison*), a species usually very sensitive to environmental contaminants. Minks (approx-

Table 14.10   Mean Percent Body Weight Changes ± SD

| Condition | O-cresol concentration (ppm) | | | |
	0	430	1400	2500
Males (n = 5)	19.5 ± 12.7	17.4 ± 11.3	13.5 ± 7.5	0.6 ± 6.7[a]
Females (n = 5)	11.3 ± 10.3	6.8 ± 6.6	−0.1 ± 5.3	−5.4 ± 6.8
	Percent change by period (sexes combined)			
Week 1 (n = 10)	9.6 ± 6.7	10.3 ± 6.6	6.9 ± 5.8	4.0 ± 6.6
Week 2 (n = 10)	3.4 ± 5.4	4.1 ± 5.7	1.1 ± 4.3	0.1 ± 4.3
Week 3 (n = 10)	1.6 ± 4.6	3.7 ± 4.6	−0.3 ± 3.2	−1.3 ± 3.5
Week 4 (n = 10)	0.8 ± 3.7	−1.0 ± 2.4	−1.0 ± 2.6	−5.2 ± 3.0
4-Week cumulative	15.4 ± 11.5	7.1 ± 9.0	6.7 ± 6.4	−2.4 ± 6.8

[a]Significantly different from control ($p < .05$) using Dunnett's test.

imately 6 months old) were randomly assigned to treatment groups (with the restriction that littermates were not assigned to the same group). For dietary studies, five males and five females were used per treatment group with 0, 430, 1400, and 2500 ppm O-creosol–spiked diets tested. Food and water were provided *ad libitum*. Body weights were measured initially and weekly thereafter for 4 weeks when the test was terminated. Percent body weight changes (from initial value) by sex, time, and group were calculated (see Table 14.10).

A mixed factorial ANOVA was performed on the percent body weight changes and revealed a significant Sex × Dose × Week interaction, $F(9, 96)$ = 3.24, $p < .01$, and a significant main effect of week, $F(3, 96) = 4.45, p < .01$. The Sex × Dose interaction, the Sex × Week interaction, the Dose × Week interaction, and the main effects of dose and sex were not significant, $p > .05$. A comparison of treatment means with control means using Dunnett's method indicated that only the male minks fed a diet of 2500 ppm O-cresol were significantly different from controls ($p < .05$). The authors concluded that the minks in all treatment groups showed a decrease in weight gain with time. In addition, they concluded that dietary levels of O-cresol up to 1400 ppm do not significantly affect weight gain in male mink and that levels up to 2500 ppm do not significantly affect weight gain in female mink.

Critique

The research hypothesis is whether diet-delivered O-cresol (0, 430, 1400, and 2500 ppm) affects the body weights of male and female minks. The experimental design used is illustrated in Figure 14.5.

The general ANOVA for this study is presented in Table 6.7. The specific ANOVA for the 2 × 2 × (4 × S) mixed factorial design used in this experiment is

Source	df	Error term
Sex	1	S/Sex, Dose
Dose	3	S/Sex, Dose
Week	3	Week × S/Sex, Dose
S/Sex, Dose	32	
Sex × Dose	3	S/Sex, Dose
Sex × Week	3	Week × S/Sex, Dose
Dose × Week	9	Week × S/Sex, Dose
Sex × Dose × Week	9	Week × S/Sex, Dose
Week × S/Sex, Dose	96	
Total	159	

The statistical test selected was appropriate. However, the authors do not indicate how the significant three-way interaction was evaluated (6.14) nor why the Dunnett test (10.6) was used to compare control body weight changes with all *O*-cresol treatments within each sex. The data for both sexes clearly indicate that

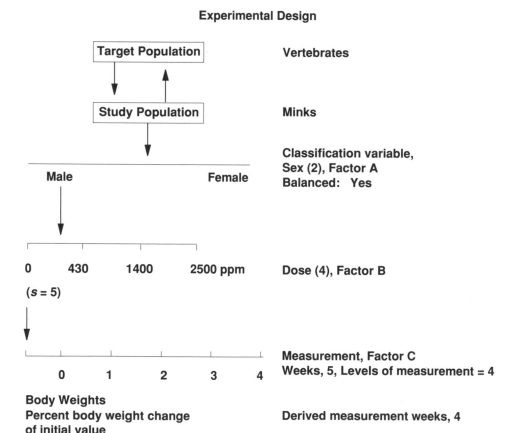

Experimental Design

Target Population — Vertebrates

Study Population — Minks

Male — Female — Classification variable, Sex (2), Factor A. Balanced: Yes

0   430   1400   2500 ppm — Dose (4), Factor B

(s = 5)

0   1   2   3   4 — Measurement, Factor C. Weeks, 5, Levels of measurement = 4

Body Weights
Percent body weight change of initial value — Derived measurement weeks, 4

Mixed Factorial Design: A x B x (C x S)

Figure 14.5   Experimental design for research problem 66.

the percent weight gain decreases as the *O*-cresol concentration increases; however, only one treatment group is reported to differ significantly from the control (male mink at 2500 ppm using the Dunnett test). A t-test comparison of the female mink at 2500 ppm (the highest dose of *O*-cresol) with the control mink indicates a significant difference between the two groups, $t(8) = 3.03, p < .02$. Also, the male control minks gained more weight than did the female control minks (0 ppm groups); consequently, body weight change during this time period should be a more sensitive measure for male than female minks. Furthermore, with the small sample size the minks within each sex probably should have been matched for initial body weights and the matched blocks of animals then assigned randomly to the four treatment groups (4.8). Hence, the authors' conclusion that ". . . levels up to 2500 ppm do not significantly affect weight gain in female mink" is not appropriate given the data presented. Also, the authors concluded that ". . . the mink in all treatment groups showed a decrease in weight gain with time" which indicates they misinterpreted the significant main effect of week given that there was a significant Sex $\times$ Dose $\times$ Week interaction. Note that if data for the Sex $\times$ Dose $\times$ Week interaction had been given in Table 14.10, you could have reconstructed approximate mean values for the other effects. When derived measures based upon initial values are used (5.25), initial values should also be presented for each group.

RESEARCH DESIGN PROBLEM 67

Cigarette smoke causes a greater airway narrowing in patients who suffer from respiratory tract infection than in noninfected people. This increased response to smoke inhalation during airway infection has been suggested to be due to an enhanced airway sensitivity to smoke irritation. Airway narrowing also becomes more severe when the patients smoke cigarettes containing a higher than normal nicotine content. Because nicotine is known to stimulate airway sensory nerve endings, this effect of nicotine may be responsible for the smoke-induced airway irritation and reflex responses in patients with respiratory tract infection. A mixed factorial A $\times$ (B $\times$ C $\times$ S) experiment was designed to test this hypothesis (see Table 14.11). Forty healthy adult guinea pigs were randomly divided into two groups (20 each). One group served as control and the other group was vaccinated with live attenuated influenza virus. Lab tests verified acute airway infections in the animals of the experimental group and no infections in the animals of the control group. Each animal was then challenged three times with a single

Table 14.11 Significant Differences Among the Various Subgroups

Control group (A₁)						Infected group (A₂)					
Prevagotomy (B₁)			Postvagotomy (B₂)			Prevagotomy (B₁)			Postvagotomy (B₂)		
Low	Med	High	Low	Med	High	Low	Med	High	Low	Med	High
5	4	3	5	5	5	5	2	1	5	5	5

puff of smoke generated from research cigarettes containing three different levels of nicotine (high, medium, and low), and airway resistance was measured. Ample recovery time was allowed between challenges and the order of the challenges was counterbalanced among animals. Following bilateral vagotomy (which denervated all pulmonary airway receptors) the same procedures of smoke challenges were repeated in all guinea pigs. An ANOVA test of the airway resistance data showed significant main effects (A, B, and C) and a significant three-way interaction (A × B × C). A post hoc test (Duncan's test) showed the comparisons presented in Table 14.11.

The low, medium, and high are the three levels of factor C, and for the 12 subgroups ($A_1B_1C_1$, $A_1B_1C_2$, . . . , $A_2B_2C_3$) the following code is used: $1 > 2 > 3 > 4 > 5$ and no significant difference exists between conditions having the same number, that is, $5 = 5$.

Based upon this data analysis, the authors concluded that (1) cigarette smoke causes an increased airway constriction in guinea pigs with influenza viral infection of the airways compared with noninfected guinea pigs; (2) a greater response (more airway resistance) is caused by cigarette smoke containing higher nicotine content, suggesting that nicotine is the primary stimulus; and (3) the increased response in infected animals is abolished by vagotomy, indicating the involvement of the vagus nerve.

Critique

The research hypothesis is whether nicotine causes the smoke-induced airway irritation and the reflexive airway narrowing observed in patients with respiratory tract infection. The general ANOVA table for the mixed factorial A × (B × C × S) experiment is presented in Table 6.9. The specific ANOVA table for this experiment is

Source	df	Error term
Infection	1	S/Infection
Pre-Post (vagotomy, V)	1	V × S/Infection
Nicotine	2	Nicotine × S/Infection
S/Infection	38	
Infection × V	1	V × S/Infection
Infection × Nicotine	2	Nicotine × S/Infection
V × Nicotine	2	V × Nicotine × S/Infection
V × S/Infection	38	
Nicotine × S/Infection	76	
V × Nicotine × S/Infection	76	
Infection × V × Nicotine	2	V × Nicotine × S/Infection
Total	239	

The statistical test selected was appropriate. The pattern of results presented in the experimental data is consistent with the authors' conclusions. Bilateral vagotomy is an irreversible experimental procedure; consequently, the prevagotomy test was always carried out first (before the postvagotomy test) in each animal. This time confound, however, would probably not affect the authors' conclusion which is only that the vagus nerve is involved in the increased response in infected animals (4.19).

RESEARCH DESIGN PROBLEM 68

Pretreatment of experimental animals with capsaicin, a principal constituent in red pepper, induces degeneration of primary sensory neurons and this pretreatment effect is greater in newborn animals than in mature animals. Because sensory nerve activity may be involved in the neurogenic inflammatory response caused by an application of pain-inducing chemical irritants to the skin, an experiment was designed to test (1) whether capsaicin pretreatment reduces the degree of the neurogenic inflammatory response and (2) whether capsaicin pretreatment is more effective when applied in the neonatal stage of life. Twelve time-pregnant Sprague-Dawley rats were used and each litter was culled to six male pups of which three were randomly assigned into three groups (12 pups per group). One group (Group I) was injected subcutaneously with capsaicin (50 μg/kg) on the second day after birth, another group (Group II) with vehicle (10% ethanol in saline), and the last group (Group III) received no treatment in the neonatal stage. A total of 36 newborn rats were kept for three months before the inflammation test. All rats in Group III were injected with capsaicin (50 μg/kg) the day before the test. The test was performed during anesthesia by painting the skin of the left hind paw with 5% mustard oil in liquid paraffin, and the degree of inflammatory response was then measured as the amount of Evans Blue dye exudation in the subcutaneous tissue. Data for each of the three groups are shown in Table 14.12.

A single-factor ANOVA revealed a significant group effect, $F(2, 33) = 9.18$, $p < .001$, and subsequent Newman-Keuls post hoc analysis showed that the response of Group I was significantly lower than that of Groups II and III (p's $<$ .05) and no difference existed between the responses of Groups II and III. Therefore, the pharmacologist concluded that (1) neurogenic inflammatory responses induced by chemical irritation of the adult rat's skin are reduced by the neonatal capsaicin pretreatment and (2) capsaicin pretreatment in adult rats is not effective.

Table 14.12 Amount of Evans Blue Dye Exudation for Treatment Groups

Treatment condition	Number of rats	Excess dye (μg) Mean $\pm$ SD
Group I	12	1.5 $\pm$ 2.1
Group II	12	23.7 $\pm$ 8.2
Group III	12	20.1 $\pm$ 9.0

Critique

The research hypothesis is whether the effectiveness of capsaicin pretreatment in reducing the neurogenic inflammatory response is related to the age of the rat when pretreatment is given. The general ANOVA table for the experiment reported is presented in Table 6.1. The specific ANOVA table is

Source	df	Error term
Group	2	S/Group
S/Group	33	
Total	35	

The single-factor ANOVA was appropriate and correct given the data presented in Table 14.12. A more sensitive statistical test may have been a randomized-blocks design because three male littermates were assigned to each of the three groups (9.4). The general ANOVA table for a randomized-blocks design is presented in Tables 4.5 and 9.3. The specific ANOVA table for this design would be

Source	df	Error term
Treatment	2	Treatment × Littermates
Littermates	11	
Treatment × Littermates	22	
Total	35	

If a significant correlation exists among the male littermates, the MS Treatment × Littermates would be smaller than MS littermates by an amount determined by the correlation (9.2, 9.4). The author ignored the litter classification and treated the data as though all the observations were independent. That is, the ss values for littermates and the Treatment × Littermates interaction were pooled and divided by 33 (the summation of df for the two sources of variation). Because the pooled value will be larger than the MS Treatment × Littermates (given that a positive correlation exists among littermates) the outcome is to produce an F-ratio smaller than it should be. Hence, the author would underestimate the level of significance (see 9.4).

In this experiment, however, a significant F-value was obtained and a smaller error source to evaluate differences among the three groups would not have resulted in a significant difference between Groups II and III given the means and standard deviations presented. The first conclusion of the author is, therefore, appropriate. But no control group exists to compare the capsaicin pretreatment in the adult rat, consequently, the author cannot assume that capsaicin pretreatment in adult rats is not effective. Furthermore, capsaicin pretreatment might have been effective if more time had elapsed between pretreatment and test in the adult animal. About 90 days elapsed between the treatment and test in the neonatal administered group yet only a day elapsed between treatment

and test in the adult administered group. To conclude that capsaicin pretreatment in the adult rat is not effective is not an appropriate conclusion given the
lack of a control group and the time difference between treatment and test.

RESEARCH DESIGN PROBLEM 69

In people with asthma, the release of endogenous mediators (e.g., prostaglandins) may be involved both in the initial bronchoconstriction which normally
occurs after exercise and in the refractory period during which repeated exercise
challenges induce less bronchoconstriction (habituation). Therefore, the purpose of this study was to determine (a) the involvement of contractile (broncho-
constrictive) prostaglandins (e.g., $PGF_{2\alpha}$) in the initial bronchoconstriction after
exercise and (b) the involvement of inhibitory (bronchodilatory) prostaglandins
(e.g., PGE_2) in the refractoriness after exercise. Five asthmatic males, who had
both exercise-induced bronchoconstriction and refractoriness after exercise,
were tested on two separate days. The two test days were separated by a 3-week
period. On both test days, the asthmatics were given an initial exercise challenge
for 5 min on a bicycle ergometer. (A work load which increased the heart rate
response to 80% predicted maximum was used on both test days.) During the
exercise the men breathed dry air at room temperature (21–23°C). The airway
resistance was measured every minute after the exercise challenge until maximal
bronchoconstriction had occurred (typically within 5 min after the challenge)
and measurements continued until the airway resistance returned to the baseline
value. The exercise challenge was then repeated using the same experimental
protocol. The men were given placebo capsules or indomethacin (inhibitor of
prostaglandins' synthesis) 100 mg per day in a double-blind randomized fashion
for 3 days before each test day. A repeated-measures ANOVA was used for statistical analysis. The responses between the first and second exercise challenges
were significantly different, $F(1, 4) = 7.81, p < .05$, but there was no significant
drug effect, $F(1,4) = 2.01$, or Drug $\times$ Exercise interaction, $F(1,4) = 2.23$. For
the placebo treatment, the airway resistance increased by 19.1% $\pm$ 4.9% (mean
$\pm$ SEM) after the first exercise challenge and the increase of resistance after the
second challenge was significantly reduced at 11.8% $\pm$ 1.5% indicating refractoriness. For the indomethacin treatment, the increase of resistance after the first
exercise challenge was 16.8% $\pm$ 4.0%, which was not significantly different from
the placebo day. In addition, the response to the second exercise challenge was
13.8% $\pm$ 3.4%, which was not different from the first challenge indicating that
refractoriness did not occur. The authors concluded, therefore, that contractile
prostaglandins do not appear to be important in the initial bronchoconstriction
after exercise, however, inhibitory prostaglandins are involved in the development of refractoriness after exercise.

Critique

The research hypothesis is whether prostaglandins in asthmatic males are
involved both in the initial bronchoconstriction following exercise and in the

reduction in this bronchoconstriction that occurs following repeated exercise periods. The general ANOVA table for the experiment is presented in Table 6.3. The specific ANOVA table for this experiment is

Source	df	Error term
Drug	1	Drug × Subject
Exercise	1	Exercise × Subject
Subject	4	
Drug × Exercise	1	Drug × Exercise × Subject
Drug × Subject	4	
Exercise × Subject	4	
Drug × Exercise × Subject	4	
Total	19	

The statistical test selected was appropriate. The description of the experimental design implies that a three-factor within-subject design was used (e.g., drug, test day, exercise), but drug and test day are really only one within-subject factor. For each male, four airway resistance measurements were evaluated (two measures from each of the two test days). The two test days were a placebo test day and an indomethacin test day, hence, a complete within-subject two-factor design was used: (A × B × S).

The authors report only a significant main effect of exercise which would not support any conclusion regarding the different roles of contractile and inhibitory prostaglandins. The involvement of prostaglandins in airway resistance would be indicated by either a significant drug effect or a significant Drug × Exercise interaction. But, neither of these comparisons were significant; consequently, post hoc tests among the four treatment conditions are not appropriate (unless these comparisons were planned comparisons, 6.10). Given that only five subjects were used in this experiment the power of any statistical test would not be very high (5.15). The finding that asthmatic males, pretreated with either a placebo or indomethacin, show a significant decrease in airway resistance on the second exercise challenge of the day indicates a robust practice effect. But this finding was not discussed. Rather, the authors concluded that inhibitory prostaglandins are involved in the development of refractoriness after exercise—a conclusion not supported by the data.

RESEARCH DESIGN PROBLEM 70

Retrograde dyes are used extensively in anatomical studies of the central nervous system (CNS), for example, a muscle is injected with a dye, sufficient time is allowed for the dye to be transported up axons to cell bodies in the animal's CNS, then the animal is sacrificed, neural tissue fixed and removed, tissue slides prepared, and cells labeled with the dye are measured. Labeled neurons indicate direct neural connections between the tissue observed and the muscle injected.

A newly developed fluorescent retrograde dye (FRD-2) was tested to determine whether it had an economical advantage over more familiar dyes such as

Fast Blue. FRD-2 was not toxic in cats or rats, was active at a concentration of 5% (as is Fast Blue), and labeled tissue brightly and clearly. Bright labeling is important because the dyes tend to fade with exposure to the UV light of the microscope. For this new dye to be competitive, however, a significant cost savings over the established dyes (which are very expensive) had to be demonstrated. Because FRD-2 cost as much to produce as other dyes, the new dye would have to produce clear, bright labeling in less time than Fast Blue. This outcome with FRD-2 would allow shorter experimental recovery time and lower animal care costs.

The costal diaphragm of the cat was used because transport of Fast Blue to the fifth cervical dorsal root ganglion takes 7 days for maximum results. In this muscle-nerve preparation injecting the left costal diaphragm with Fast Blue results in about 90 percent of observed labeled cells being in the left dorsal root ganglion, and the other 10 percent in the right dorsal root ganglion. Twenty cats (2.5–3 kg) were assigned randomly to receive similar injections into the muscle of the left costal diaphragm of either 5% Fast Blue or FRD-2 in a concentration of 5% ($n = 10$ per group). The cats in each treatment group were then randomized as to recovery time ($n = 2$ per time) of 1, 3, 5, 7, or 9 days. Because of the length of surgery (for injection), only one cat was done daily and a month was required to collect all the data. The order of surgery was blocked and counterbalanced for both the dye and the time of recovery so that conditions occurred evenly throughout the 1-month experimental period. All surgery was performed by a technician who did not know the dye injected, and all cats received the same post-op care. Cats were sacrificed the morning of the appropriate day, all perfusions being done using a standard protocol. All tissues were post-fixed and cut into 16-μm sections on a cryostat. All sections were prepared and cut by a single technician, and all tissue observations were made by another technician; neither technician knew the prior history of the animal. The average number of clear, labeled, nucleated cells was obtained for the two cats in each condition. A nonparametric test indicated that all effects were nonsignificant ($p > .05$). The investigators concluded that because their new dye is not transported significantly faster than Fast Blue from the diaphragm of the cat to the dorsal root ganglion it is probably not a good market risk on the basis of reduced experimental costs.

Critique

The research hypothesis is whether the dye (FRD-2) would result in clear, bright labeling of neurons significantly quicker than the dye Fast Blue. Given the small number of cats in each group ($s = 2$) and the fact that a nonparametric test was used (5.22) the power of the statistical test would be extremely low (5.12). Notice that differences between the two dyes would not be expected to occur in the cats sacrificed 7 or 9 days after dye injection (transport of Fast Blue takes 7 days for maximum result). Also, no difference would be expected to occur in cats sacrificed on day 1; therefore, significant effects would have been expected to occur only between 2 to 6 days after dye injection. Thus, the recovery times selected did not provide a very sensitive test of the research question. Placement of all cats into a 2-day recovery design, that is, day 3 and day 6 after dye injection, would have increased the power of the statistical test. If the number of labeled cells from each cat was used as datum (and there were no zero counts), a between-subject 2 × 2 factorial design (4.13) could have been used which would also have increased the power of the statistical test. In this suggested design, five cats would be in each of the four subgroups. The general ANOVA table is presented in Table 6.2 and the specific ANOVA table for this suggested design would be

Source	df	Error term
Dye	1	S/Dye, Recovery
Recovery	1	S/Dye, Recovery
Dye × Recovery	1	S/Dye, Recovery
S/Dye, Recovery	16	
Total	19	

RESEARCH DESIGN PROBLEM 71

The present study investigated ^{3}H-dihydromorphine binding in various brain regions of young and old male and female rats. Twelve young female, twelve young male, twelve old female, and twelve old male Sprague-Dawley rats were randomly selected from a breeding colony. The young animals were 60 to 70 days old and the old animals were 24 to 26 months old. The rats were decapitated and the following brain areas were removed: frontal poles, anterior cortex, diencephalon, hippocampus, and midbrain. A receptor binding assay was performed separately for each of these brain areas. The data from these assays were analyzed by a 2 (Age) × 2 (Sex) × 5 (Brain Area × S) mixed factorial ANOVA. The analysis showed that there was a significant Age × Sex × Brain Area interaction, $F(4, 220) = 6.01, p < .01$. Analysis of the interaction using the Tukey HSD test showed that although young and old males and young females did not differ in binding in frontal and anterior cortex, old females showed less binding in the frontal poles than in the anterior cortex. The authors concluded that a sex-specific, age-related deficit in binding in the frontal poles occurs in rats.

Critique

The research question is whether ^{3}H-dihydromorphine binding in various brain regions is affected by the sex and age of the animal. A 2 (Age) × 2 (Sex) × 5 (Brain Area × S) mixed factorial design was used to analyze the data. But, a repeated-measures factor was not present in the present experiment (4.16). Different brain regions were measured for each animal which is *not* the same as repeated measures taken from the same region from the same animal (1.5, 4.10, 4.16, 4.21). Therefore, the data should not be combined into one ANOVA because separate receptor binding assays were done for five different brain regions. In receptor binding studies, differences across brain regions are also difficult to interpret because of typical time-confounding and sensitivity of the assay procedure for different levels of the receptors in various brain regions. In this situation, a MANOVA procedure (6.17) would be appropriate if sample sizes were sufficiently large so that any pattern effects could be evaluated.

The random selection of animals from the breeding colony would permit littermates to be assigned to the same treatment condition (Chapter 9). These correlated measures (9.2, 9.5) would affect subsequent F-ratios; consequently, a restriction should be placed on the random sampling procedure, namely, no littermates are assigned to the same treatment condition.

RESEARCH DESIGN PROBLEM 72

Angiotensin II (AII) is present in the central nervous system (CNS) of the terrestrial gastropod, *Limax maximus*. Injection of AII at 2×10 mM concentration initiates drinking (contact rehydration behavior) in *Limax*. Contact rehydration is one of a number of behavior regulatory responses to dehydration in this moist-skinned gastropod. Another response of importance in water regulation is increased locomotor activity in dry conditions which results in the animal spending less time in the dry area and thus, presumably, avoiding desication. Therefore, a biologist wanted to determine whether the increase in locomotion induced by drying conditions was also affected by AII administration in *Limax*.

Thirty animals were randomly assigned to three groups ($s = 10$ per group): a vehicle control group, a drug group given an injection of 2×10 mM AII (a concentration known to be sufficient to initiate contact rehydration behavior), and a drug-drug group given both the AII injection of 2×10 mM and Saralasin at 2×10 mM (Saralasin is an AII antagonist and the concentration used inhibits contact rehydration behavior). All animals in each group were tested on activity wheels using an identical experimental protocol. Each animal was run for 3 days on the wheels under controlled temperature and light cycle. On day 1 all animals were injected and tested on wet wheels (saturated with water). On day 2 all animals were transferred to dry wheels ($< 5\%$ R.H.) and injected with their respective treatments. On day 3 all animals were transferred to wet wheels once again and injected. The injection times for each group were identical. The wheel activity of each animal was continuously monitored. At the end of the experiment the activity record of each animal was counted and a mean value for the 10 animals in each group was obtained (see Table 14.13).

A subsequent ANOVA found a significant group effect, $F(2, 27) = 3.42$, $p <$

Table 14.13 Average Activity Wheel Counts (M ± SEM) for the Three Groups of Animals Across Days

	Day 1	Day 2	Day 3
Control	80 (± 3)	150 (± 5)	84 (± 4)
AII	84 (± 4)	280 (± 10)	87 (± 6)
AII + Sar	87 (± 3)	175 (± 3)	83 (± 7)

.05; a significant day effect, $F(2, 54) = 8.31, p < .001$; and a significant inter-action, Day $\times$ Group, $F(4, 54) = 5.34, p < .01$. Post hoc Neuman-Keuls tests revealed that the AII group had a significantly greater increase in locomotor activity on day 2 than either of the other two groups and that the increase seen in the control versus AII + SAR group on day 2 was not significantly different. Therefore, the biologist concluded that an increase in dehydration-induced loco-motion upon injection of AII occurs in *Limax* and this increase is blocked by administration of AII antagonist Saralasin. The biologist also suggested that the data are consistent with an endogenous release of AII under dehydration stress and that AII might be a regulator of the entire water regulatory repertoire of *Limax*.

Critique

The research hypothesis is whether endogenous angiotensin II would affect the activity increase in *Limax maximus* caused by exposure to drying conditions. The general ANOVA table for the experiment is presented in Table 6.4. The spe-cific ANOVA table for the 3 (Group) $\times$ (3, Day $\times$ S) mixed factorial experiment is

Source	df	Error term
Group	2	S/Group
Day	2	Day $\times$ S/Group
S/Group	27	
Group $\times$ Day	4	
Day $\times$ S/Group	54	Day $\times$ S/Group
Total	89	

The statistical test selected was appropriate. The conclusions of the author are valid. The suggestions of the author are general speculations based upon the obtained data and are not regarded as the major conclusions of the experiment.

RESEARCH DESIGN PROBLEM 73

SD-413A is a steroid derivative which modulates both male and female sex ste-roid activity. In the rat, SD-413A enhances the effects of both estrogen and tes-tosterone and, therefore, may be a useful therapy for individuals suffering from hormonal imbalances associated with decreased sex hormone activity. The clearance (removal of the drug from the body) of SD-413A has been determined in rats but not in humans. In rats SD-413A is well absorbed when given orally, and is metabolized primarily ($> 95\%$) by the liver into inactive products.

To compare these rat findings with data from humans, 30 male and 30 female humans were assigned equally to two treatment groups, one receiving SD-413A orally and the other intravenously. Individuals in both groups had their dosages normalized for body weight. Administration of oral doses in gelatin capsules fol-lowed overnight fasting, and subjects were required to refrain from eating for 4 h following administration. Gelatin capsules had previously been shown to dissolve completely within 45 min after ingestion. In the same manner, intravenous doses were administered following an overnight fast, and these subjects also refrained from food for 4 h after the start of the IV. The IV itself was given over a 45-min period. At regular intervals, plasma levels of the parent drug were determined and plotted to obtain clearance estimates for each subject. Analysis of stool samples in the oral administration group showed no parent compound was present.

A Sex × (Route × Subject) mixed factorial ANOVA was used to evaluate the clearance data. The analysis showed no significant main effect of route nor was the Route × Sex interaction significant. The main effect of sex was significant, $F(1, 56) = 14.97, p < .001$. The researchers concluded that the clearance estimates were not different for route of administration (which was expected given no parent compound in stools). Because the main effect of sex was significant, the researchers also concluded that the drug produced a differential effect on clearance in male compared with female humans.

Critique

The research hypothesis is not stated explicitly. Apparently, the research hypothesis is whether SD-413A given orally or intravenously produces different clearances in males and females. A single measure, clearance rate, was used for each subject even through plasma levels of the parent drug were measured at regular intervals to obtain the clearance estimate. The general ANOVA table for the experiment is presented in Table 6.2. The specific ANOVA table for this experiment is

Source	df	Error term
Route	1	S/Route, Sex
Sex	1	S/Route, Sex
Route × Sex	1	S/Route, Sex
S/Route, Sex	56	
Total	59	

This statistical test was appropriate for a 2 × 2 factorial design. The authors, however, reported that a mixed factorial ANOVA (4.21, Table 6.4) was used to analyze the data. The specific ANOVA table for a Sex × (Route × Subject) mixed factorial design (Table 6.4) for a sample size of 15 (male, female) would be

Source	df		Error term
Sex	1	(1)	S/Sex
Route	1	(1)	Route × S/Sex
S/Sex	28	(58)	
Sex × Route	1	(1)	Route × S/Sex
Route × S/Sex	28	(58)	
Total	59	(119)	

The df values in parentheses ( ) are those that would be correct if a sample size of 30 per group (male, female) was used and two clearance measures (oral and IV treatment) obtained from each subject, that is, 60 subjects $\times$ 2 measures = $120 - 1 = 119$ total degrees of freedom (5.17, 6.5). The reported F-value for the main effect of sex had 1 and 56 df which indicates that a 2×2 factorial design (Table 6.2) was used to analyze the data and the reported design is mistakenly described as a mixed factorial. The confusion regarding sample size is based upon an interpretation of what the authors meant by the statement that ". . . 30 males and 30 females were assigned equally to the two treatment groups. . . ." Notice that the report did not provide the direction of the significant main effect of sex. In short, the authors' conclusion is correct (a significant main effect of sex) but this conclusion is meaningless because the direction of the effect is not presented. The conclusion of the authors is simply a restatement of the F-ratio, that is, a significant sex difference exists.

RESEARCH DESIGN PROBLEM 74

A positive correlation between resting metabolic rate and the ventilatory response to hypoxia (low atmospheric oxygen partial pressure) has been reported in men but not in women. Increasing the metabolic rate by exercise may alter the hypoxic ventilatory response (HVR) and the purpose of the present experiment was to determine if increasing metabolic rate by exercise influenced HVR differently in men and women.

The HVR for 12 women and 12 men was measured at rest, during mild exercise, and during moderate exercise. Exercise measurements were taken in the midmorning for the women and in the midafternoon for the men. Control (rest) values for both groups were measured before their exercise phase of the experiment (see Table 14.14).

A mixed factorial ANOVA was done and a significant sex main effect, $F(1, 22) = 4.58, p < .05$; a significant exercise main effect, $F(2, 44) = 5.31, p < .01$; and a significant Sex $\times$ Exercise interaction, $F(2, 44) = 6.11, p < .01$ were found. A Tukey test was used to analyze the significant Sex $\times$ Exercise interaction with the following results: (a) women did not increase their HVR during mild exercise whereas men did ($p < .05$), (b) the change in HVR from rest to mild exercise was significant in men but not in women ($p < .05$), and (c) mod-

Table 14.14 Mean (M) and Standard Deviation (SD) of Hypoxic Ventilatory Response (HVR) for Males and Females During Exercise

Group	Rest	Mild exercise	Moderate exercise
Women	114 ± 19	119 ± 18	963 ± 96
Men	113 ± 13	163 ± 17	599 ± 67

erate exercise caused the HVR to increase in both sexes ($p < .01$) with women having a higher HVR than men during moderate exercise ($p < .01$).

The authors concluded that a gender difference exists in the influence of metabolic rate during exercise on the respiratory response to hypoxic environments and, therefore, on central ventilatory control.

Critique

The research hypothesis is whether exercise affects differently the hypoxic ventilatory response in men and women. The general ANOVA table for this experiment is presented in Table 6.4. The specific ANOVA table for this experiment is

Source	df	Error term
Sex	1	S/Sex
Exercise	2	Exercise $\times$ S/Sex
S/Sex	22	
Sex $\times$ Exercise	2	Exercise $\times$ S/Sex
Exercise $\times$ S/Sex	44	
Total	71	

The statistical test selected was appropriate. However, a time confound exists in this between-subject experiment (4.19) as the men were tested later in the day than the women. Physiological responses to exercise do differ with time of day and this time confound could be responsible for the sex difference reported. A critical discussion of exercise cycles and sex differences might have explained away this time confound but a simple counterbalancing procedure (4.20) would have eliminated the design problem, that is, one-half of the males tested during midmorning and one-half of the females tested during midafternoon. Error variance may be increased with this counterbalancing procedure but a significant effect could be generalized across times. An analysis using time as a factor would also provide additional information but the small sample size ($n = 6$) would have to be considered.

Metabolic rates were not measured in this study and, therefore, rate changes in the two sexes induced by exercise cannot be determined. The descriptive terms of mild and moderate exercise are not precise and would probably not be the same for both males and females.

RESEARCH DESIGN PROBLEM 75

Opioid peptides may act as brain neurotransmitters and the amygdala is rich in both opiate receptors and enkephalins. The amygdala, a limbic system structure, appears to participate in memory processes, particularly for aversive experiences. Therefore, an experiment was done to determine whether the amygdala opioid peptide system was involved in the learning and memory of an aversively motivated task. Male rats were surgically implanted with guide cannulae positioned at the dorsal surface of the amygdala ($n = 30$) or positioned in the basal ganglia ($n = 20$) approximately 1.0 mm dorsal to the amygdala (the latter group served as a control). Ten male rats received no surgery. All rats were about the same age and weight.

Following 1 week of post-operative recovery all rats were trained in a passive avoidance task. On day 1, each rat was placed in the lit compartment of a two-compartment apparatus. As the rat stepped into a dark compartment through an open door it received a footshock (1 mA, 2 sec). Retention of passive avoidance was measured 24 h later (day 2) when each animal was placed again in the lit compartment and time to enter the dark compartment was recorded. Longer latencies on day 2 (i.e., time between start of trial and entry into the dark compartment) indicate better memory of the previous aversive event. Immediately following the training trial on day 1, animals were injected bilaterally through the implanted cannulae with either the opiate agonist levorphanol, the opiate antagonist naloxone, or Krebs-Ringer phosphate vehicle solution.

Cannulae placements were determined histologically for all operated animals at the end of the experiment. Cannula tip placements were rated as unacceptable if they were (1) more than .5 mm dorsal or ventral to the dorsal surface of the amygdala, (2) more than .2 mm anterior or posterior to the coronal plane at bregma, (3) lateral to the external capsule or with any medial damage to the optic tract. Only animals with bilaterally acceptable cannulae placements were included in the data analysis (see Table 14.15).

A Mann-Whitney U test (two-tailed) performed between the unoperated and vehicle-injected control groups revealed no significant difference ($p > .10$). Therefore, the data from these two groups were pooled into a single control group for the purpose of further statistical analysis. In Table 14.15, the following letter symbols indicate:

(a) Independent Mann-Whitney U tests (two-tailed) revealed that each of these groups did not differ from the pooled control group data ($p > .10$).

(b) A Mann-Whitney U test (two-tailed) between this group and the pooled control data revealed a significant difference ($p < .002$).

Table 14.15 Retention Latencies on Day 2

Group	n	Median (sec)	Interquartile range (sec)
Control groups			
Unoperated	10	189	105–427
Vehicle injected	10	172	147–351
Basal ganglia			
Levorphanol (5.0 nmol)	8	148[a]	123–350
Naloxane (2.5 nmol)	7	211[a]	150–300
Amygdala			
Levorphanol (5.0 nmol)	7	22[b]	17–50
Naloxane (2.5 nmol)	8	600[c]	486–600

(*c*) A Mann-Whitney U test (two-tailed) between this group and the pooled control data revealed a significant difference ($p < .02$).

From these comparisons, the authors concluded that, when delivered to the amygdala, levorphanol impaired performance, and naloxone improved performance of the male rat on the passive avoidance task. The authors also suggested that the opioid peptide system in the amygdala may be involved in memory processes for aversive events, although further research is necessary to elucidate this possibility.

Critique

The research hypothesis is whether levorphanol (an opiate agonist) and naloxone (an opiate antagonist) when applied to the dorsal surface of the amygdala affects the passive avoidance learning of the male rat. Multiple Mann-Whitney U tests were performed but the slight increase in familywise error would not change the conclusions (6.9, 10.1). Because of the unequal sample size the nonparametric Kruskal-Wallis test could not be used (11.6), but the unequal *n*'s in the comparisons should not have any significant effect on the Mann-Whitney U test (11.5).

RESEARCH DESIGN PROBLEM 76

The amount of sugar in the diet has been suggested to be correlated with behavioral problems in hyperactive children. To test this hypothesis, mothers of 108 hyperactive children kept a daily record of the food intake of their children for 1 week. Detail and accuracy were emphasized and the mothers were instructed not to alter the child's normal diet during the recording week. The amount of sugar (g/day) was estimated from these dietary records, and children were assigned to one of the following three groups based upon their sugar consumption:

High sugar consumption	320–400 g/day ($n = 36$)
Moderate sugar consumption	250–300 g/day ($n = 42$)
Low sugar consumption	Less than 225 g/day ($n = 30$)

These three groups did not differ significantly on family income, mothers' level of education, occupational status for the head of the household, family size, or sex. Also, none of the children were on medication during the experiment.

The children were videotaped through a one-way mirror while playing alone in a playroom during two 45-min sessions. The tapes were scored on three behavioral categories by two trained observers who did not know the group classification of the child. The categories were destruction/aggression (i.e., hitting, kicking, attempts to damage objects), restlessness (i.e., repetition of arm, leg, head, or finger movements), and quadrant crossings (i.e., number of times child moved from one quadrant of the room to another). Analyses of variance with repeated measures were done on each of the three measures (Table 14.16).

Table 14.16 Mean Behavioral Measures for Groups and ANOVA Tables

Sugar consumption group	Incidence of destruction/ agression (mean for session)		Restlessness rating (mean for session)		Quadrant crossings (mean for session)	
	1	2	1	2	1	2
High	6.2	7.1	9.6	9.8	29.8	32.4
Moderate	4.8	6.1	5.9	5.3	21.0	19.4
Low	7.4	4.9	5.0	5.6	18.9	22.9

Source of variance	F-values	F-values	F-values
Group	1.09	6.78[a]	7.46[a]
Session	.78	.97	.66
Group × Session	.56	.89	1.18

[a] $p < .01$

Post hoc Newman-Kuels tests showed that for restlessness and quadrant cross-ings the high sugar consumption group was significantly different from both the moderate and low groups ($p < .05$), and there was no difference between the moderate and low sugar consumption groups.

The authors concluded that although decreasing the sugar consumption of hyperactive children would not significantly reduce aggressive/destructive behavior, it would significantly reduce hyperactivity as measured by restlessness and quadrant crossings.

Critique

The research question is whether dietary sugar intake is correlated with behav-ioral problems (aggression, restlessness, and activity) in hyperactive children. The general ANOVA for the study is presented in Table 6.4. The specific ANOVA table for the study is

Source	df	Error term
Group	2	S/Group
Session	1	Session × S/Group
S/Group	105	
Group × Session	2	Session × S/Group
Session × S/Group	105	
Total	215	

Because of the unequal group size, the df formulas for equal sample size can-not be used to calculate df's. Although the scale of measurement (5.3) used for the destruction/aggression category may be ordinal, ANOVAs on the number of repetition counts and quadrant crossings can easily be defended. However, this study is not an experiment because sugar consumption was not manipulated by the researcher (4.1, 4.4). Hence, a cause-and-effect relation between sugar consumption and hyperactivity is not valid for this classification study (4.2). Restricting a hyperactive child's diet (to decrease sugar consumption in the high group) might exacerbate behavioral problems. The research question was to determine whether a correlation between the amount of dietary sugar and behavioral problems existed in hyperactive children. An association was found but the authors concluded that by manipulating dietary sugar the hyperactivity of the child could also be affected. This conclusion implies a cause-and-effect relation which is inappropriate.

RESEARCH DESIGN PROBLEM 77

Granulocytes and macrophages, cells of great importance in the body's immune response, are derived from a common, undifferentiated precursor cell in the organs of the body involved in immune responsiveness (e.g., spleen and liver). These undifferentiated precursor cells (progenitor cells) differentiate into both granulocytes and macrophages when exposed to a low-molecular-weight glycoprotein called the granulocyte-macrophage colony-stimulating factor (GM-CSF). The progenitor cells found throughout the body are genetically identical as they are derived from a common stem cell early in development. Because differing immune responses result in the preferential production of granulocytes or macrophages (yet both are postulated to be controlled by GM-CSF release) a change in the concentration of the chemical signal (GM-CSF) may elicit preferential differentiation from the same progenitor cells within an organ.

To determine whether preferential granulocyte or macrophage production was caused by the concentration of GM-CSF released in different immune responses, progenitor cells (selected randomly from 30 mice) were randomly assigned to agar plates (four cells chosen from each mouse, one cell from each animal was assigned to each of the four groups tested, $n = 120$ total cells with 30 cells in each treatment group). The four treatment groups used were (1) high concentration (2500 units) GM-CSF, (2) low concentration (50 units) GM-CSF, (3) vehicle alone, and (4) no perturbation at all. In each plate the cell cycle time, cell density (number of cells within a cluster derived from the same progenitor cell), and cell identity (i.e., whether cells within individual clusters were granulocytes or macrophages) were recorded.

Two percent of the cells in the vehicle plate produced clusters of granulocytes or macrophages and 5 percent of the cells in the non-injection plate produced clusters of either granulocytes or macrophages. The mean number of cells per cluster in the vehicle-only plate was 32 ± 2 (mean $\pm$ SEM), and the cell cycle time was 24 ± 6 h. The mean cell density per cluster in the non-injection plate was 37 ± 7 and the cell cycle time was 20 ± 9 h. In contrast, the high GM-CSF plate had a short cell cycle (3.5 ± 2.5), high mean cell density (2500 ± 100), and 68 percent of the clusters were composed entirely of granulocytes. The low GM-CSF plate had a longer mean cycle time (10 ± 2.0), lower cell density per cluster

(70 ± 15), and 70 percent of the clusters were composed entirely of macrophages.

The authors found a significant difference between plates in the composition of the clusters (chi-square = 27.4, $p < .001$) with the high GM-CSF producing mostly granulocytes, the low GM-CSF producing mostly macrophages, and neither of the controls producing significant levels of either. From these results the authors concluded that the differentiation of progenitor cells was determined, at least in part, by the concentration of GM-CSF present and that high concentrations of GM-CSF result in granulocytes and low concentrations of GM-CSF result in macrophages. Furthermore, the authors concluded that granulocytes have a shorter cell cycle time and greater density per cluster as they differentiate compared with macrophages.

Critique

The research hypothesis is whether the concentration of GM-CSF determines preferentially granulocyte or macrophage production. The general ANOVA table for the randomized-blocks design used in this study is presented in Tables 4.5 and 9.3. The specific ANOVA table for this experiment is

Source	df	Error term
Cells	29	
Treatment	3	Cells × Treatment
Cells × Treatment	87	
Total	119	

This statistical test could be used to determine whether significant treatment effects existed for cell cycle time, cell density, and cell identity (number). If the main effect of treatment was significant, subsequent multiple comparisons tests would be required to determine significant differences among the four treatment means (6.8, Chapter 10).

The statistical analyses used, however, were individual chi-square (11.2) tests and this nonparametric statistical analysis of the raw data supported the authors' conclusions (5.22, 11.1). The descriptive statistics (means and standard errors of the means) also support the authors' conclusion. The standard error of the mean should be converted to the standard deviation to determine the variability in each of the sample treatment groups (5.2).

RESEARCH DESIGN PROBLEM 78

Sodium (Na^+) plays a key role in the management and possibly the etiology of hypertension (HTN). An altered Na^+ transport system in red blood cells (RBCs) may exist in the hypertensive person compared with the normotensive person. To test this hypothesis, blood was obtained from five newly diagnosed hypertensive patients without prior medical management (diastolic blood pressure, bp > 100 mmHg and with a family history for HTN) and from five normotensive

Table 14.17 Mean ^{22}Na Influx ($\pm$ Standard Deviation, SD) in the Two Groups

Group	(μM/L cells/h) $\pm$ SD
HTN	637 $\pm$ 132
Normotensive	470 $\pm$ 105

patients (diastolic bp $<$ 85 mmHg, matched for weight, age, and sex to the HTN group and with no family history for HTN). Cells were isolated and triplicate ^{22}Na influx studies were performed on all blood samples under identical conditions using a single-blind procedure (Table 14.17).

A between-subject ANOVA was used for statistical analysis and the group effect was not significant, $F(1, 8) = 4.90$, $p > .05$. The authors concluded that ^{22}Na influx in RBCs does not differ significantly between hypertensive and normotensive patients and, consequently, sodium transport differences do not contribute to the pathophysiology of hypertension.

Critique

The research hypothesis is whether a difference in ^{22}Na influx occurs in the red blood cells of hypertensive patients compared with normotensive patients. The general ANOVA table for this study is presented in Table 6.1. The specific ANOVA table for this study is

Source	df	Error term
Group	1	S/Group
S/Group	8	
Total	9	

The statistical test selected was appropriate. The t-test which is used normally to test for a significant difference between the means of two groups is a special case of the F-ratio (5.18). However, the power of the statistical test (between-subject ANOVA, 1.5) is low given the small sample size (5.13). The authors appear to be proving the null hypothesis which is logically impossible (5.5). In this study an $F(1, 8)$ value of 5.32 would be required for $p < .05$ and an F-value of 4.90 was obtained. It is likely, therefore, that by increasing sample size and thereby increasing the power of the statistical test (5.15) a significant difference between the two groups would be obtained. Because classification variables were used to select the two groups (4.2), a significant difference between the two groups would have to be interpreted cautiously.

RESEARCH DESIGN PROBLEM 79

Evidence for mimicry of expressions has been reported in studies in which the tension levels in the facial muscles of people are measured while they are shown photographs of various facial expressions. When the people saw an angry face, for instance, their facial muscles mimicked the anger as measured by EMG's. There is a belief that married couples, through mimicry of expressions, eventually begin to look alike. To test this hypothesis, college students were presented a random array of 48 photographs of faces, with the backgrounds blacked out. The students were instructed to match each man with the woman who most closely resembled him. Two dozen of the photographs were of couples when first married and another two dozen were of the same couples 25 years later.

The young couples were judged by the college students to have only a chance similarity to each other whereas a significant resemblance was found between the couples who had been married a quarter-century ($p < .05$). The authors concluded that the increase in facial similarity observed in the present study was the result of shared emotions during a lifetime. Thus, people often unconsciously mimic the facial expressions of their spouses in a silent empathy and that, over the years, sharing the same expressions shapes the faces similarly. The authors also suggested that shared facial expressions bring on identical emotions because facial muscles are involved in regulating blood flow to the brain. Hence, a given facial expression may trigger the brain neurotransmitters that evoke the associated feeling. Consequently, when people mimic their spouses' facial expressions, they also evoke the same emotions, thereby empathizing all the better.

Critique

The research hypothesis is whether photographs of old married individuals are more likely to be matched with their correct spouses than are photographs of the same individuals taken when they were 25 years younger. Common life experiences over years could alter facial muscles and wrinkle patterns leading to an increased resemblance. For example, similar diets and activities (walking, running, etc.) over the years and the deposits of fatty tissues may contribute to the resemblance. Hence, mimicking of facial expressions or experiencing similar emotions may not be involved in the increased similarity of married couple's faces observed in this study. The explanations of facial tensions, differential blood flow to the brain, and associated feelings are speculations and should not be confused with the authors' primary conclusion that ". . . the increase in facial similarity . . . was the result of shared emotions during a lifetime."

The generalization of the findings beyond the specific set of photographs used might also be of concern in the present study. It would be important to know how the photographs were selected and by whom because a bias may have been introduced before the study was done by a selection of photographs by the experimenters or by the married couples themselves. For example, only one or two photographs might have been available for selection when the couples were young and many may have been available right before the study was started. The couples may have selected the best photograph from a wide selection of pictures before the study. The best photograph may have been the one that both of the individuals looked the best as judged by the individuals. Both may have similar facial expressions because they both now respond to the photographer's jokes in the same way. In this case, therefore, the selection of the sample of photographs may have affected the outcome of the study.

RESEARCH DESIGN PROBLEM 80

Acute and subacute methylmercury toxicity has been found in many species. However, the effects of long-term chronic ingestion of methylmercury, at levels which do not produce overt toxicity, have not been determined. The effect of prolonged ingestion of low levels of methylmercury was studied in 60 male and 60 female weanling Wistar rats (60–70 g) fed diets containing mercury in doses of 0, .002, .01, .05, or .25 mg Hg per day. Rats were observed daily for signs of toxicity and body weights were measured at 3, 6, 12, 18, and 26 months. After 26 months the study was terminated and all animals sacrificed. Samples of blood, liver, and kidney from the 12 rats in each group were analyzed for total mercury concentration.

No overt signs of toxicity were observed during the study period. Differences between the means (treated-control and male-female) were assessed using t-tests (two-tailed) maintaining an overall significance level of 5 percent for all comparisons within each time-sex category through the use of the Bonferroni inequality. Results showed that, in general, mean body weights of treated rats were lower than controls and the male rats weighed more than the female rats. Both male and female rats receiving .05 and .25 mg Hg/day had reduced weights ($p < .05$) at 12, 18, and 26 months compared with their respective controls. Mean mercury concentrations ($\pm$ SEM) for the various tissue samples after 26 months are presented in Table 14.18.

Statistical analysis showed that all treatment groups had significantly higher ($p < .05$) mercury levels than their respective controls for each tissue analyzed. There were no sex-related differences within the control group tissues; however, there were significant differences ($p < .05$) between the two sexes for mercury in the kidney at all treatment doses. The authors concluded that in future studies with methylmercury kidney concentrations should be monitored because they were usually higher than for any other tissue tested and might be the most appro-

Table 14.18 Mercury Concentrations for Tissues from the Groups (Mean Hg Concentration $\pm$ SEM)

Dose mg/day	Sex	Number of rats	Whole blood	Liver	Kidney
0	Male	12	.10 ± .04	.11 ± .02	.36 ± .06
	Female	12	.17 ± .07	.07 ± .01	.23 ± .02
.002	Male	12	.52 ± .04	.31 ± .02	2.04 ± .20
	Female	12	.92 ± .11[a]	.82 ± .15[a]	5.11 ± .47[a]
.010	Male	12	4.61 ± .47	1.80 ± .15	8.3 ± .50
	Female	12	5.32 ± .36	2.02 ± .11[a]	13.9 ± 1.1[a]
.050	Male	12	29.8 ± 2.8	7.92 ± .60	26.7 ± 3.0
	Female	12	36.1 ± 2.8	9.36 ± .63	45.4 ± 1.8[a]
.250	Male	12	107.8 ± 9.9	36.9 ± 3.6	30.2 ± 2.4
	Female	12	124.5 ± 6.9	42.9 ± 1.5	59.5 ± 4.1[a]

[a]Significant difference between sexes ($p < .05$) for a given dose.

priate predictor of methylmercury toxicity. In addition, the authors also concluded that if methylmercury toxicity is related to kidney concentration then females should be more sensitive than males because they accumulate more there.

Critique

The research hypothesis is whether chronic ingestion of low levels of methylmercury produces different effects in male and female rats. The general ANOVA table for this experiment is presented in Table 6.7. The specific ANOVA table for the 2 (Sex) $\times$ 5 (Dose) $\times$ 5 (Day $\times$ Subject) mixed factorial design is

Source	df	Error term
Sex	1	S/Sex, Dose
Dose	4	S/Sex, Dose
Day (Months)[a]	4	Day $\times$ S/Sex, Dose
S/Sex, Dose	110	
Sex $\times$ Dose	4	S/Sex, Dose
Sex $\times$ Day	4	Day $\times$ S/Sex, Dose
Dose $\times$ Day	16	Day $\times$ S/Sex, Dose
Sex $\times$ Dose $\times$ Day	16	Day $\times$ S/Sex, Dose
Day $\times$ S/Sex, Dose	440	
Total	599	

[a]Number of days would be more precise than months for length of treatment as the days in months vary.

This statistical test would be approximate for body weight measurements. Three 2 (Sex) $\times$ 5 (Dose) factorial ANOVA analyses would be done to evaluate the total mercury concentrations in the blood, liver, and kidney (but see 6.17). The general ANOVA table for these analyses is presented in Table 6.2. The specific ANOVA table for these analyses is

Source	df	Error term
Sex	1	S/Sex, Dose
Dose	4	S/Sex, Dose
Sex $\times$ Dose	4	S/Sex, Dose
S/Sex, Dose	110	
Total	119	

In these analyses the within-subject component (days) has been eliminated because only *one* measure is taken for *each* tissue sample. Rather than use an overall ANOVA followed by appropriate multiple comparison tests (10.1) the authors used the Bonferroni t-test (10.7). But, this test becomes very conservative when many pairwise comparisons are made, that is, with an increase in the number of comparisons the Bonferroni t-procedure overestimates the true probability of making a Type 1 error (5.10, 5.11). Fortunately, most of the comparisons were significant (Table 14.18).

Unfortunately, this experiment is confounded because the concentration of

Hg fed daily was not normalized for body weight changes over time. Because females did not gain as much weight as males (but were fed the same concentrations of Hg) it is not surprising that they accumulate more Hg in their kidneys compared with males. In fact, all tissues showed the same sex trend but differences were not always significant between sexes (see Table 14.18). Also, the increase in tissue concentration with increasing dose is confounded because animals at higher doses had significantly lower body weights than their respective controls (and also lower body weights than animals at lower doses).

RESEARCH DESIGN PROBLEM 81

A newly developed drug, gepirone, has anxiolytic properties (reduction in anxiety) similar to the commonly prescribed drug diazepam (Valium). Diazepam also increases appetite and decreases spontaneous locomotor activity in rats. A previous study comparing the effects of diazepam and gepirone on food intake in rats found that at equal doses, Valium increased food intake whereas gepirone decreased food intake. Hence, the two drugs have similar anxiolytic properties but produce different effects on appetite.

To determine whether gepirone had any effect on locomotor activity 30 male rats were randomly assigned to two groups: a drug-treated group that received gepirone (3 mg/kg, IP) and a saline-control group. Activity was monitored in a sound-attenuating chamber equipped with 14 infrared emitters and detectors, 8 being spaced at 10-cm intervals along the length of the chamber and 6 along the width of the chamber at a height of 5 and 15 cm above the grid floor. The design allowed for an estimate of both horizontal activity (i.e., running and walking) and vertical activity (i.e., rearing or jumping). The animals were injected with their appropriate drug 10 min prior to the start of a 2-h activity monitoring test in the chamber.

A t-test on vertical activity showed that there was no difference between the two groups, $t(28) = 1.62$, NS. A t-test on horizontal activity showed that the gepirone-treated group was significantly less active than the saline-control group, $t(28) = 1.71$, $p < .05$, one-tailed. The pharmacologist concluded that 3 mg/kg gepirone, like diazepam, decreases spontaneous locomotor activity (running and walking) in male rats.

Critique

The research hypothesis is whether gepirone affects locomotor activity in rats. The general ANOVA table for this experiment is presented in Table 6.1. The specific ANOVA table for this experiment is

Source	df	Error term
Drug	1	S/Drug
S/Drug	28	
Total	29	

The t-test is a special case of the F-ratio (5.18), and the statistical test used was appropriate. Because there was no a priori reason that gepirone would only produce hypoactivity (decrease activity), a one-tailed test is not appropriate (5.20). Indeed, the research hypothesis reported in the brief was to determine what effect (if any) gepirone had on locomotor activity in rats. This research hypothesis is nondirectional; hence, the pharmacologist's conclusion based upon a significant difference between the two groups on a directional test should be rejected. Obviously, the research hypothesis could be rephrased after the data were collected to ". . . determine whether gepirone, like diazepam, decreases spontaneous locomotor activity. . . ." For this reason, the use of a one-tailed t-test is viewed with skepticism by most reviewers (5.20).

RESEARCH DESIGN PROBLEM 82

A pharmacologist interested in weight control wanted to determine whether a new drug (BK346) affected the body weights of rats. In the experiment 15 male and 15 female adult rats were randomized into control, low-dose (1 mg/kg), and high-dose (10 mg/kg) groups ($n = 5$ male and 5 female per group).

Each rat was weighed on day 1, and daily IP injections of BK346 or vehicle were begun at 9 A.M. All further injections were also given at 9 A.M. Food and water were available *ad lib* and food intake was monitored by housing animals in single cages and weighing food presented and recovered for each 24 h. Body weights were measured weekly for five weeks and rats receiving 1 mg/kg of BK346 showed no change in weight, whereas the rats receiving 10 mg/kg of the drug lost weight. All control animals gained weight. Analysis of the body weight data indicated a significant main effect of dose, $F(2, 24) = 3.47, p < .05$, and a significant Dose $\times$ Week interaction, $F(8, 96) = 2.10, p < .05$. The main effects of week and of sex and all of the other interactions were not significant. A separate analysis of the food intake data failed to reveal any significant relationships, although rats on 10 mg/kg·day tended to eat less than the others.

The pharmacologist concluded that because of the significant Dose $\times$ Week interaction, the drug's effect on body weight of rats would be unpredictable over time and for this reason the drug could not be reliably used for controlling body weight.

Critique

The research hypothesis is whether the drug BK346 affects differentially body weight changes in male and female rats. The general ANOVA table for this experiment is presented in Table 6.7. The specific ANOVA table for this 2 (Sex) $\times$ 3 (Dose) $\times$ 5 (Body Weight $\times$ Subject) mixed factorial design is

Source	df	Error term
Sex	1	S/Sex, Dose
Dose	2	S/Sex, Dose
Week	4	Week × S/Sex, Dose
S/Sex, Dose	24	
Sex × Dose	2	S/Sex, Dose
Sex × Week	4	Week × S/Sex, Dose
Dose × Week	8	Week × S/Sex, Dose
Sex × Dose × Week	8	Week × S/Sex, Dose
Week × S/Sex, Dose	96	
Total	149	

The statistical test selected was appropriate. However, the pharmacologist misinterpreted the significant Dose × Week interaction (6.12, 6.13) by assuming that an A × B interaction implies that the data across weeks are unreliable. The research hypothesis is evaluated by first determining whether the Sex × Dose × Week interaction is significant. This interaction was reported to be not significant; consequently, the significant Dose × Week interaction indicates that the dose changes across weeks are similar in males and females. A graphic plot of the averaged 15 means would provide information for the proper interpretation of the Dose × Week interaction. A trend analysis (6.16) of body weight changes across the five weeks of the experiment may be a more reasonable analysis for interpreting the significant Dose × Week interaction than numerous post hoc pairwise mean comparison tests (10.1).

RESEARCH DESIGN PROBLEM 83

In the adult animal, visual cortical neurons have orientation preferences for stimuli presented in their retinal receptive fields. In the mature cat, for example, some neurons (about 10% of the sample) respond selectively to vertical bars and other neurons (about 10% of the sample) respond selectively to horizontal bars. The other neurons (80% of the sample) respond to bars tilted to other degrees.

To determine whether postnatal visual pattern experience produces these neuronal orientation preferences a neurophysiologist randomly assigned 30 kittens to three visual rearing conditions. Optical devices were placed over the eyes of each kitten before normal eye opening occurred. With these devices, a plus (+) pattern was presented continuously to 10 kittens, a vertical bar (|) pattern to another 10 kittens, and a horizontal bar (–) pattern to the remaining 10 kittens.

All kittens wore these devices for at least 3 months and were kept healthy by daily handling and feeding. Standard neurophysiological procedures were then used to determine the responsiveness of individual visual cortical neurons when each kitten was exposed in a counterbalanced order to vertical (V) and horizontal (H) bars. The H or V preference orientation of each neuron was determined before another neuron was sampled. Microelectrode recordings were taken from as many neurons as possible in each kitten by using systematic and extensive

Table 14.19   Orientations for Rearing Groups

Rearing group	Number of kittens	Mean number of neurons per cat responding selectively to bars ± SD	
		Vertical bar	Horizontal bar
+ Group	10	24.6 ± 2.1	25.8 ± 1.8
| Group	10	25.8 ± 2.0	1.9* ± 0.1
− Group	10	1.8* ± 0.2	26.1 ± 2.0

penetrations of the left visual hemisphere. (The bars were presented simultaneously to both the left and right eyes during these recordings.) Because only one kitten could be tested daily, the scheduling of kittens in the three rearing groups was counterbalanced and all kittens wore their devices until recordings were taken. Furthermore, the neurophysiologist doing the recordings did not know the prior history of the kitten.

At the end of the experiment the data presented in Table 14.19 were available. A 3 × 2 mixed factorial ANOVA indicated a significant group effect, $F(2, 27) = 5.69, p < .01$, and a significant Group × Orientation interaction, $F(2, 27) = 14.61, p < .001$. The main effect of orientation was not significant, $F(1, 27) = 1.34$. Newman-Keuls post hoc tests of the significant Group × Orientation interaction indicated that those means with the * were not significantly different from each other but both were significantly different from all other means. None of the other means differed significantly from each other. From these findings the neurophysiologist wanted to conclude that postnatal pattern experience was necessary for any orientation preferences to be observed in visual cortical neurons. Being careful, however, the neurophysiologist concluded that exposure to either vertical or horizontal bars during postnatal development was necessary for visual cortical neurons of the young cat to have either vertical or horizontal orientation preferences.

Critique

The research hypothesis is whether postnatal exposure to a vertical line and a horizontal line is necessary for visual cortical neurons to have vertical and horizontal orientation preferences. The general ANOVA for the 3 × 2 mixed factorial design used in this experiment is presented in Table 6.4. The specific ANOVA for this experiment is

Source	df	Error term
Group (G)	2	S/Group
Orientation (O)	1	O × S/Group
S/Group	27	
G × O	2	O × S/Group
O × S/Group	27	
Total	59	

The statistical test selected was appropriate. However, when kittens are reared viewing a plus (+) pattern about 50 neurons are observed in the visual cortex, half of which respond to a vertical bar and half of which respond to a horizontal bar (see Table 14.19). In contrast, the kittens in each of the bar-reared groups had only around 25 neurons in their visual cortex that responded to their respective rearing orientation. This difference among the three groups is the basis for the reported significant group effect, $F(2, 27) = 5.69, p < .01$. The question that must be answered is what happened to the other 25 neurons in both of the two bar groups compared with the plus (+) pattern group? A selective loss of neurons based upon treatment conditions (4.12) occurred and whether this loss could affect the author's conclusions must be determined. A selective loss may imply that without adequate visual stimulation certain cortical neurons may die *or* may not become large enough for reliable neurophysiological measurements to be taken. If the latter alternative is correct, the author's interpretation is wrong because exposure to the bars would not be necessary for cortical neurons to have orientation preferences. Postnatal exposure would only be necessary to increase neuronal size so that reliable recordings with microelectrodes could be made from neurons that already had specific orientation preferences. Suppose that the following data from the same experiment were obtained:

Group	Vertical bar (mean ± SD)	Horizontal bar (mean ± SD)
+ Group	24 ± 2.1	25 ± 1.8
∣ Group	48 ± 2.0	1.9 ± .1
– Group	1.8 ± .2	47 ± 2.0

From these data, it is evident that the Group × Orientation interaction (6.13) would be significant but neither main effect (group, orientation) would be significant (6.7). From these data, the neurophysiologist could conclude that exposure to either vertical or horizontal bars during postnatal development was necessary for visual cortical neurons of the young cat to have either vertical or horizontal orientation preferences. Hence, although the two-way interaction (A × B) serves a critical role in the analysis of a two-factor design (6.13), a significant main effect and the pattern of mean results are also important in deciding what conclusions may be made.

RESEARCH DESIGN PROBLEM 84

D-652 is a new beta-blocker drug (i.e., inhibits heart rate increases due to sympathetic tone) which has an extended half-life of 24 h, a time significantly greater than the 6-h half-life of the commonly used beta-blocker propranolol. The next phase in D-652 development was to verify its predicted increased potency over propranolol, a prediction based upon a structural comparison of the two drugs.

To test this hypothesis, 50 Sprague-Dawley rats were obtained from a university colony (290–300 g; 25 males, 25 females). In all rats, during an initial 2-day

Table 14.20   Mean (M) Heart Rates ($\pm$ SD) for the Three
Drug Conditions

Drug	Females (M $\pm$ SD)		Males (M $\pm$ SD)	
	Pre	Post	Pre	Post
Vehicle	98(6)	106(7)	97(7)	105(6)
D-652	96(4)	63(10)	95(5)	51(7)
Propranolol	85(7)	59(6)	81(4)	49(6)

period baseline heart rate was determined, vehicle was injected IP on each day
and heart rate again determined 2 h following the injection (heart rate was the
average rate per minute after 30 min of monitoring). This procedure was
repeated for 2 days with D-652 (1 mg) being injected and then again for 2 more
days with propranolol (equal molar dose as D-652) being injected (see Table
14.20).

A mixed factorial ANOVA was used for statistical analysis [2 $\times$ (3 $\times$ 2 $\times$
25)]. A significant Sex $\times$ Drug $\times$ Time interaction was observed, $F(2, 96) =$
3.99, $p < .025$. Post hoc multiple comparisons tests revealed postheart rates to
be significantly different between males and females for both D-652 and propranolol, $p < .01$. In addition, pre– and post–heart rates were significantly different for D-652 and propranolol ($p < .001$) but not for vehicle. Post–heart rates
between propranolol and D-652 were not significant.

The authors concluded that D-652 and propranolol are equal in potency for
lowering heart rate. In addition, they concluded that males are more responsive
to beta-blockers than females which could represent increased resting sympathetic tone in males.

Critique

The research hypothesis is whether D-652 has a greater effect than propranolol
on the heart rates of male and female rats. The general ANOVA table for this
experiment is presented in Table 6.9. The specific ANOVA table for this 2 $\times$ (2
$\times$ 2 $\times$ S) mixed factorial design is

Source	df	Error term
Sex	1	S/Sex
Drug	2	Drug $\times$ S/Sex
Time	1	Time $\times$ S/Sex
S/Sex	48	
Sex $\times$ Drug	2	Drug $\times$ S/Sex
Sex $\times$ Time	1	Time $\times$ S/Sex
Drug $\times$ Time	2	Drug $\times$ Time $\times$ S/Sex
Drug $\times$ S/Sex	96	
Time $\times$ S/Sex	48	
Drug $\times$ Time $\times$ S/Sex	96	
Sex $\times$ Drug $\times$ Time	2	Drug $\times$ Time $\times$ S/Sex
Total	299	

Although not stated explicitly the measurements taken during each of the 2-day drug periods must have been averaged. The degrees of freedom for the significant Sex × Drug × Time interaction, $F(2, 96)$, indicates that averaged values were used. If the day values were not averaged then a 2 (Sex) × 3 (Dose) × 2 (Day) × 2 (Time) mixed factorial design would have been used with repeated measures on the last three factors, that is, a 2 × (3 × 2 × 2 × S) design (6.15).

The statistical test reported was appropriate. However, many problems exist with this brief. A carry-over treatment confound is apparent in this mixed factorial design (4.19, 4.22). As reported, D-652 has a half-life of 24 h and propranolol was given to the same animal just 24 h after the last injection of D-652; consequently, at least 25 percent of the original D-652 dose was still present in the animal at the time of its propranolol injection. Notice that the mean heart rates of the rats before propranolol was injected were lower that the preinjection values for either the vehicle or D-652 days. A counterbalancing procedure (4.20) would not eliminate the carry-over treatment confound in this experiment. A counterbalancing procedure would only result in greater experimental variability as one-half of the animals would be studied under the combined influence of two drugs and the other half only under the influence of one drug (given the 6-h half-life of propranolol). A substantial time period would have to be used between the counterbalanced treatment periods to avoid this type of carry-over effect (4.19).

It is not clear what comparisons are being made to evaluate the significant three-way interaction (6.14). Actually a significant two-way Drug × Time interaction is being evaluated in some of the comparisons but a significant Drug × Time interaction was not reported (6.13).

RESEARCH DESIGN PROBLEM 85

The opioid peptide system in the amygdala appears to be involved in learning and memory of aversively motivated tasks (i.e., opiate agonists such as levorphanol impair performance and opiate antagonists such as naloxone improve performance). The aim of the present study was to determine whether these drug-behavioral effects would generalize to appetite-motivated tasks.

Rats were surgically implanted bilaterally with guide cannulae positioned at the dorsal surface of the amygdala ($n = 30$) and were then randomly assigned to one of three drug conditions: levorphanol 5.0 nmol, naloxone 2.5 nmol, or Krebs ringer solution. Following one week of postoperative recovery all animals were trained in a Y-maze task. The maze had a start box located at the base of the Y and goal boxes located at the end of the branches (arms) of the Y. Rats usually show a natural preference for turning down one of the arms. On the first day, both arms were baited with a food reward and the rat's preferred arm was determined. On the subsequent acquisition days, only the nonpreferred arm was baited with food, and the rats had to learn to go to that arm. Entries into the preferred (unbaited) arm were considered errors. The rats were given 10 trials a day for 4 consecutive days, and were infused with their appropriate drug 15 min before training.

At the end of behavioral training cannulae placements were determined his-

Table 14.21   Mean Number of Errors for the Three Groups

		Days			
Group	n	1	2	3	4
Krebs	6	7.1	4.9	4.8	4.1
Levorphanol	5	6.2	6.1	5.2	4.4
Naloxone	9	5.8	5.7	3.7	1.8[a]

[a]Significant from other two groups, $p < .05$.

tologically for all operated animals. Cannula tip placements were rated as unacceptable if they were (1) more than .5 mm dorsal or ventral to the dorsal surface of the amygdala, (2) more than .2 mm anterior or posterior to the coronal plane at bregma, (3) lateral to the external capsule or with any medial damage to the optic tract. Only animals with bilaterally acceptable cannulae placements were included in the data analysis, and the mean number of errors for each group is shown in Table 14.21.

Mean errors were analyzed using a 3 (Drug) $\times$ 4 (Day) ANOVA with repeated measures for unequal n. The main effect of drug was not significant, $F(2, 17) = .69$. The effect of day was significant, $F(3, 51) = 13.9, p < .01$, and the Drug $\times$ Day interaction was significant, $F(6, 51) = 2.30, p < .05$. To analyze the interaction, post hoc comparisons using Duncan's multiple range test were made between the means for each group on each of the 4 days. The results showed that there was no difference among treatment means of any of the groups on days 1–3. However, on day 4 the naloxone group made fewer errors than both the levorphanol group and the Krebs ringer group ($p < .05$). The levorphanol and Krebs groups did not differ significantly.

The authors concluded that neither drug produced a strong effect on acquisition performance, because the main effect of treatment was not significant. However, naloxone did improve acquisition performance significantly as this group made fewer errors than the other two groups on the last day of testing.

Critique

The research hypothesis is whether levorphanol would decrease and naloxone increase maze performance in the rat where food is used as a reinforcer. The general ANOVA table for this experiment is presented in Table 6.4. The specific ANOVA table for this 3 $\times$ (4 $\times$ S) mixed factorial design is

Source	df	Error term
Drug	2	S/Drug
Day	3	Day $\times$ S/Drug
S/Drug	17	
Drug $\times$ Day	6	Day $\times$ S/Drug
Day $\times$ S/Drug	51	
Total	79	

The statistical test selected was appropriate. The df formula (6.5) for an equal sample size cannot be used for this unequal sample size experiment. Because this experiment had unequal sample size, relatively small samples, and had a within-subject component, the assumption of homogeneity of variance must be considered (4.18). The reported Drug $\times$ Day interaction, which includes the within-subject component, was just significant at the $p < .05$ level. In this case, therefore, if violation of the homogeneity assumption occurred a correction of the biased F-test should be done (9.6) and with the correction it is likely that the Drug $\times$ Day interaction would not be significant.

The authors used the Duncan Multiple Range test (10.2) to evaluate differences between pairs of mean but the Duncan test does not adequately control for familywise error rate (10.1) and is only appropriate, in some cases, if the group sizes are equal. Furthermore, in the report this multiple comparison test was used to evaluate mean differences on each of the 4 days (day 1–day 4). The reported significant difference exists among at least one pair of the numerous comparisons that are possible with 16 means that cannot be attributed to a drug effect or a day effect (6.12, 6.13). Hence, the authors' statistical analysis appeared to be a desperate attempt to produce a significant finding (6.11).

RESEARCH DESIGN PROBLEM 86

Paraquat is a bipyridinium herbicide with widespread agricultural uses. The persistence and usage pattern of paraquat make it likely that both birds and mammals would be exposed to any toxic environmental effects of this herbicide. Therefore, to determine the effect of chronic dietary exposure to paraquat on bird behavior, 50 young (2 months old) male bobwhite quail were randomly assigned to either 25 or 100 ppm dietary treatment groups (25 birds per group). Prior to introducing treated diets, all quail were acclimated for 1 week to a control diet (0 ppm) after which the initial behavioral testing was conducted. The quail first learned to discriminate between two geometrical patterns and were then given several reversal tests (the correct pattern was reversed and became the incorrect pattern). Acquisition or reversal tests ended when a bird reached a criterion of 18 correct responses in 20 trials for three consecutive testing sessions. The percent errors and total number of trials were used as measures of performance and learning. Following this initial behavioral testing, each group of quails received its assigned treatment diet for 60 days, and the behavioral testing was then repeated. After completion of this testing, all birds were sacrificed and histological examinations of various body organs and tissues were done.

Separate ANOVAs were run for percent errors and total number of trials. Neither of these ANOVAs indicated a significant group effect, $F(1, 48) = 1.02$ and 1.15 or a Group $\times$ Age interaction, $F(1, 48) = 1.21$ and 1.36. However, for both variables measured there were significant main effects of age with increases in both the percent errors, $F(1, 48) = 4.70$, and total number of trials, $F(1, 48) = 4.08$, after the 60 days of treatment compared with initial values ($p < .05$). No treatment-related gross or histopathological lesions were found. Based upon these results, the authors concluded that paraquat in the diet at 25 and 100 ppm affected the discrimination performance of male bobwhite quail despite an absence of apparent histopathological abnormalities.

Critique

The research hypothesis is whether a chronic 60-day dietary exposure to different doses of paraquat (25 or 100 ppm) would affect the subsequent discrimination learning of bobwhite quail. The general ANOVA table for this experiment is presented in Table 6.4. The specific ANOVA table for this 2 (Group) $\times$ 2 (Age $\times$ Subject) mixed factorial design is

Source	df	Error term
Group	1	S/Group
Age	1	Age $\times$ S/Group
S/Group	48	
Group $\times$ Age	1	Age $\times$ S/Group
Age $\times$ S/Group	48	
Total	99	

The statistical test selected was appropriate. But, the experiment contains a time confound as a concurrent control group is not available to compare with the two paraquat treatment groups (1.2). Therefore, the effect of treatments versus the effect of age alone cannot be determined (4.4). Because the quail were young at the beginning of the test, their discrimination performance would be expected to change as they became older regardless of paraquat treatment. On some behavioral tests young animals do perform better than older animals, a result which occurred in this study.

RESEARCH DESIGN PROBLEM 87

Because of its chemical structure, alpha-1-acid glycoprotein (AAG) may be effective as a drug treatment for tricyclic antidepressant toxicity caused by an overdose of medication for depression. To determine the effects of AAG administration on desipramine (DMI) distribution in the body (a drug used to treat depressive patients), 60 Wistar rats were randomly divided into three equal groups. On the morning of the study, all 60 rats were injected intraperitoneally with 30 mg/kg DMI (⅔ of toxic dose). Fifteen minutes later the rats were injected (IV) with one of the following treatments: saline (S), 2.2 mg/kg bovine serum albumin (BSA), or 2.2 mg/kg AAG in BSA. Blood samples were drawn every 15 min for the next hour. The serum DMI concentration data were analyzed by a mixed factorial ANOVA: 3 $\times$ (4 $\times$ 20). The analysis showed no significant Treatment $\times$ Time interaction, $F(6,171) = 1.32$, or time effect, $F(3,171) = 2.13$, but the treatment effect was significant, $F(2, 57) = 7.76, p < .001$. A Newman-Keuls test revealed the rats treated with AAG had higher serum DMI levels than the rats in the other two groups ($p < .01$). The rats in the vehicle and saline groups did not differ significantly in serum DM1 levels. The researchers concluded that AAG is an effective treatment to redistribute DMI from tissues to serum in Wistar rats and may be useful in controlling tricyclic antidepressant toxicity in humans.

Critique

The research hypothesis is whether AAG affects desipramine distribution in the rat's body. The general ANOVA table for the $3 \times (4 \times 20)$ mixed factorial design is presented in Table 6.4. The specific ANOVA for this experiment is

Source	df	Error term
Treatment	2	S/Treatment
Time	3	Time × S/Treatment
S/Treatment	57	
Treatment × Time	6	Time × S/Treatment
Time × S/Treatment	171	
Total	239	

The statistical test selected was appropriate and the authors' conclusion is also appropriate.

RESEARCH DESIGN PROBLEM 88

In many gastropods, intracellular injection of cyclic nucleotides (e.g., cAMP and cGMP) produces transmembrane conductance changes in neurons. Although this conductance effect may be caused by the cyclic nucleotide's activation of a protein kinase (which phosphorylates a membrane channel gate protein thus opening a membrane ionic channel and changing the conductance), the effect of cyclic nucleotide injection could also be produced by a change in intracellular pH. Therefore, the effects of intracellular injection of cAMP and cGMP on membrane conductance and intracellular pH in neurons of the mollusc *Archidoris montereyensis* were measured to determine if conductance changes were correlated with intracellular pH changes.

Membrane potentials of identified neurons from randomly selected *Archidoris* were recorded intracellularly under voltage clamp conditions. A single neuron was used from each animal ($n = 14$ animals). Neurons were randomly assigned to one of two groups (7 neurons/group). The neurons in one group received injections of varying concentrations of cAMP while neurons in the other group received injections of cGMP (both administrated in standard vehicle solutions). Each neuron in each group was monitored for changes in intracellular pH (by using a second pH-sensitive microelectrode and by absorbance changes in the dye Arsenazo III) and conductance (via voltage clamp circuit). The doses of nucleotide used were .1, .5, 1.0, 1.5, 2.0, 2.5, 5.0, 10 μM. The protocol for each neuron was (*a*) a 20-min baseline measurement was taken prior to any injection then the lowest dose of nucleotide was injected (picoliter quantities) and the pH and conductance were monitored for 20 min, (b) after 20 min the neurons were allowed to stabilize for an additional 20 min (after 40 min all neurons had returned to baseline for all concentrations used), and (c) after this second period of 20 min the next higher dose of nucleotide was injected and the procedure was repeated.

A mixed factorial ANOVA was run on the pH data and on the conductance data. For the pH data no significant group effect was found (cAMP vs. cGMP) but a significant dose effect was found, $F(7, 84) = 4.09$, $p < .001$. The Group × Dose interaction was not significant. A trend analysis was run on the dose data and a significant linear trend was found ($p < .01$). The conductance data showed the same statistical results: the main effect of group and Group × Dose interaction were not significant and the main effect of the dose, $F(7, 84) = 5.13$, $p < .001$, was significant. A significant linear trend also existed for the conductance data ($p < .01$).

The authors concluded that the conductance change found in these neurons was associated with a change in intracellular pH and suggest that pH changes could be the primary mechanism by which intracellular injections of cyclic nucleotides affect membrane conductance in many molluscan neurons.

Critique

The research hypothesis is whether intracellular injections of cAMP and cGMP affect membrane conductance and intracellular pH in neurons of the mollusc *Archidoris montereyensis*. The general ANOVA table for the mixed factorial used in this experiment is presented in Table 6.4. The specific ANOVA table for the 2 (Group) × 7 (Dose × Subject) mixed factorial design for this experiment is

Source	df	Error term
Group	1	S/Group
Dose	7	Dose × S/Group
S/Group	12	
Group × Dose	7	Dose × S/Group
Dose × S/Group	84	
Total	111	

The statistical test selected was appropriate. The authors' conclusions are restatements of the major results, that is, intracellular injections of cAMP and cGMP affect both membrane conductance and intracellular pH. No vehicle injection control was used in this experiment and the vehicle *per se* may have caused the significant changes in membrane conductance and intracellular pH. Standard vehicle solutions were used and these solutions would have been used in previous intracellular injection studies which showed membrane conductance changes. The time confound inherent in always increasing the doses of the nucleotides could have been eliminated by counterbalancing (4.19, 4.20) but this confound *would not* invalidate the authors' conclusions. Both conduction and pH changed together (linear trends) and even if the actual doses were different than those given (because of carry-over effects), the conclusions of the authors would still be valid. The intracellular injections of cyclic nucleotides which produce neuronal conductance change could be producing their effects by changes in pH. Notice that if the authors had concluded that cyclic nucleotides affect membrane conductance by changing intracellular pH, this conclusion would be inappropriate.

RESEARCH DESIGN PROBLEM 89

Kainic acid, a rigid dicarboxylic acid, is a convulsant with unique properties. Small amounts of kainic acid (KA) injected directly into the hippocampus cause massive, simultaneous discharge of many neurons (epileptiform activity). Because the effect of KA administration mimics the symptoms of epilepsy, KA injection has been used as a model paradigm to study the physiology of epileptigenesis. The sensitivity of the hippocampus to KA application has been found to be much greater than the amygdala (or any other limbic structure of the brain). The purpose of the present study was to determine if the three distinct regions of the hippocampus (CA_1, CA_3, and dentate gyrus) had the same sensitivity to KA application and if the effects of KA application on these three regions were similar.

Hippocampal brain slices were obtained from four male albino rats (220–320 g). The slices were randomly assigned to three groups with the neurons in the slices being recorded from CA_1 (group 1), CA_3 (group 2), and dentate gyrus (group 3). Ten slices were used for each recording group. For each brain slice the effect of KA application was determined on spontaneous activity and evoked responses, and microelectrodes recorded the activity of individual neurons from each region. Three different doses of KA (.5, 1.0, and 1.5 μM) were applied to each slice and spontaneous activity was monitored for 10 min. After this baseline recording the evoked responsiveness of each neuron was monitored for 10 min. Evoked responsiveness was determined by stimulating an area of the slice known to send monosynaptic connections to the particular regions of the hippocampus (i.e., the CA_1 neurons were tested under monosynaptic stimulation from Schaffer-collateral commissure afferents, SC-C, and the CA_3 and dentate neurons were tested under monosynaptic stimulation of either the perforant pathway, PP, or the mossy fibers, MF). The responsiveness of the neurons to two different stimulation intensities (.2 Hz at 5 and 10 V) was determined. A sample protocol was (1) one slice was chosen and the specified region of the hippocampus recorded from, (2) a baseline measure was taken for 10 min, (3) after this .5 μM KA was applied and spontaneous activity was monitored for 10 min, (4) after 10 min evoked responsiveness was determined by stimulating through another microelectrode located at the appropriate location (e.g., the SC-C for CA_1 region neurons) at .2 Hz and 5 V stimulation, (5) the mean response for 10 min was recorded, (6) after this the same area was stimulated at 10 V and .2 Hz for another 10-min trial. All stimulation intensities were tested for the three KA doses (KA was continuously infused during the stimulation trials) and the order of stimulation intensity was counterbalanced. Ten minutes between each manipulation was sufficient to allow the variables measured to return to baseline.

The data for the averaged evoked activity during the 10-min trial were analyzed with a factorial ANOVA. There was a significant Group × Dose × Stimulation interaction, $F(4, 162) = 10.2, p < .01$. Post hoc comparisons using Scheffé's test indicated that the spontaneous activity of the CA_3 region of hippocampus was more sensitive to KA application (i.e., had a maximal response at the lowest dose) than the other two regions (maximal at highest dose). Furthermore, the CA_3 region showed higher averaged evoked activity than the other two regions at both stimulation intensities ($p < .01$). The evoked activities of CA_1 and dentate did not differ.

The authors concluded that different regions of the hippocampus respond differently to evoked activity upon KA application and that CA_3 had a greater sensitivity to KA application than did the other two hippocampal regions. The authors also suggested that a synapse-mediated effect of KA on hippocampus neurons appeared to be the best explanation for the observed data.

Critique

The research hypothesis is whether the application of kainic acid to brain tissue slices affects differentially the spontaneous activity and evoked responses of neurons in CA_1, CA_3, and the dentate gyrus of the hippocampus. The general ANOVA table for this experiment is not presented in the text because of the difficulty in attempting to understand a four-way interaction (6.15). The levels of the factors in this experiment are group (3), dose (6), frequency (5), stimulation (10), and subjects (5), an A × (B × C × D × S) mixed factorial design. Four-way interactions are difficult to interpret (6.15) and the presentation of the statistical analysis makes it difficult to determine what pair comparisons are made. The massive number of comparisons needed probably warranted using the conservative Scheffé test (10.5). This post hoc test, however, is very susceptible to Type II error thus many pairwise differences could potentially be missed. The authors probably selected a conservative test so that only the largest differences would be significant between pairs of means. The statistical power of their tests, however, would be low (5.15). The number of independent observations was not presented in this report. Thirty hippocampal brain slices were obtained from male rats but only four rats were used. The problems involved in the use of correlated observations (9.2, 9.5) must be considered because numerous brain slices were taken from each rat. Overall, however, the authors' conclusions appear to be reasonable given the very restricted interpretation that the CA_3 region had a greater sensitivity to KA application than did the other two hippocampal regions.

RESEARCH DESIGN PROBLEM 90

Endogenous opiates may be involved in stress responses because in some cases painful stimuli result in stress-induced analgesia and this analgesia can be

Table 14.22 Effect of Naloxone (NAL) on Open-Field Behavior of Drug-Treated Rats

Treatment group	N	Horizontal activity	Rearing	Defecation
		(median and interquartile range)		
Saline	15	116 (112–133)	13 (11–21)	0 (0–1)
Nal (.5 mg/kg)	15	103 (90–114)[a]	9 (5–15)[a]	0 (0–3.5)
Nal (1.0 mg/kg)	13	84 (62–104)[b]	7 (4.5–11)[b]	3 (0–4)[a]
Nal (2.0 mg/kg)	13	122 (86–124)	9 (5–11)	3 (0–4)[a]
Nal (4.0 mg/kg)	15	109 (99–115)[a]	11 (9–14)	1 (0–4)

[a] $p < .05$
[b] $p < .005$

blocked by the opiate antagonist naloxone. The aim of the present experiment was to determine whether endogenous opiates would reduce the nonpainful stress produced by exposing rats to a novel open field. To test this hypothesis, naloxone hydrochloride (doses ranging from 0–4.0 mg/kg SC) was given to rats prior to being placed in an open-field situation. The test arena was equipped with two rows of photobeams, with the lower bank positioned 3 cm above the floor and the upper bank 12.5 cm above the floor. Interruption of the lower beams provided a measure of horizontal activity, while interruption of the upper beams provided a measure of rearing. In addition to these activity measures, a measure of defecation was also recorded. The animals were injected with the appropriate drug dose 15 min before behavioral testing. For the test, each animal was placed individually into the arena for a 2-min observation period. This brief test period was selected to maximize novelty and minimize habituation. Comparisons between vehicle- and naloxone-treated rats were performed using the Mann-Whitney U test. The data obtained and the statistical analyses are presented in Table 14.22.

Although a simple dose-response relationship was not established, naloxone-treated groups did have significantly reduced levels of locomotor activity and rearing, and an increase in defecation. Based upon these results the authors concluded that naloxone decreases emotionality in the rat and that opioid peptides are released under conditions of nonpainful stress.

Critique

The research hypothesis is whether naloxone hydrochloride (from .5–4.0 mg/kg SC) given to rats before exposure to a novel open field would affect activity and the amount of defecation. The research hypothesis being tested is not whether opioid peptides are released under conditions of nonpainful stress; consequently, the authors cannot conclude from the data presented that ". . . opioid peptides are released under conditions of nonpainful stress." Indeed, it is questionable whether emotionality is being measured by activity changes in novel open fields. Opioid systems are involved in activity and defecation of rats (i.e., opiate agonists increase activity and induce constipation). Therefore, the authors' finding may be explained by the effects naloxone may have on other systems independent of stress or emotionality. Hence, the relation between the research hypothesis and treatment conditions is not appropriate (1.1, 1.2). In every situation you must determine what the experimenter did and not accept at face value what the experimenter said was done. A potential problem also exists with familywise error rate given the number of Mann-Whitney U tests (11.5) used in data analysis. Using a nonparametric (11.1) test for repeated pair comparisons presents the same problem as using multiple t-test comparisons (5.19) with three or more groups.

RESEARCH DESIGN PROBLEM 91

Animal bioassays for carcinogenesis normally use very high dose levels of chemicals to detect potential toxic effects with relatively small numbers of animals. Unfortunately, this procedure makes it difficult to predict toxic responses at lower environmental dosage levels. To determine more precisely the shape of the tumor dose response curve, a large-scale, long-term, low-dose study was conducted. Female mice ($n = 20,880$ BALB/c) were randomly assigned (with equal numbers in each group) at weanling to meal diets (Purina 5010C) containing 0, 15, 30, 45, 60, 75, 100, or 150 ppm of 2-acetylaminofluorene (2-AAF), a known bladder carcinogen. Animals were sacrificed after 9, 12, 14, 15, 16, 17, 18, 24, and 33 months on their respective diets. Upon death detailed necropsies were performed and all findings recorded. To ensure a consistent evaluation, a pathologist who did not know the group classification of the animal reviewed all the bladder carcinomas and a strict definition and classification of tumors were used.

Bladder carcinomas were found in all treatment groups except the controls and the 30 ppm 2-AAF group. Beyond 635 days, a sharp increase in bladder tumors occurred at 75, 100, and 150 ppm of 2-AAF with incidences exceeding 10 percent. The shape of the dose-tumor curve at low doses was of particular interest and the tumor incidence results for the 0–60 ppm groups at different times are presented in Table 14.23.

A trend analysis of the dose-tumor response curve showed a highly significant linear trend, $p < .005$. A nonparametric comparison of the tumor incidences indicated that the percent of animals with bladder tumors in the 30-, 45-, and 60-ppm groups differed significantly ($p < .01$) from that of the 0- and 15-ppm 2-AAF groups (see Table 14.23).

Table 14.23 Percent Occurrence of Mice with Bladder Tumors

Dose (ppm)	Time (days)			
	1–543	544–635	636–938	939–1001
0	.0000	.0000	.0000	.0000
15	.0000	.0000	.0000	.0000
30	.0000	.0006	.0028	.0085
45	.0000	.0010	.0055	.0355
60	.0000	.0020	.0093	.0909

The authors indicated that the dose response for urinary bladder tumors with a shallow trend at low doses and sharp increases at higher doses suggests a "threshold"-type response. They concluded that because the 15-ppm group had a zero tumor incidence over the entire experiment, the threshold dose for 2-AAF probably lies between 15 and 30 ppm in the diet for female BALB/c mice.

Critique

The research hypothesis is not explicitly stated but appears to be whether bladder carcinomas are dependent upon the dose and the duration of exposure to 2-acetylaminofluorene (2-AAF). The authors state that the aim of the experiment was to determine ". . . more precisely the shape of the tumor-dose response curve." The statistical analyses of the data are difficult to understand, but Table 14.23 presents the percentage of occurrence of bladder tumors in the 20 subgroups each one with 1044 mice. The 15-ppm group had zero tumor incidence and the statistical trend analysis of the data (6.16) would be affected by the absence of variance in this group.

Notice that in the beginning of the report the authors reported that "Bladder carcinomas were found in all treatment groups except the controls and the 30-ppm 2-AFF group" but at the end stated that ". . . the 15-ppm group had a zero tumor incidence over the entire experiment." The data presented in Table 14.23 indicate that the latter statement is correct. Unfortunately, numerical inconsistencies often appear in published papers. With revisions, retyping of drafts and quick proofreading, errors are easy to make and sometimes cannot be identified. The careful reader will make sure that no discrepancies exist between numbers given in tables or graphs and those presented in the text, that numbers or percentages in tables do add up to the required totals, and so forth.

In spite of some problems in the statistical analysis and presentation of the data, the authors' weak conclusions are appropriate. The threshold dose for 2-AAF to produce bladder carcinomas appears to be between 15 and 30 ppm in the diet for female BALB/c mice.

RESEARCH DESIGN PROBLEM 92

Twelve patients with essential hypertension were given mild aerobic exercise training for 20 weeks. The time course of changes in resting blood pressure (BP) and plasma catecholamines (CA) of these patients were monitored. Depressor responses of both systolic and diastolic pressure were found, and after 5 weeks of exercise BP stabilized at a significantly lower level. Adjustment of work load in response to increased physical fitness at the tenth week produced further reduction of BP especially in diastolic. After exercise therapy a significant reduction in CA levels was observed. A reduction in systolic/ diastolic (mean) pressures by more than 20/10 mmHg was seen in 50 percent of patients after 10 weeks and in 78 percent ($p < .001$) after 20 weeks of exercise. Patients who achieved an effective BP fall after 10 weeks of training ($n = 6$) were compared with the rest ($n = 6$). This analysis revealed that the CA levels of patients showing a BP drop were significantly lower, $t(10) = 52.1$, $p < .001$, than that of patients who did not have an effective BP fall. Further analysis revealed that mean BP was significantly lower after 20 weeks when compared to 10 weeks, $t(10) = 43.2$, $p < .01$. The authors concluded that exercise therapy is a potent nonpharmacological tool for the treatment of essential hypertension. They also suggested that diminished sympathoadrenergic activity might be responsible for the fall in BP.

Critique

The research hypothesis is whether mild aerobic exercise training for 20 weeks will reduce blood pressure and plasma catecholamine levels in patients with essential hypertension. The general ANOVA table for this experiment is presented in Table 4.5. The specific ANOVA table for this single-factor within-subject design is

Source	df	Error term
Weeks	19	Weeks × Subject
Subject	11	
Weeks × Subject	209	
Total	239	

This statistical test would be appropriate. A significant weeks effect could then be further analyzed by trend analysis (6.16) which would provide a sensitive analysis of the time changes. Although numerous t-tests were done in the reported experiment, the increase in familywise error would not affect the conclusions given the reported significance levels (5.19).

In some of the reported statistical tests the authors split their sample into two groups: those patients showing significant BP falls after 10 weeks and those patients not showing this BP fall. The general ANOVA table for this analysis is presented in Table 6.4. The specific ANOVA table for this (2) × (10 × 6) mixed factorial design is

Source	df	Error term
Group	1	S/Group
Weeks	9	Weeks × S/Group
S/Group	10	
Group × Weeks	9	Weeks × S/Group
Weeks × S/Group	90	
Total	119	

This post hoc analysis must be interpreted with caution. The groups became classification variables (4.2) as the patients separated themselves (self-selection) into the two groups. Because cause-and-effect relations cannot be determined in correlational studies (4.1), the authors were correct in not making any strong conclusions based upon this post hoc analysis. Actually, this analysis was not required given the research hypothesis. The data indicated that a significant reduction in both BP and CA occurred in patients with essential hypertension following 20 weeks of mild aerobic exercise training.

RESEARCH DESIGN PROBLEM 93

A measure of epileptic seizure activity in rats is known as "wild running" which appears to be associated with stimulation of the inferior collicular nucleus. In this nucleus, an aspartic acid–sensitive excitatory neuron has been identified and postulated to be involved in "wild running." Therefore, to determine whether an aspartic acid antagonist would affect "wild running" 30 male rats were randomly and equally assigned to one of two treatment groups. Treated rats were given a preselected dose of the antagonist twice a day over a 2-week period and untreated rats were given vehicle. All animals had a PE cannula inserted surgically into the area of the inferior collicular nucleus (proper placement of cannula was ascertained by histological procedures at the end of the study). Once a day, at least 4 h after dosing, a challenge dose of 5 μL of aspartic acid was administered via the cannula. Within 15 min seizures were evident, and the duration of the wild running was recorded. The mean duration (in seconds) across the 2-week period is presented in Table 14.24.

The ANOVA run on the data showed a significant drug effect, $F(1, 28) = 7.73$, $p < .01$, a significant day effect, $F(13, 364) = 2.35$, $p < .01$, but no significant Drug $\times$ Day interaction, $F(13, 364) = 1.93$. Because the Drug $\times$ Day interaction was not significant the authors concluded that across days the aspartic acid antagonist was not effective in the dose given, and suggested that further dose-response relationships be determined before other experiments were done.

Critique

The research hypothesis is whether an aspartic acid antagonist would affect "wild running" in rats. The general ANOVA table for this experiment is pre-

Table 14.24 Mean (M) $\pm$ SD Duration (sec) for Days 1, 7, and 14

Groups	Days[a]		
	1	7	14
Control	110(11)	65(10)	35(9)
Drug	80(8)	45(8)	25(6)

[a]Only the first, middle, and last day's results are presented.

sented in Table 6.4. The specific ANOVA table for this A × (B × S) mixed factorial design is

Source	df	Error term
Drug	1	S/Drug
Day	13	Day × S/Drug
S/Drug	28	
Drug × Day	13	Day × S/Drug
Day × S/Drug	364	
Total	419	

The statistical test selected was appropriate. The authors, however, did not understand the meaning of an A × B interaction (6.12, 6.13). Because the Drug × Day interaction was not significant, the significant group effect indicates that the aspartic acid antagonist had a significant averaged effect across the treatment days (Table 6.17, Figure 6.1). As may be seen in Table 14.24 the antagonist produced a significant decrease in the duration of wild running. Also, the significant day effect indicates that the duration of wild running decreases across days (Table 14.24). A trend analysis (6.16) of this significant day effect could be used to evaluate this change in behavior across the treatment days.

RESEARCH DESIGN PROBLEM 94

Evidence exists that stallions can distinguish between mares in estrus and mares in anestrus by detecting pheromones secreted by the estrus mare. To test this hypothesis, five padded holding stocks were constructed in a normal outdoor breeding paddock and either a gelding, a stallion, a pregnant mare, a mare in estrus, or a mare in anestrus were placed individually in the stocks. All animals were dark bay in color with no distinguishing markings and were placed in a different stock each day. Twenty healthy quarterhorse stallions (8 to 12 years old) were randomly assigned to two treatment groups. All the stallions selected were successful breeders and had aggressive libidos. For 5 straight days, individually and in a random order, the stallions were turned loose in the paddock. For each trial a graduate student recorded the first animal the stallion attempted to mount and the position of that animal in the paddock. Because of the design of the stocks, the stallion could not breed the animal and the animal could not kick the stallion. Stallions in group A ($n = 10$) were simply turned loose in the paddock. Stallions in group B ($n = 10$) were turned loose while wearing a standard racing blinker with full cups, thus allowing them to hear and smell but not to see. Horses not able to see quickly adjusted and their mounting behavior was not affected. The data were recorded as the percent of stallions in each group that on their first attempt made incorrect choices (see Table 14.25).

A mixed factorial ANOVA was used to analyze the data and indicated no significant group effect, $F(1, 18) = 2.13$, no significant day effect, $F(4,72) = 1.98$, and no significant Group × Day Interaction, $F(4,72) = 2.10$.

The researchers concluded that because group B stallions were not signifi-

Table 14.25 Mean Percent Incorrect Choices on First
Mount

			Test day		
Group	1	2	3	4	5
Normal	90	90	8C	90	90
Blinded	90	100	90	100	90

cantly different than group A stallions in their choices that stallions can detect
pheromones secreted by estrus mares, at least in the quarterhorse animals studied.

Critique

The research hypothesis is whether stallions can distinguish between a mare in
estrus and other nonestrus horses (gelding, stallion, pregnant mare, and a mare
in anestrus). The general ANOVA table reported for the experiment is presented
in Table 6.4. The specific ANOVA table reported for the experiment is

Source	df	Error term
Group	1	S/Group
Day	4	Day × S/Group
S/Group	18	
Group × Day	4	Day × S/Group
Day × S/Group	72	
Total	99	

The data do not support the conclusion made by the authors. Giving the mean
percent of incorrect choices on first mount is an odd presentation of the data. At
first glance all horses appeared to do very well but a 90 percent means only a 10
percent correct choice. Also, the scale of measurement (5.3) indicates that a nonparametric rather than a parametric test would be more appropriate (5.22, 11.1)
because on each trial the score of each animal was either correct or incorrect.
Because there were five possible choices, one correct and four incorrect, the
expected probability for a correct choice would be .20 on the first mount. The
design used in this experiment is not very efficient. A choice between a mare in
estrus and a mare in anestrus would have tested the proposed research hypothesis. The expected frequency would then be .50 and a nonparametric test could
be used to evaluate the data.

RESEARCH DESIGN PROBLEM 95

In humans a relationship between stress, the immune system, and various diseases has been postulated. Therefore, a study was done to determine the degree

of conditioned suppression of natural killer (NK) cells using a taste aversion procedure with morphine as the unconditioned stimulus. Thirty female C57 black mice were used in this study in which a sweet-tasting substance (.5% sodium saccharin, the conditioned stimulus, CS) was paired with a subcutaneous injection of the unconditioned stimulus, US, 50 mg/kg of morphine sulfate. Following this phase, the conditioned suppression of NK cell cytotoxicity was determined.

Besides the conditioning group [CS-US . . . (CS, test)], four other groups ($n =$ 6) were used and included a saline (SAL) control group for behavioral control which required a subcutaneous injection of physiological saline [CS-SAL . . . (CS, test)], a backward-paired group to control for any residual effects of saccharin and/or morphine [US-CS . . . (CS, test)], a double US group to determine the magnitude of the conditioned response relative to the unconditioned response [CS-US . . . (US, test)], and an unstimulated group as a "normal" population for immunologic comparison [0–0 . . . (0, test)].

Three days after the conditioning phase of the experiment, mice in the CS-US-CS, CS-SAL-CS, and US-CS-CS groups were given 15-min access to the saccharin solution (CS, test) and then immediately injected with saline. The mice in group CS-US-US received 15-min access to water and then immediately injected with morphine. The six mice in the unstimulated group [0–0 . . . (0, test)] were not disturbed.

One and one-half hours after the test injections, all mice were sacrificed via cervical dislocation and spleens removed for immunologic assay using a standard NK cell assay procedure. In this assay, effector:target ratios of 100:1, 50:1, and 25:1 were used and the target cells were YAC-1 cells. Chromium release was measured by a gamma counter and reflected the degree of lysis of YAC-1 cells by the natural killer cells. From these counts percent cytotoxicity was determined for each mouse at each of the three effector:target ratios.

The mean data for the various groups are presented in Table 14.26. An analysis of variance (ANOVA) with repeated measures indicated a significant effector:target ratio, $F(2,50) = 6.85$, $p < .01$. Post hoc multiple comparison tests revealed that the three ratios were each significantly different from each other. The main effect of group, $F(4,25) = 2.41$, and Group $\times$ Ratio interaction, $F(8,50) = 1.23$, were not significant. From this data, the authors concluded that their taste aversion conditioning procedure did not significantly affect the per-

Table 14.26 Mean and Standard Deviation of Percentage of Cytotoxicity of Groups Across the Three Effector:Target Ratios

| Groups | Effector:target ratios | | |
	100:1	50:1	25:1
CS-US-CS	15 ± 3	7 ± 2	3 ± 1
CS-SAL-CS	28 ± 4	14 ± 3	6 ± 2
US-CS-CS	29 ± 5	15 ± 3	7 ± 2
CS-US-US	25 ± 3	13 ± 2	5 ± 1
Unstimulated	27 ± 4	14 ± 3	8 ± 2

cent of cytotoxicity even though the immunologic assay was sensitive enough to detect significant differences among the three effector:target ratios.

Critique

The research hypothesis is whether conditioned suppression of natural killer (NK) cells occurs with a saccharin (CS)–morphine (US) taste aversion procedure. The general ANOVA table for the $A \times (B \times S)$ mixed factorial design is presented in Table 6.4. The specific ANOVA table for the $5 \times (3 \times 6)$ mixed factorial experiment is

Source	df	Error term
Group	4	S/Group
Ratio	2	Ratio × S/Group
S/Group	25	
Group × Ratio	8	Ratio × S/Group
Ratio × S/Group	50	
Total	89	

The overall F-ratio (6.8) for group was not significant (5.9) and this finding is consistent with the authors' conclusion. However, the data presented in Table 14.26 indicate that the conditioning group (CS-US-CS) was different from the other four groups, which were not different from each other. These latter groups were various control groups for the conditioning group. As the number of control groups increases in an experiment so does the likelihood of the overall F-ratio for group being nonsignificant. Essentially, the more nondifferences (controls) that are built into an experiment, the smaller the MS treatment becomes (4.24). In this case (Table 14.26), the F-ratio for the group comparison indicates that all control groups performed as expected, no significant difference among the controls.

Normally, it is not wise to interpret nonsignificant statistical outcomes (6.11, 6.20). However, the main effect of group, $F(4,25) = 2.41$, was at about the .08 level of significance. Given this level of significance, the number of control groups used, and the descriptive data presented in Table 14.26 a significant conditioned suppression of natural killer cells did occur in this taste aversion experiment. A planned comparison between the conditioning group and all the control groups (using the Scheffé test, 10.5) may be appropriate in this situation. Although the authors did not provide information of the strength of conditioning (comparison of saccharin drinking during test), the data in Table 14.26 indicate that conditioning occurred. Double-blind control procedures (4.26) would also have controlled for experimenter bias.

RESEARCH DESIGN PROBLEM 96

The increased demand for skin blood flow during mild exercise in a hot environment may be met by an increased cardiac output, a redistribution of blood

Table 14.27 Mean ± SD of Rectal Temperature, Heart Rate, and Cardiac Output

	Rectal temperature	Heart rate	Cardiac output
Thermoneutral	37.7 ± .1°C	91 ± 9 beats/min	13.0 ± .11 L/min
Dry heat	38.4 ± .3°C	129 ± 12 beats/min	14.0 ± .61 L/min

flow, or by both mechanisms. To determine the contribution of cardiac output to increased blood flow during heat stress, six unacclimated trained men (30–35 years old) walked on a treadmill at 30 percent of their maximal oxygen consumption (mild exercise) for 3.5 h (7 exercise periods of 30 min with 5-min breaks) once in a thermoneutral environment condition (ambient temperature = 20.8 ± .9°C) and once in dry heat (ambient temperature = 39.9 ± .1°C). Exercise conditions were given on two separate days and the treatment conditions were counterbalanced. At the end of these 3.5-h exercise periods heart rate, rectal temperature, and cardiac output were measured (see Table 14.27).

Heart rate was the only parameter that was significantly different in the two environment conditions, treatment effect $F(1, 5) = 37.18$, $p < .001$. Although not statistically significant, an increase in both rectal temperature and cardiac output occurred in the dry heat conditions. Therefore, the authors concluded that cardiovascular adjustment to mild exercise in dry heat is achieved by an increase in either heart rate or cardiac output.

Critique

The research hypothesis is whether significant differences occur in body temperature, heart rate, and cardiac output when exercising trained men are exposed to normal and "heat" stress environments. The general ANOVA table for this experiment is presented in Table 4.5. The specific ANOVA for this complete within-subject experiment is

Source	df	Error term
Treatment	1	Treatment × Subject
Subject	5	
Treatment × Subject	5	
Total	11	

The statistical test selected was appropriate. Three separate ANOVAs were performed, one for heart rate, another for rectal temperature, and the last for cardiac output. The authors cannot conclude, however, that an increase in cardiac output is a major contributor to cardiovascular adjustment in dry heat because cardiac output was not significantly different between the two conditions. Furthermore, the authors did not measure changes in blood flow to various areas of the body and, therefore, do not know the contribution the redistribution of blood flow may have made to cardiovascular adjustment. An increase in heart rate and a redistribution of blood flow may be important cardiovascular adjustments to mild exercise in dry heat but other processes (not measured) may also be involved.

RESEARCH DESIGN PROBLEM 97

L-Glutamic and L-aspartic acids are putative excitatory neurotransmitters in the mammalian central nervous system. The purpose of the present study was to determine the mechanism underlying the excitatory action of these putative transmitters, specifically to determine if the depolarization (excitation) produced by these substances was mediated *via* tetrodotoxin (TTX)-sensitive Na^+ channels.

Cultured mouse spinal cord neurons were randomly assigned to one of three groups: (1) a group bathed in 50 μM L-glutamate, (2) a group bathed in 50 μM L-aspartate, (3) a group bathed in vehicle alone (same vehicle was used for each amino acid used). Thirty neurons were assigned to each treatment group. The concentrations of amino acid used normally elicited excitation (depolarization) in these neurons and all neurons were tested under the following protocol. Each neuron was first given 10 constant-current pulses of known magnitude for 20 min delivered through a microelectrode inserted intracellularly. From the magnitude of the membrane potential changes evoked by this injection, the conductance of the membrane was calculated (by Ohm's law). Following this 20-min baseline measurement each neuron was bathed in TTX for 20 min and the 10 current pulses were again given in the presence of TTX . The concentration of TTX used would block any TTX-sensitive Na^+ channels present in these cells. Following this TTX exposure, the neurons were washed for 20 min and the conductance was again measured for 20 min by the current pulse method. Because the conductance of the membrane is a direct measure of its excitability this protocol would determine if the excitation due to these two amino acids was due to TTX-sensitive Na^+ channels.

A mixed factorial ANOVA was run on the data and a significant group effect was found, $F(2, 87) = 4.98$, $p < .01$. No significant interaction or other main effect was found. A post hoc Newman-Keuls test revealed that the neurons treated with L-glutamate had conductances greater than the L-aspartate–treated or control neurons whereas no differences existed between the conductance of control and L-aspartate–treated neurons. Because an increase in conductance results in an increase in excitation the neuropharmacologists concluded that L-glutamate excites spinal neurons through a different mechanism than L-aspartate, and that L-aspartate excitation is probably dependent, at least in part, on TTX-sensitive Na^+ channels while L-glutamate excitation is not.

Critique

The research hypothesis is whether L-glutamate and L-aspartate affect the depolarization of neurons by changes in tetrodotoxin (TTX)-sensitive Na^+ channels.

The general ANOVA table for this experiment is presented in Table 6.4. The specific ANOVA table for this experiment is

Source	df	Error term
Group	2	S/Group
Test	2	Test × S/Group
S/Group	87	
Group × Test	4	Test × S/Group
Test × S/Group	174	
Total	269	

This analysis was appropriate and used all the data collected. The three groups of neurons ($n = 30$) were given a 20-min pretreatment, a 20-min treatment, and a 20-min posttreatment, that is, membrane conductance was measured before, during, and after TTX exposure. Hence, the complete design was a mixed factorial 3 (group) × (3, measurement × 30, subject) design.

If the authors had not included either the baseline or recovery membrane conductance measure in their ANOVA then the within-subject factor would have been eliminated (4.21). Hence, the specific ANOVA for this type of analysis would be

Source	df	Error term
Group	2	S/Group
S/Group	87	
Total	89	

The general ANOVA table for this reduced between-subject design is presented in Tables 4.5 and 6.1. The complete mixed factorial design, however, allows a comparison of baselines before treatments, a comparison of treatment effects, a comparison of recovery effects, and so forth.

From the df's presented for the significant group effect (2, 87) it is not possible to determine which ANOVA was used. However, the authors indicate no significant interaction or other main effect was found which indicates that all the data collected was used in the analysis. Indeed, the authors reported that a mixed factorial ANOVA was used to analyze the data; consequently, a within-subject component was included in the analysis (Table 6.4).

A significant group effect was reported but this indicates only that the L-glutamate group value (averaged membrane conductance for before, during, and after treatment) was different than the L-aspartate or control group averaged values. Baseline values could have been different or treatment values could have been different or recovery values could have been different. The Group × Test interaction (6.13) is important for the proposed research question, yet this interaction was not significant. Hence, the statistical analysis and results do not justify the authors' conclusions.

RESEARCH DESIGN PROBLEM 98

To test a newly discovered respiratory depressant drug (RD-14) 10 cats (2–3 kg) randomly selected from a university animal care facility were anesthetized, and had tracheal cannulae inserted, as well as cannulae inserted into the femoral artery and vein. A blood pressure reading was taken from the arterial line, and RD-14 was injected into the venous line (IV). Pneumotachographic measurements were taken for tidal volume and respiratory rate, and all measurements were recorded continuously and at a high speed on a polygraph.

Because the drug caused a slight concentration-dependent change in the pH of the vehicle (from 7.45 to 7.35) four cats received only vehicle which was adjusted to the pH of the solution of RD-14 at the various concentrations used. The other six cats were given doses of cither 0 μg (vehicle alone at pH 7.45), .1 μg, .5 μg, 1 μg, 1.5g, or 2.0 g of RD-14 IV. All five cats receiving RD-14 had a period of apnea after injection, but vehicle injections did not produce apnea. The length of apnea was measured, and ranged from 30 to 60 sec before the cats spontaneously began to breathe again. An ANOVA comparing baseline data taken just before the apnea appeared to data after treatment for the two groups showed a significant drug effect, $p < .01$, a significant measurement effect, $p < .01$, and a significant Drug $\times$ Measurement interaction, $p < .001$. The authors interpreted the interaction on the basis of the vehicle injections having no effect on respiration whereas the drug always depressed respiration. Because of the short duration of the apnea, the authors also concluded that RD-14's effect on receptor sites is rapidly reversed.

Critique

Although not stated explicitly, the research hypothesis was whether RD-14 would affect tidal volume and respiratory rate in cats. With only one cat in most of the drug-dose groups, an ANOVA with dose as a factor could not be done. Because all five of the cats that received the drug had apnea whereas none of the five cats receiving vehicle solutions had apnea, the conclusion of the authors is appropriate. Because the df's (5.17) for the F-ratios (5.18) are not given, the ANOVA table cannot be reconstructed. The appropriate statistical test would have been to have two groups: vehicle control group, $n = 5$, and drug (.1μg–2.0 mg) group, $n = 5$. Notice that the estimate of within-subject variability would increase because of the different doses included in the experimental group (5.16). However, significant F-ratios were reported and the power of the test was adequate (5.12). In this situation a mixed factorial ANOVA could be used to analyze the data (6.4). The specific ANOVA table for this analysis would be

Source	df	Error term
Group	1	S/Group
Measurement	1	Measurement × S/Group
S/Group	8	
Group × Measurement	1	Measurement × S/Group
Measurement × S/Group	8	
Total	19	

The data reported were probably averaged duration of the interbreath interval for each cat under each treatment and measurement condition. Hence, because of the significant apnea reported for the drug-injected cats, the duration of their interbreath interval would be significantly higher than the vehicle-injected control cats. Although post hoc multiple comparison tests (6.9, 10.1) were not done, the reported individual data indicate that the authors' conclusions were appropriate.

RESEARCH DESIGN PROBLEM 99

The artificial sweetener aspartame (APM) is hydrolyzed in the gut to yield aspartic acid, phenylalanine, and methanol. L-Phenylalanine has been reported to affect lactation in rats when incorporated at a level of 5 to 7 percent in the diet. To determine if APM might also affect lactational performance a pair-feeding experimental design was used to distinguish between a direct effect of the sweetener and the effect of food restriction. Sixty female rats and their litters (culled to eight pups) were randomly assigned to 10 groups (5 treatment groups and 5 matched control groups) of similar average body weights (6 dams and 48 pups per group). The five treatment groups were fed either 1, 2, 4, 7.5, or 14 percent (W/W) APM in laboratory chow *ad libitum*. The five paired control group dams were fed an amount of basal diet (no added APM) equivalent to the amount of test diet consumed by the paired treatment group dams during the preceding 24-h period. Pups fed by suckling only. Body weights were recorded on days 1, 6, 8, 10, 12, 16, and 21 of lactation for all dams and pups.

A mixed factorial ANOVA was performed on the pup body weight data. There was a significant Day × APM concentration interaction, $F(24, 1316) = 3.95, p < .001$, and significant main effects for day, $F(6, 329) = 4.62, p < .001$, and concentration, $F(4, 235) = 3.89, p < .01$. Pups of dams given APM at levels of 1, 2, and 4 percent in the diet had similar mean body weights throughout the lactational period but these weights were significantly higher ($p < .01$) after day 6 than the weights of pups from dams given 7.5 percent or 14 percent APM in the diet. Therefore, the investigators concluded that aspartame in amounts of 7.5 percent or greater in the diets of lactating dams has a detrimental effect on weight gain of their offspring during the first 21 days of lactation.

Critique

The research hypothesis is whether aspartame added to the diet of lactating female rats would affect the body weights of their pups. This experiment is an example of a nested design because littermates are included in the same treatment condition (9.3, Table 9.2). Because littermates are probably more similar than nonlittermates (i.e., a significant correlation exists among littermates), ignoring the littermate classification results in an error term that is numerically less than it should be, thereby leading to inflated F-ratios (9.5). Also, the authors never distinguished between the effects of the sweetener and any effect on food restriction (differences in food consumption at different levels of APM in the diet) because individual treatments were never compared with their paired controls. This analysis cannot be done using only one ANOVA directly but rather requires multiple comparisons of treatment and control means for each day and percent APM in the diet. A more appropriate analysis would be by using trend analysis or by converting the weight data to growth rates (6.16). Differences in growth rates between the paired controls and treatments could be assumed to be due only to APM in the diet because the amount of food consumption in the two groups was equated. In the report a mistake exists in the degrees of freedom (6.5); for the Day $\times$ Concentration interaction they should be (54, 2820) and for the main effect of day the df's should be (6, 2820) assuming an A $\times$ (B $\times$ S) design where A = APM concentration and B = day was used (see Table 6.4).

RESEARCH DESIGN PROBLEM 100

Long sleep (LS) and short sleep (SS) mice were selectively bred for ethanol-induced sleep times and the aim of the present study was to determine whether the effect of sodium barbital over time was also different for each strain. Six mice were used to generate dose versus sleep-time curves. From the curves, the ED60 (that dose required to produce a 60-min sleep-time) was obtained. Previous research had shown the dose selected to be appropriate for obtaining ED60. Three sets of six mice of each strain were used to obtain three independent estimates of the ED60 for each strain. The same six mice in each group were used every other day (to allow cumulative effects of the barbital to wear off) to again obtain estimates of the ED60, using a diagram-balanced design for the administration of the dose of barbital. The study was continued over the course of 9 days—giving a total of 5 days by 3 independent ED60 estimates by 2 strains = 30 data points. Data obtained are presented in Table 14.28 (mean ED60 $\pm$ SD).

The authors concluded that the doses of sodium barbital required to produce ED60's in these two strains of mice were different. Also, they concluded that the increasing effect of sodium barbital was probably because the effects of sodium barbital did not wear off by the time the next injection was given. A significant interaction was not found, but the authors concluded that this was probably due to the low power of the statistical tests given the very small sample size.

Table 14.28 Millimoles per Kilogram of Sodium Barbital Required for ED60

Day	Strain LS ($n = 3$)	Strain SS ($n = 3$)
1	$1.26 \pm .093$	$.86 \pm .093$
3	$1.19 \pm .037$	$.75 + .028$
5	$1.14 \pm .024$	$.64 \pm .028$
7	$1.09 \pm .037$	$.53 \pm .062$
9	$1.04 \pm .112$	$.50 \pm .028$

Main effect of strain: $F(1, 4) = 558.1, p < .001$
Main effect of time: $F(4, 16) = 50.16, p < .001$
Strain $\times$ Time: $F(4, 4) = 2.12, p > .10$

Critique

The research hypothesis is whether sodium barbital affects differently repeated sleep induction in mice selectively bred for long and short ethanol-induced sleep times. The general ANOVA for the $2 \times (5 \times 3)$ mixed factorial design is presented in Table 6.4. The specific ANOVA Table for the reported experiment is

Source	df	Error term
Strain	1	S/Strain
Days	4	Days $\times$ S/Strain
S/Strain	4	
Strain $\times$ Days	4	Days $\times$ S/Strain
Days $\times$ S/Strain	16	
Total	29	

The Strain $\times$ Time interaction was evaluated with an F-ratio having 4 and 4 df's; whereas, the correct df's would be 4 and 16. With these correct df's an F-value of 3.01 would be required for $p < .05$. If the error mean square was based upon within-subject variance divided by 4, rather than by 16, then the correct F-value would be much higher than reported and would be significant (5.17, 6.5).

POSTSCRIPT

To make substantial contributions to their scientific disciplines, biological scientists strive to translate important research questions into appropriate treatment conditions, to obtain accurate and valid measures of significant biological processes, to perform well-designed experiments which provide unequivocal data, and to integrate their data with current knowledge. In these endeavors, errors are inevitable. Indeed, the only way to avoid errors in science is to avoid doing experimental and theoretical work.

The experiment is the inferential tool in biological research in which decisions (inferences, estimates) are made about large groups (populations) from the limited data obtained from small groups (samples). The research design problems presented include most of the experimental design and statistical errors that appear frequently in the biological literature. Because of the diversity of biological research it is impossible to give a single set of hard and fast rules for determining whether an experiment is properly conceived, correctly controlled, adequately analyzed, and properly interpreted. Nevertheless, a few guidelines deserve to be stated again.

For any given research question the experimental design should be a well-conceived plan for data collection, analysis, and interpretation which will provide, if the research question has been translated into appropriate treatment conditions, a tentative answer to the proposed question. A well-designed experiment is one in which the treatment conditions selected and manipulated by the researcher are not confounded by subject-, environment-, or time-related extraneous variables. And conversely, a poorly designed experiment is one in which treatment conditions are unknowingly confounded with one or more of these extraneous variables. If both accurate and valid measurements of significant biological processes are obtained in a well-designed experiment an important contribution to scientific knowledge is likely.

A well-designed experiment will include methods of data analysis that make the two statistical errors of inference as small as possible for the data to be collected and the comparisons to be made. The selection of the statistical methods to test a research hypothesis is a very important part of the experimental design. A liaison exists between experimental design and statistical inference which, if properly exploited, will increase greatly the likelihood of making correct decisions. Conversely, a bad experimental design will not consider statistical analysis and inference until after data are collected. In such cases, statistical methods will often be selected for convenience rather than for being the most appropriate and powerful for the proposed research question.

Most of the research design problems presented are *simplified and distorted* summaries of published experiments. An excellent way to obtain a good research design problem is to select a well-written abstract and insert malevolently a design or statistical error. Because the research design problems do not reflect accurately the experimental methods of the published article and often distort the author's conclusions, citations to original articles are not given. Although the research design problems no longer represent the original experimental conditions or the results or the interpretations of the authors, a vague resemblance may still remain. An apology is extended to those authors who sense that their experimental efforts have first been distorted and then criticized.

The more you are exposed to both good and bad experimental designs the better your own scientific output should become. Therefore, in reviewing experimental work in your scientific discipline if a particularly enlightening general design or statistical problem is encountered would you please send me the reference to the article. An abstract of the research design problem along with a cross-referenced critique would be helpful but a reference will suffice. Also, if any of your critiques are substantially different from those presented in this book, please send your critique to me at the Department of Physiology and Biophysics, Medical Center, University of Kentucky, Lexington, KY 40536-0084. Remember, errors will be made but the self-correcting nature of scientific exchange can eliminate most errors.

REFERENCES

Altman, D. G. (1980a). Statistics and ethics in medical research: I. Misuse of statistics is unethical. *British Medical Journal, 281,* 1181–1184.

———. (1980b). Statistics and ethics in medical research: III. How large a sample? *British Medical Journal, 281,* 1336–1338.

———. (1982). Statistics in medical journals. *Statistics in Medicine, 1,* 59–71.

Armitage, P., and Berry, G. (1987). *Statistical Methods in Medical Research.* Blackwell, Oxford, U.K.

Atkinson, A. C. (1987). *Plots, Transformations, and Regression: An Introduction to Graphical Methods of Diagnostic Regression Analysis.* Oxford University Press, Oxford, U.K.

Bailar, III, J. C., and Mosteller, F. (1986). *Medical Uses of Statistics.* Massachusetts Medical Society, Waltham, Mass.

Beckman, R. J., and Cook, R. D. (1983). Outliers. *Technometrics, 25,* 119–163.

Bland, M. (1987). *An Introduction to Medical Statistics.* Oxford University Press, Oxford, U.K.

Bolles, R. C. (1988). Why you should avoid statistics. *Biological Psychiatry, 23,* 79–85.

Borenstein, M., and Cohen, J. (1988). *Statistical Power Analysis: A Computer Program.* Lawrence Erlbaum Associates, Inc., Hillsdale, N.J.

Botstein, D., and Fink, G. R. (1988). *Yeast:* An experimental organism for modern biology. *Science, 240,* 1439–1442.

Bourke, G. J., Daly, L., and McGilvray, J. (1985). *Interpretation and Uses of Medical Statistics.* Blackwell Scientific Publications, Oxford, U.K.

Brent, E. E. (1989). *Statistical Navigator* TM: *An Expert System to Assist in Selecting Appropriate Statistical Analyses, Version 1.1.* The Ideal Works, Inc., Columbia, Mo.

Calabrese, E. J. (1983). *Principles of Animal Extrapolation.* John Wiley, New York.

Chambers, J. M., Cleveland, W. S., Kleiner, B., and Tukey, P. A. (1983). *Graphical Methods for Data Analysis.* Wadsworth, Belmont, Calif.

Cleveland, W. S., and McGill, R. (1984). Graphical perception: Theory, experimentation, and application to the development of graphical methods. *Journal of the American Statistical Association, 79,* 531–554.

Cody, R. P., and Smith, J. K. (1987). *Applied Statistics and the SAS Programming Language.* Elsevier Science Publishing Co., Inc., New York.

Cohen, C. (1986). The case for the use of animals in biomedical research. *New England Journal of Medicine, 315,* 865–870.

Cohen, J. (1988). *Statistical Power Analysis for the Behavioral Sciences,* 2nd *ed.* Lawrence Erlbaum Associates, Inc., Hillsdale, N.J.

———. (1990). Things I have learned (so far). *American Psychologist, 45,* 1304–1313.

Conover, W. J. (1980). *Practical Nonparametric Statistics,* 2nd ed. John Wiley, New York.

Cooper, H. M., and Rosenthal, R. (1980). Statistical versus traditional procedures for summarizing research findings. *Psychological Bulletin, 87,* 442–449.

Cornfield, J., and Tukey, J. W. (1956). Average values of mean squares in factorials. *Annals of Mathematical Statistics, 27,* 907–949.

Cremmins, E. T. (1982). *The Art of Abstracting*. ISI Press, Philadelphia, Pa.

Dallal, G. E. (1988). DESIGN: *A Supplementary Module for* SYSTAT *and* SYGRAPH. SYSTAT, Inc., Evanston, Ill.

Dawid, I. B., and Sargent, T. D. (1988). *Xenopus laevis* in developmental and molecular biology. *Science, 240*, 1443–1447.

Day, R. A. (1988). *How to Write and Publish a Scientific Paper*. ISI Press, Philadelphia, Pa.

Day, S. J., Hutton, J. L., and Gardner, M. J. (1990). Workshop on teaching statistics to medical undergraduates. *Statistics in Medicine, 9*, 1011–1078.

Denenberg, V. H. (1979). Analysis of variance procedures for estimating reliability and comparing individual subjects. In E. B. Thomas (ed.), *Origins of the Infant's Social Responsiveness* (pp. 339–348). Erlbaum, Hillsdale, N.J.

———. (1984). Some statistical and experimental considerations in the use of the analysis-of-variance procedure. *American Journal of Physiology, 15*, R403–408.

DiStefano, J. J., and Landow, E. M. (1984). Multiexponential, multicompartmental, and noncompartmental modeling: I. Methodological limitations and physiological interpretations. *American Journal of Physiology, 246*, R651–R664.

Dixon, W. J. (ed.) (1983). *BMDP-Statistical Software: 1983*. University of California Press, Berkeley, Calif.

Dubin, S., and Herr, A. (1986). Determining experimental sample size: A computer-assisted statistical approach. *Lab Science*, November/December, 35–39.

Dworkin, B. R., and Miller, N. E. (1986). Failure to replicate visceral learning in the acute curarized rat preparaton. *Behavioral Neuroscience, 100*, 299–314.

Elston, R. C., and Johnson, W. D. (1987). *Essentials of Biostatistics*. F.A. Davis Company, Philadelphia, Pa.

Elwood, J. M. (1988). *Causal Relationships in Medicine: A Practical System for Critical Appraisal*. Oxford University Press, Oxford, U.K.

Engleberg, J. (1983). Integrative physiology: On mapping the organism. *The Physiologist, 26*, 142–144.

Everitt, B. S. (1989). *Statistical Methods for Medical Investigations*. Oxford University Press, Oxford, U.K.

———, and Dunn, G. (1983). *Advanced Methods of Data Exploration and Modelling*. Gower, London, U.K.

Feinstein, A. R. (1988). Scientific standards in epidemiologic studies of the menace of daily life. *Science, 242*, 1257–1263.

Follath, F. (1988). Alternatives to animal experimentation. *Experientia, 44*, 807–877.

Friedman, H. H., and Friedman, L. W. (1980). A new approach to teaching statistics: Learning from misuses. *New York Statistician, 31*(4–5), 1–3.

Gaito, J. (1980). Measurement scales and statistics: Resurgence of an old misconception. *Psychological Bulletin, 87*, 564–567.

Gale, W. A. (1985). *Artificial Intelligence and Statistics*. Addison-Wesley, Reading, Mass.

Games, P. A., Keselman, H. J., and Rogan, J. C. (1981). Simultaneous pairwise multiple comparison procedures for means when sample sizes are unequal. *Psychological Bulletin, 90*, 594–598.

Garfinkel, D., and Fegley, K. A. (1984). Fitting physiological models to data. *American Journal of Physiology, 246*, R641–R650.

Gehlbach, S. H. (1988). *Interpreting the Medical Literature: Practical Epidemiology for Clinicians*. 2nd ed. Macmillan Publishing Co., New York.

Gerbarge, E. S., and Horwitz, R. I. (1988). Resolving conflicting clinical trials: Guidelines for meta analysis. *Journal of Clinical Epidemiology, 41*, 503–509.

Gilbert, N. G. (1989). *Biometrical Interpretation: Making Sense of Statistics in Biology*, 2nd ed. Oxford University Press, Oxford, U.K.

Glantz, S. A. (1987). *Primer of Biostatistics*. 2nd ed. McGraw-Hill, New York.

————, and Slinker, B. K. (1990). *Primer of Applied Regression and Analysis of Variance*. McGraw-Hill, New York.

Godfrey, K. (1986a). Simple linear regression in medical research. In J. C. Bailar, III, and F. Mosteller (eds.), *Medical Uses of Statistics* (pp. 170–204). New England Journal of Medicine, Mass.

————. (1986b). Comparing the means of several groups. In J. C. Bailar, III, and F. Mosteller (eds.), *Medical Uses of Statistics* (pp. 205–234). New England Journal of Medicine, Mass.

Govindarajulu, Z. (1987). *Statistical Techniques in Bioassay*. S. Karger Publishers, Inc., New York.

Hand, D. J. (1984). Statistical expert systems: Design. *The Statistician, 33*, 351–369.

————. (1985). Statistical expert systems: Necessary attributes. *Journal of Applied Statistics, 12*, 19–27.

Hedges, L., and Olkin, I. (1985). *Statistical Methods for Meta-Analysis*. Academic Press, New York.

Hoaglin, D. C., Mosteller, F., and Tukey, J. W. (eds.) (1982). *Understanding Robust and Exploratory Data Analysis*. John Wiley, New York.

Hochberg, Y., and Tamhane, A. C. (1987). *Multiple Comparison Procedures*. John Wiley, New York.

Hofacker, C. F. (1983). Abuse of statistical packages: The case of the general linear model. *American Journal of Physiology, 245*, R299–R302.

Holland, B. S., and Copenhaver, M. D. (1988). Improved Bonferroni-type multiple testing procedures. *Psychological Bulletin, 104*, 145–149.

Hooke, R. (1980). Getting people to use statistics properly. *The American Statistician, 34*, 39–42.

————. (1983). *How to Tell the Liars from the Statisticians*. Marcel Dekker, Inc., New York.

Howell, D. C. (1987). *Statistical Methods for Psychology*, 2nd ed. Duxbury Press, Boston, Mass.

Hulley, S. B., and Cummings, S. R. (1988). *Designing Clinical Research: An Epidemiologic Approach*. Williams and Wilkins, Baltimore, Md.

Huth, E. J. (1982). *How to Write and Publish Papers in the Medical Sciences*. ISI Press, Philadelphia, Pa.

Jaccard, J., Becker, M. A., and Woods, G. (1984). Pairwise multiple comparison procedures: A review. *Psychological Bulletin, 96*, 589–596.

Jaenisch, R. (1988). Transgenic animals. *Science, 240*, 1468–1474.

Jaffe, A. J., and Spirer, H. F. (1987). *Misused Statistics: Straight Talk for Twisted Numbers*. Marcel Dekker, Inc., New York.

Johnson, B. T. (1989). *DSTAT: Software for the Meta-Analytic Review of Research Literatures*. Lawrence Erlbaum Associates, Inc., Hillsdale, N.J.

Kachigan, S. K. (1986). *Statistical Analysis: An Interdisciplinary Introduction to Univariate and Multivariate Methods*. Radius Press, New York.

Katz, M. J. (1985). *Elements of the Scientific Paper*. Yale University Press, New Haven, Conn.

Kenyon, C. (1988). The nematode *Caenorhabditis elegans*. *Science, 240*, 1448–1452.

Keppel, G. (1982). *Design and Analysis: A Researcher's Handbook*, 2nd ed. Prentice-Hall, Englewood Cliffs, N.J.

————. (1991). *Design and Analysis: A Researcher's Handbook,* 3rd ed. Prentice-Hall, Englewood Cliffs, N.J.

————, and Zedeck, S. (1989). *Data Analysis for Research Designs: Analysis of Variance and Multiple Regression/Correlation Approaches*. W. H. Freeman, New York.

King, F. A., Yarbrough, C. J., Anderson, D. C., Gordon, T. P., and Gould, K. G. (1988). Primates. *Science, 240,* 1475–1482.

Landow, E. M., and DiStefano, J. J. (1984). Multiexponential, multicompartmental, and noncompartmetnal modeling. II. Data analysis and statistical considerations. *American Journal of Physiology, 246,* R665–R677.

Lembeck, F. (1989). *Scientific Alternatives to Animal Experiments*. Ellis Horwood Limited, Chichester, U.K.

Light, R., and Pillemer, D. (1984). *Summing Up: The Science of Reviewing Research*. Harvard University Press, Cambridge, Mass.

Lindman, H. R. (1974). *Analysis of Variance in Complex Experimental Designs*. W. H. Freeman, San Francisco, Calif.

Luey, B. (1987). *Handbook for Academic Authors*. Cambridge University Press, Cambridge, U.K.

Magasanik, B. (1988). Research on bacteria in the mainstream of biology. *Science, 240,* 1435–1439.

Mann, C. (1990). Meta-analysis in the breech. *Science, 249,* 476–480.

Marks, R. (1982a). *Analyzing Research Data*. Lifetime Learning Publications, Belmont, Calif.

————. (1982b). *Designing a Research Project*. Lifetime Learning Publications, Belmont, Calif.

Mayer, L. C., Horwitz, R. I., and Feinstein, A. R. (1988). A collection of 56 topics with contradictory results in case-control research. *International Journal of Epidemiology, 17,* 680–685.

Mead, R. (1988). *The Design of Experiments: Statistical Principles for Practical Applications*. Cambridge University Press, Cambridge, U.K.

Michael III, M., Boyce, W. T., and Wilcox, A. J. (1984). *Biomedical Bestiary: An Epidemiologic Guide to Flaws and Fallacies in the Medical Literature*. Little Brown and Co., Boston, Mass.

Miké, V., and Stanley, K. E. (1982). *Statistics in Medical Research: Methods and Issues, with Applications in Cancer Research*. John Wiley, New York.

Miller, R. (1985). Multiple comparisions. In S. Kotz and N. L. John (eds.), *Encyclopedia of Statistical Sciences*, Vol. 5 (pp. 679–689). John Wiley, New York.

Morgan, P. (1986). *An Insider's Guide for Medical Authors and Editors*. ISI Press, Philadelphia, Pa.

Mullen, B. (1989). *Advanced Basic Meta-Analysis*. Lawrence Erlbaum Associates, Inc., Hillsdale, N.J.

Murphy, E. A. (1985). *A Companion to Medical Statistics*. John Hopkins University Press, Baltimore, Md.

Murry, G. D. (1990). How should we approach the future. *Statistics in Medicine, 9,* 1063–1068.

Myers, J. L., and Well, A. D. (1991). *Research Design and Statistical Analysis*. HarperCollins, New York.

Nicholl, C. S., and Russell, R. M. (1990). Analysis of animal rights literature reveals the underlying motives of the movement: Ammunition for counter offensive by scientists. *Endocrinology, 127,* 985–989.

Oakes, M. (1986). *Statistical Inference: A Commentary for the Social and Behavioural Sciences*. John Wiley, Chichester, U.K.

Rideout, V. C. (1991). *Mathematical and Computer Modeling of Physiological Systems*. Prentice-Hall, New York.

Riegelman, R. K., and Hirsch, R. P. (1989). *Studying a Study and Testing a Test: How to Read the Medical Literature*. Little, Brown and Co., Boston, Mass.

Rosenthal, R. (1984). *Meta-Analytic Procedures for Social Research*. Sage, Beverly Hills, Calif.

Rosner, B. (1990). *Fundamentals of Biostatistics*, 3rd ed. Duxbury Press, Boston, Mass.

Rosnow, R. L., and Rosenthal, R. (1989). Statistical procedures and the justification of knowledge in psychological science. *American Psychologist, 44*, 1276–1284.

Rubin, G. M. (1988). *Drosophilia melanogaster* as an experimental organism. *Science, 240*, 1453–1459.

Runyon, R. P. (1985). *Fundamentals of Statistics in the Biological, Medical, and Health Sciences*. Duxbury Press, Boston, Mass.

Ryan, T. A., Joiner, B. L., and Ryan, B. F. (1982). *Minitab Reference Manual*, Duxbury Press, Boston, Mass.

Sackett, D. L. (1979). Bias in analytic research. *Journal of Chronic Disease, 32*, 51–63.

Schlesselman, J. J. (1982). *Case-Control Studies: Design, Conduct, Analysis*. Oxford University Press, New York.

Schmidt, C. F. (1983). *Statistical Graphics*. John Wiley, New York.

Scott, E. M., and Waterhouse, J. M. (1986). *Physiology and the Scientific Method: The Design of Experiments in Physiology*. Manchester University Press, Manchester, U.K.

Shott, S. (1990). *Statistics for Health Professionals*. W.B. Saunders Co., Philadelphia, Pa.

Siebert, W. M. (1978). Contributions of the communication sciences to physiology. *American Journal of Physiology, 3*, R161–R166.

Slinker, B. K., and Glantz, S. A. (1988). Multiple linear regression is a useful alternative to traditional analyses of variance. *American Journal of Physiology, 225*, R353–R367.

Sokal, R. R., and Rohlf, F. J. (1981). *Biometry: The Principles and Practice of Statistics in Biological Research*. W. H. Freeman and Co., New York.

Stevens, J. (1986). *Applied Multivariate Statistics for the Social Sciences*. Lawrence Erlbaum Associates, Inc., Hillsdale, N.J.

Tufte, E. R. (1983). *The Visual Display of Quantitative Information*. Graphics Press, Cheshire, Conn.

———. (1990). *Envisioning Information*. Graphics Press, Cheshire, Conn.

Tukey, J. W. (1977). *Exploratory Data Analysis*. Addision-Wesley, Reading, Mass.

Vaisrub, N. (1985). Manuscript review from a statistician's perspective. *Journal of the American Medical Association, 253*, 3145–3147.

Varmus, H. (1988). Retroviruses. *Science, 240*, 1427–1434.

Velleman, P. F., and Hoaglin, D. C. (1981). *Applications, Basics, and Computing of Exploratory Data Analysis*. Duxbury Press, Boston, Mass.

Wachter, K. W. (1988). Disturbed by meta-analysis. *Science, 241*, 1407–1408.

Wainer, H. (1984). How to display data badly. *The American Statistician, 38*, 137–147.

Wallenstein, S., Zucker, C. L., and Fleiss, J. L. (1980). Some statistical methods useful in circulation research. *Circulation Research, 47*, 1–9.

Walter, S. D. (1980). Berkson's bias and its control in epidemiologic studies. *Journal of Chronic Disease, 33*, 721–725.

Wilcox, R. R. (1987a). New designs in analysis of variance. *Annual Review of Psychology, 38*, 29–60.

———. (1987b). *New Statistical Procedures for the Social Sciences: Modern Solutions to Basic Problems*. Lawrence Erlbaum Associates, Inc., Hillsdale, N.J.

Wilkerson, A. M. (1991). *The Scientist's Handbook for Writing Papers and Dissertations*. Prentice-Hall, New York.

Wilkinson, L. (1990). SYSTAT: *The System for Statistics*. SYSTAT, Evanston, Ill.

Williamson, J. W., Goldschmidt, P. G., and Colton, T. (1986). The quality of medical literature: An analysis of validation assessments. In J. C. Bailar, III, and F. Mosteller (eds.), *Medical Uses of Statistics* (pp. 370–391), New England Journal of Medicine, Mass.

Winer, B. J. (1971). *Statistical Principles in Experimental Design*. McGraw-Hill, New York.

Wise, D. L. (ed.) (1990). *Bioinstrumentation: Research, Developments, and Applications*. Butterworth, Boston, Mass.

Wolf, F. M. (1986). *Meta-Analysis: Quantitative Methods for Research Synthesis*. Sage, Beverly Hills, Calif.

Woodward, W. A., Elliott, A. C., Gray, H. L., and Matlock, D. C. (1988). *Directory of Statistical Microcomputer Software*. Marcel Dekker, Inc., New York.

Yates, F. E. (1978). Good manners in good modeling: Mathematical models and computer simulations of physiological systems. *American Journal of Physiology, 234,* R159–R160.

Zar, J. H. (1974). *Biostatistical Analysis*. Prentice-Hall, Englewood Cliffs, N.J.

Zolman, J. F., and Peretz, B. (1987). Motor neuronal function in old *Aplysia* is improved by long-term stimulation of the siphon/gill reflex. *Behavioral Neuroscience, 101,* 524–533.

INDEX